FOUNDATIONS OF
MODERN NEUROLOGY

A CENTURY OF PROGRESS

Robert B Aird

Jan. 7, 1999

FOUNDATIONS OF MODERN NEUROLOGY

A CENTURY OF PROGRESS

ROBERT B. AIRD, M.D.
Professor of Neurology Emeritus
University of California
San Francisco, California

Raven Press   New York

Raven Press, Ltd., 1185 Avenue of the Americas, New York, New York 10036

Library of Congress Cataloging-in-Publication Data

Aird, Robert B. (Robert Burns), 1903-
    Foundations of modern neurology: a century of progress/Robert B. Aird
        p.   cm.
   Includes bibliographical references and index.
ISBN 0-7817-0112-0
1. Neurology—History   I. Title.
[DNLM: 1. Neurology—history—essays. 2. Neurosciences—history—essays. WL
11.1 A298f   1994]
RC338.A45   1994
616.8'09—dc20
DNLM/DLC
for Library of Congress   93-2568
                                                                CIP

9 8 7 6 5 4 3 2 1

To those neurologists and neuroscientists who utilized
the new scientific techniques of the early decades of the 20th century
to establish modern neurology and its allied fields
on a firm and independent basis

Contents

Section 5: OTHER ASPECTS OF NEUROLOGY

Acknowledgments

The collection of the necessary background data for these essays has been a tedious task and at times very frustrating. I am indebted to Nancy Zinn, the Archivist of the UCSF Library, for help on this. Her ability at the computer and knowledge of her vast historical collection considerably expedited my work at frustrating points. I am also grateful to Professor Olle Höök of Uppsala, Sweden, for his collection of data and guidance on the most difficult chapter, Neurological Rehabilitation. Gary Topping aided in obtaining bits of data on several neuroscientists. Only 25 of the 107 individuals used to illustrate the many aspects of the flowering of neurology are still alive. Their cooperation in sending me their *curricula vitae* and bibliographies is warmly acknowledged. This is also true of the personal communications of several others listed in the references. Likewise, I am grateful to the American Medical Association for authorizing the use of material in an article that I wrote in 1988 at the request of Dr. Robert Joynt for the Archives of Neurology.

Marilyn Stubblebine was a great help in the medical editing of the essays, and I am also grateful for the review and suggestions of John Nicholson. As an objective critic, he helped my muddling through the inevitable quagmire of subjective evaluations that were involved in writing these essays. My young friend, Erik Hilt, helped resolve a number of computer problems. In addition, Professors Guenter Risse, Jack Pressman, and Francis Schiller of the Department of the History of the Health Sciences have reviewed portions of the manuscript and made suggestions. This has also been true of Professors Michael Bishop, David Cox, Herbert Boyer, and Stanley Prusiner. It is a pleasure to acknowledge the help and encouragement of all those mentioned.

Preface

The purpose of this series of essays is to give recognition to that generation of neurologists and neuroscientists who firmly established modern neurology and its related fields as independent disciplines. The first group, the "Founders of Neurology" is discussed in Chapter 1. The next group of neurologists, who worked between the 1930s and the 1960s, developed the neurological field into its present, more complex and modern form. This became aparent to me while summarizing the early history of the Neurology Department at the University of California, San Francisco (UCSF), undertaken at the request of my successor, Robert A. Fishman. The preceding generations of neurologists and neuroscientists, the so-called founders, were a fine group, but they were not neurologists or neuroscientists in the modern sense. They invariably combined their neurological activities with some other specialty, had teaching appointments, or had some other means of support. It was impossible for the field of neurology to develop in its modern form until the scientific techniques of improved neurological diagnosis, therapy, and research had become established in the early decades of the present century. My account, therefore, describes the scientific developments that made the flowering of neurology possible and presents some of the leading neurologists and neuroscientists who accomplished it. In particular, it is the teachers and research workers of that period who should be recognized. They are the ones who adapted the new scientific techniques to the neurological field and trained the great influx of young men and women in the next generation. Their role in establishing neurology and the neurosciences on a firm basis was not easy and, in some respects, was more complex and difficult than the pioneering efforts of the so-called founders. In discussing this point with others, the misconceptions involved appear to be fairly widespread and well justify this attempt to correct them.

I have been encouraged to undertake this considerable task, not only because of its importance, but also because of the remarkable response to the article "Some Reminiscences," which I wrote in 1988 at the request of Dr. Robert Joynt, editor of *Archives of Neurology*. Initially, I hesitated to undertake the 1988 article because I wondered about the value of such an effort and was busy with other projects. However, the response to this article made it obvious that personal experiences that highlighted the distinctive aspects of the characters and events of a former day are of value and of interest to others. This experience also suggested that a summary of the events and characters involved in the flowering period of neurology, plus my personal contacts and reactions, might be of greater interest than a dry, detailed report, even though organized in a scholarly fashion.

Many requests have been received to extend my reminiscences, but I have not felt that this was justified when based on my own career, which is the sequential theme that held the article in the *Archives* together. However, it is conceivable that the broader theme of the "flowering of neurology" can serve this purpose. Discussions with neurological friends and a medical historian encouraged me to explore this possibility.

A third factor concerns the broad contacts provided by my career in neurology. My early training at Cornell, Harvard, Rochester, the University of California in San Francisco, and the University of Pennsylvania provided rich contacts. These were especially rich in the fields of neurology, neurosurgery, roentgenography, and neurophysiology. As the former head of a department of neurology and the developer of a visiting professor program, which involved essentially all the leading neurologists and many outstanding neuroscientists of the flowering period, I have had unusual contacts of value for the proposed project. In many instances, the contacts so established involved relationships that lasted over decades. My research interests have been of particular value in extending my contacts with many neuroscientists. I believe it is because of these facts that I have been urged to pursue this project.

How well I accomplished the task, of course, is another matter. The project has been a daunting one, which has involved much library research and endless care in collecting the necessary background data. Although my personal contacts hopefully add color and interest to the story, the project involved far more than this. The scientific background, which accounts for the flowering, and the methods employed by the leaders to achieve the flowering constitute the essential framework of this historical commentary.

Because the project involves a selection of leaders to illustrate how the advances in many related fields were made, the pitfalls of the undertaking are obvious. Endless arguments can be launched as to the relative worthiness of others whom I have not selected. This, however, is aside from the point of my account. My objective is to show how the modern field of neurology developed in the mid-20th century when its scientific underpinnings became sufficiently available to make this possible. The individuals selected to illustrate this development were not necessarily the most outstanding or popular leaders. They have been selected because of their illustrative value, their colorfulness as individuals, and my ability to develop an interesting account.

As emphasized in my *Archives* article, another problem of this approach concerns the subjective evaluations involved, which may reflect more on the author than those considered. Because of this, I have felt that it was important to include the background and circumstances of my contacts. The pitfall involved in this is that I may have overdone it and interjected my activities, reactions, and opinions beyond what was necessary. As indicated in the Acknowledgments, I have used an outside, objective critic to evaluate this aspect of the project. Oral history and essays of this type are all right when many sources of information are on tap but become precarious when only one opinion is available. I am hoping that readers will give me the benefit of their reactions, especially those who knew the leaders whom I have used to illustrate the various aspects of the flowering of neurology. Should the approach used in these essays merit a second edition, such help would be invaluable and enable me to improve it considerably. This would be especially true for the few leaders included, whom I did not know personally. Only in this way can one's subjective reactions and enthusiasms be put into perspective and tempered to advantage.

In spite of the several pitfalls that my approach involves, my hope is that these essays will serve to arouse the browsing interests of neurologists and others to read further about this exciting period of neurology. To this end, references to additional sources of reading have been appended to each chapter.

Robert B. Aird, M.D.
Professor of Neurology Emeritus
University of California, San Francisco

FOUNDATIONS OF MODERN NEUROLOGY

A CENTURY OF PROGRESS

The Flowering of Neurology

Background

The Founders of Neurology, a book compiled and edited by Haymaker and Schiller, properly includes that early group of neurologists and neuroscientists who laid the groundwork for all other advances in the field of neurology (1). Their selection involved such early workers as Willis and Hensig, born in the 17th century, and 14 others, born in the 18th century. Despite the considerable background documented in *The Founders of Neurology*, neurology did not come into its own as an independent clinical discipline until well after World War II. Before then, it was generally agreed that neurologists could not make a living except if they held academic appointments or combined neurology with general practice or some other specialty. An analysis of *The Founders of Neurology* clearly verifies this. At one point, I wondered if perhaps Amand Duchenne was an early exception to this. He lived a lonely life in Paris and, as Raymond Adams has written, "gained his livelihood from private practice . . . adequate to supply his limited needs" (1). Even in this instance, however, it seems obvious that his "private practice" was not primarily of a neurological character.

Another feature characterized this early stage of neurology. It was largely limited to the descriptive phases of the subject and clinicopathological correlations. Because of this, it has remained for a later generation to delineate more fully the diagnostic and essentially all the therapeutic, rehabilitative, and preventive measures that now characterize the field of neurology. Except for a few neurological surgeons and one neuropathologist, there are only about 12 neurologists and neuroscientists considered in the 146 biographies in *The Founders of Neurology* who overlapped into the period of the flowering of neurology (approximately 1935 to 1965) and who might properly be included in this account.

The developments that explain the full flowering of neurology can be traced to a number of scientific advances that had their inception in the first three decades of the present century (2). These can be listed under the following headings:

1. *More precise diagnostic techniques*, including (a) roentgenographic methods (skull x-rays, pneumoencephalography, and myelography) for visualization of the outlines of the central nervous system; (b) electroencephalography (EEG), evoked responses, telemetry and allied techniques for the physiological study of brain function; (c) electromyography (EMG) for the physiological study of muscle and motor function; (d) arteriography for the study of the cardiovascular system and the blood supply of the central nervous system (CNS); (e) radioactive isotope studies for the visualization of lesions of the CNS and study of the neurochemistry of the CNS; (f) cytological, serological, and chemical studies of cerebrospinal fluid; (g) the Wassermann test for the identification of syphilis and other subsequent serological tests and skin reactions; and (h) computer tomographic techniques (computed axial tomographic scans, magnetic resonance imaging, and positron tomography), which are now giving a further impetus to the diagnostic aspects of neurology.
2. *Improved forms of therapy*, including (a) sedatives, hypnotics, and tranquilizers for hyperactive and psychotic states; analgesics and other forms of treatment for painful conditions; and ergotamine for migraine; (b) antiepileptics; (c) CNS stimulants; (d) immunization for smallpox, diphtheria, typhoid, and influenza; (e) vaccine therapy for poliomyelitis and tetanus; (f) correction of nutritional, vitamin, hormonal, and metabolic deficiencies and disorders; (g) antibiotics for bacterial infections; (h) penicillamine and other chelating agents for toxic conditions; (i) parasympatholytic (cholinergic-blocking) agents, corticosteroids, and other recent approaches to the treatment of myasthenia gravis; (j) anticholinergic agents, levodopa, and other dopamine agonists for parkinsonism; (k) antiallergic agents; (l) skeletal muscle relaxants; (m) prosthetic devices; and (n) the techniques of rehabilitative neurology.
3. *Improved research techniques for the study of neurological conditions*, including (a) radioactive isotopes (labeled metabolites and electrolytes) for the study of normal and abnormal physiological conditions that finally result in pathologic conditions; (b) neurophysiological recording (improved transistor amplifiers, polygraphic recording techniques, depth recording, and telemetry) for studying nervous system function and also EMG for study of the neuromuscular system; (c) neurochemical techniques, including the study of the central neurotransmitters; (d) electron microscopy; (e) computer tomography; and (f) improved immunological and genetic methods of study.

These lists of scientific techniques are by no means exhaustive but serve to indicate the principal developments that have afforded neurology a broad basis as an independent medical discipline. It would be tedious and counterproductive to the purpose of this account to elaborate on the background of the development for all the technical advances listed. However, it is important that we understand the close interdependence of the scientific advances, that is, how the techniques we use were developed, how they became incorporated into daily practice, and how important they are to our diagnostic and therapeutic armamentarium. This is a big order, but a few examples and enough background can be given to convey the desired perspective

It was the newly developed technique of EEG and the advances achieved in antiepileptic drug therapy that afforded the initial great impetus to clinical neurology. These advances occurred during the late 1930s and World War II (as discussed in Chapter 2). As other techniques of neurological study and therapy grew in number and complexity, the need for specialized training in medical neurology gradually increased. Related disciplines, such as neurophysiology, neurochemistry, and neuroimaging, greatly added to our understanding of the etiology and underlying mechanisms involved in neurological disorders. Their development in the early and middecades of the present century paralleled the developments in clinical neurology, were based on the same new scientific techniques, and in general, only slightly preceded the clinical developments. Related clinical fields, such as neurosurgery, pediatric neurology, and neurological rehabilitation, likewise participated with neurology in the broad and in-depth advances that were made over the past 60 to 70 years. As in most other aspects of modern medicine, it can truthfully be said that much more was learned about the nervous system and neurological disorders in this period than in all previous history. This fact emphasizes the importance of what may properly be called the flowering period of neurology, as opposed to the earlier descriptive period. Pathology, of course, is very important, inasmuch as it constitutes the end result of disease processes. Nevertheless, the future lies in understanding the pathophysiological aspects of neurochemistry and the infections and toxic processes that lead to pathology because such knowledge is vital to early diagnosis and the undertaking of appropriate therapeutic and preventive measures. Furthermore, the complex aspects of these subjects and the effectiveness of its therapeutic advances now clearly establish neurology as an independent clinical specialty.

THE EMERGENCE OF NEUROLOGY FROM THE OLD NEUROPSYCHIATRY

The emergence of neurology from its earlier association with neuropsychiatry, however, was not as smooth as might be gathered from the previous comments (3). Human affairs, complicated by biases, ambitions, and the restraining and delaying tactics of the status quo, invariably confused and curbed all changes. At best, the adoption of advances approximated a muddling-through process.

In an oversimplified portrayal of this earlier linkage, two major elements and trends can be traced. With the rise of psychiatry, led by Sigmund Freud and his psychoanalytic methods, which provided a remunerative basis for this specialty, what may be termed a *functional* phase of neuropsychiatry became established around the time of World War I. The "founders of neurology," on the other hand, continued in their fragmented status in what may be termed the *organic* phase of neuropsychiatry. Under the mantle of *neuropsychiatry*, both groups managed a loose hegemony, initially characterized by the predominance of psychiatry. That neurology, as a medical discipline, should be cast in this guise stemmed from the very practical fact that, prior to the development of an expanded scientific basis for neurology, the organically inclined neurologists still could not make a living without combining neurology with some other specialty (usually psychiatry), general practice, or teaching appointments. In the old days, the latter were very limited because most of the medical school instruction was covered by volunteer physicians in practice.

Much lip service was given to neurology by the older neuropsychiatrists who primarily depended on their psychiatric practice for a living and who generally were in charge of the teaching departments of neuropsychiatry in medical schools. The adoption of new developments in neurology was often delayed, and as a result, the training of the younger generation was frequently inadequate. At a later stage, the independent status of neurology was delayed in many instances by the influence and vested interests of the older neuropsychiatrists. As a younger generation of neurologists slowly emerged from the organic phase of the older neuropsychiatry, they rebelled against the neuropsychiatric impediments to their new, independent status and called for a separation of neurology and psychiatry. The organization of the American Academy of Neurology immediately following World War II in part reflected this trend. However, the movement for a separation has largely subsided with the academic development (aided by great National Institutes of Health [NIH] support) of strong teaching departments of neurology and the independent course that neurology has pursued during the past 40 years.

It was from this background that the American Board of Neurology and Psychiatry developed in 1934. One of my experiences on the Board as an associate examiner in neurology may be worth recounting because it will serve to give some flavor of the neuropsychiatry of 50 years ago.

I was presented with a middle-aged applicant who was a psychiatrist in a large California mental institution. I later was informed that his salary could be considerably enhanced if he passed the American Board of Neurology and Psychiatry examination. However, this necessitated that he pass the neurological portion of the board examination as well as the psychiatric examination. The doctor's background in neurology was meager, and he appeared to be fully conscious of this. A previous examination in neuropathology had markedly transformed his countenance and bearing. He appeared to be terrified; this was associated with profuse perspiration and trembling movements. I spent several minutes in an attempt to reassure him and calm him down. Finally, I selected the easiest patient available for him to examine. The patient was a man whose partial blindness was due to early optic atrophy caused by a pituitary tumor. The patient presented with the typical visual defect and the ophthalmoscopic and roentgenographic findings of this condition. The psychiatrist unfortunately failed to elicit a history of visual difficulties or to detect his visual defect. He also failed to use an ophthalmoscope in his examination and did not recognize the sellar erosion in the skull films. When he could not find anything wrong, I handed him one of the hospital ophthalmoscopes and gently urged him to examine the patient's eye grounds. This seemed to aggravate his disturbance. I was stunned when he directed the light of the ophthalmoscope into his own eye. At the same time, it became obvious that his accentuated tremor would now make a proper examination impossible. However, before I could think of another approach to help him, he started describing a choked disc and protruding optic nerve head. The disc, of course, was flat and showed definite optic pallor, but the doctor jumped to the conclusion that his patient had a brain tumor that produced increased intracranial pressure and papilledema.

His fabrication of findings struck me as a questionable form of conduct for a physician. I decided to consult the head examiner, an eminent neuropsychiatrist of the older generation. After hearing the story, he concluded, "Oh, he's just an old psychiatrist. He can't do any harm. We'll have to let him through, providing he can pass the psychiatric part of the exam." In an exaggerated form, this typified the attitude and practice in the older board examinations. On the other hand, the psychiatric examiners usually held the neurologists to a strict accounting; this was sometimes biased by the particular psychiatric school of thought of the examiner. In general, however, this uneven approach was ameliorated by the parenthetical designation of passing as being either in psychiatry, neurology, or both. No doubt present-day board examinations follow a more rigorous and even course.

The problems that neurology endured as it slowly emerged from its initial ties with neuropsychiatry involves many complex factors and is difficult to illustrate by any single case history. However, because the neuropsychiatric situation at University of California, San Francisco (UCSF), one-half century ago, was especially complicated, it is one of the best examples to illustrate the problems (3).

Prior to 1948, the School of Medicine in San Francisco was the only medical school in the University of California system. Like most of the medical schools in the early 20th century, it was struggling to improve its status. Following the Flexner report and World War I, the School of Medicine of the University of California went through a reorganization that had considerable promise.

In most medical schools during the 1930s and 1940s, the teaching of neurology was handled by neuropsychiatrists who served as part-time staff members in small divisions of departments of medicine, and so it was at UCSF, where the careers of the head neuropsychiatrist had started well before World War I. Furthermore, the integration of teaching from neuroanatomy on through neurology and neurosurgery was poor. I can speak with authority on this situation at UCSF because I was the representative of the curriculum committee that investigated the problem. Our situation may have been worse than most because, following the 1906 earthquake, the preclinical subjects were taught in Berkeley, although the clinical work, including pathology, remained in San Francisco. Another problem at UCSF concerned the strong development of neurosurgery under Dr. Howard C. Naffziger, Chair of the

Department of Surgery and head of neurosurgery, from 1928 to 1952, while neurology remained a stepchild of neuropsychiatry in the Department of Medicine. The result of this lopsided development was that most of the patients with neurological problems were being referred to neurosurgery with the neuropsychiatric group serving primarily as psychiatrists. Neurology did not have any beds in the hospital and did not have a full-time staff member to represent it. The operating budget was miniscule, and research facilities were lacking. By default, neurosurgery had preempted the field. This circumstance was unfortunate, not only in that neurosurgeons rather than neurologists evaluated a high percentage of neurological problems, but also in that the follow-through care required for neurological patients was not provided.

The establishment of the Langley Porter Neuropsychiatric Institute, San Francisco, in 1940, further complicated the situation. Although the institute was planned to ensure the integration of the neurological sciences—with beds for neurology, neurosurgery, and psychiatry and provisions for an EEG laboratory, a neuropathologic setup, and surgical facilities for neurosurgery—its original design was totally subverted. In large part, this was due to the dependence of the institute on the California Department of Institutions for its support rather than on the university. The Department of Institutions was mainly interested in the training of psychiatrists to staff the state psychiatric hospitals. The end result was a strong setup in psychiatry, with neurology and neurosurgery being squeezed out. Dr. Naffziger, who had powerful connections, strongly opposed this development but failed to stem it. Furthermore, the new director refused to incorporate the old part-time neuropsychiatrists into the institute, leaving them as neurologists in the Department of Medicine. In addition, this confusing situation was complicated by World War II.

Special committee investigations and recommendations led to a separation of neurology from medicine, as already had occurred with psychiatry. This, however, was strongly opposed by Professor William Kerr, Chair of the Department of Medicine, who threatened to resign if neurology was separated from medicine. Dr. Charles Aring, who had been brought in as an outside consultant, came to an understanding with Dr. Kerr and was induced to stay on and start the new Department of Neurology in July 1946. Unfortunately, the tiny spin-off from medicine did not have the necessary provisions for a viable department; Aring left early in 1947.

Much to my surprise, following a search committee study, I was offered the position. As a research worker, I had no aspirations for a clinical administrative post, and because investigation quickly showed the inadequacies of the setup, I refused the offer. This led to further major adjustments and, finally, plans for independent departments of neurology and neurosurgery were developed that would place them on an equal footing, with Naffziger heading the Department of Neurological Surgery and I as the head of the Department of Neurology. The potential for the development of neurology under this plan was quite different from the earlier, inadequate spin-off from the Department of Medicine.

I had planned to write a book on the clinical effects of impaired blood–brain barrier function, which would include my own research, previously published in various journals and congress proceedings. Another project was to make a comparative study, using the same patients, between the relative localizing abilities of my system of EEG with that of Herbert Jasper's.* Both projects would have to be given up, along with much of my other research. It was with considerable regret, therefore, that I finally agreed to head the development of the new department. Someone had to protect the interests of neurology, and in retrospect, I believe Dean Francis Scott Smyth was right, I was the only certified neurologist in the University of California, and the only one at that time who stood a good chance of doing it.

A complete reorganization of the teaching program followed with better integration of neurology with neuroanatomy, neurophysiology, neurosurgery, and the x-ray division (at that time a subdivision of surgery, in which I had worked part-time for 10 years, as discussed in Chapter 7). Care was taken to handle the postgraduate needs of both medicine and psychiatry. A neurological postgraduate training program was started. Our clinical and research facilities were greatly increased with the completion of the new medical sciences building, Moffitt Hospital, and the two research towers. Clinical services at Fort Miley Veterans Administration Hospital and San Francisco Hospital were developed. Furthermore, in the 1950s, grants from the NIH greatly expanded our training and research setup (2).

Such was neurology's poor inheritance from the old neuropsychiatry, however, that impediments to its full development still existed. In spite of the cooperation of Naffziger and several other perceptive physicians, perhaps stimulated by Smyth, the old pattern of referrals lingered on. Worse than this was the fact that, for the first 12 to 15 years of the department, well-trained neurological personnel were not available. This was partly overcome by my recruitment of Dr. Donald Macrae, a highly trained neurologist from the National Hospital, Queen Square, London, who was an excellent teacher. Robert Wartenberg, a refugee from Nazi Germany, who had been in the old neuropsychiatric setup under medicine, but who had been supported by outside refugee funds, also received an appointment. Other certified neurologists were slowly added to the staff.

A third problem concerned the great isolation of the West Coast from the main neurological centers of the East. Before the days of adequate air travel, a week was required to make the trip east and return by train. This, in combination with the limited number of qualified neurologists, presented a major problem to the development of the new department. This was further aggravated by the residuals of the political nonsense that had preceded the separation of the Department of Neurology from the Department of Medicine and the transformation of the Langley Porter Institute.

Considering the confusing neuropsychiatric background of neurology, it was obvious that neurology needed to establish its identity and that a public relations effort would be helpful in this respect. Accordingly, I initiated the Visiting Professor of Neurology Program that, during a period of 17 years, imported over 40 of the most

---

*Without significant comparative studies, Jasper's 10-20 system was later adopted by the International EEG Society as the international system of EEG, as discussed in Chapter 2.

distinguished English-speaking neurologists in the world (2,3). Funds for presentations were obtained with honoraria provided by medical societies, the Veterans
Administration, and the Extension Division of the medical school. This was supple-
mented by gifts from grateful patients and whatever I could eke out of the department's budget. Because the trips from the East, and especially from Europe, were
expensive and involved much time, the great majority of visitors spent 2 or 3 weeks
with us and many stayed 4 to 6 weeks. In addition to their participation in extension
division courses in neurology and talks before medical societies, the visitors were
incorporated into our daily schedule of teaching, neurological rounds, and conferences. The program attracted great attention locally and, finally, was effective in the
solution of the problems mentioned. However, it was not until the advent of
dependable transcontinental air travel and the great surge of trained personnel
(resulting from the expanded training programs in neurology of the 1950s and
1960s) that our problems were finally resolved.

Because of my primary interests in research, I played an unwilling administrative
role in these developments and withdrew as soon as possible in 1966. Nineteen
years of my career, however, had to be devoted to this effort. It was the only way at
that crucial period of growing pains of the medical school, following World War II,
that the interests of neurology could be protected and furthered.

Although our situation at the UCSF was more exaggerated than in most medical
schools for the reasons mentioned, the problems involved in the transformation of
the old divisions of neuropsychiatry into superior departments of neurology were
basically similar to those in the great majority of medical schools in the period from
1930 to 1960. Many others besides myself were caught in this turbulent period.
This late and labored development of neurology is not fully understood by many of
the young neurologists, an ignorance that makes them less appreciative of the
superb training and better opportunities now afforded them.

ROLE OF THE NIH IN THE DEVELOPMENT OF NEUROLOGY

Following World War II, support for neurology and its subspecialties became
available in the United States along with greatly increased support for many other
medical specialties. In the case of neurology, this initially took the form of service
and training centers in the Veterans Administration, which was richly supported
after World War II. The full development of research and training programs, however, had to await the establishment of the NIH, which initially included the
National Institute of Neurological Diseases and Blindness (NIND&B) (4,5). From
minimal support in 1950, the budget of the NIND&B quickly expanded to over
$125 million annually. This may appear trivial now, but discounting the great infla-
tion of more recent years and the almost complete lack of support before then, this
seemed like a stupendous "bursting of the dams" at that time. With this stimulus
and still extra support, nearly 40 additional independent departments of neurology

were developed in the next 20 years in the teaching hospitals and medical schools of the United States (4,5). Before the NIND&B was established in 1947, approximately 30 residency positions in neurology existed in a few teaching hospitals, and this number was increased to over 1,000 within the next 20 to 25 years. The number of full-time neurological staff members increased from 69 in 1950 to 319 in 1970, and departmental budgets during this same period expanded 30-fold.

Corresponding to the great increase of personnel and research involved in these developments, new journals and specialty societies appeared. These included the American Epilepsy Society (*Epilepsia*), the American EEG Society (*International Journal of EEG and Clinical Neurophysiology* and others), and especially the American Academy of Neurology with its "green journal" and the expansion of the American Neurological Association (*Archives of Neurology* and, later, *Annals of Neurology*). Many paramedical organizations also developed at this time; their contributions to public education, improved patient care, and support of research were notable. This was especially true for such conditions as multiple sclerosis and the neuromuscular disorders. The impact of this growth was felt internationally and, particularly, in the United Kingdom, Scandinavian countries, and Japan. The great size and wealth of the United States inevitably made it the leader in postwar events and, along with advances in other fields of medical science, resulted in English assuming—in considerable measure—the proportions of an international language.

Although the earlier foundations of neurology cannot be discounted, the period from the mid-1930s to the mid-1960s constituted a particularly exciting era. It was during this relatively brief period of some 30 years that neurology came into its own, as we know it today. By the end of World War II, it had become apparent that a scientific basis for neurology had finally emerged. This and the turmoil of the war, with its disruptions and its new innovative spirit, were the factors that led to the formation of NIH. It was this timely combination of potential and support that turned the tide and resulted in the flowering of neurology. In their more advanced and complex forms, the resulting neurological developments of this era matched the earlier remarkable advances in the late 19th and early 20th centuries of anesthesia, asepsis, and modern surgery.

REFERENCES

1. Haymaker, W., and Schiller, F. *The Founders of Neurology*, 2nd ed. Springfield, IL, Charles C. Thomas, 1970.
2. Aird, R.B. *The History of Neurology*. San Francisco: University of California, San Francisco, 1979.
3. Aird, R.B. Some reminiscences. *Arch. Neurol.*, 45:1145—1155, 1988.
4. Office of Resource Analysis, National Institutes of Health. *Resources for Biomedical Research and Education.* Bethesda, MD, National Institutes of Health, 1969.
5. National Research Council Committee, National Institute of Neurology and Communicative Diseases and Stroke. *Manpower Needs for Teaching and Research in Basic Neurologic and Communicative Sciences. Present Status and Future Needs.* monograph no. 20. Bethesda, MD, National Institutes of Health, 1977.

The Role of Epilepsy in the Early Flowering of Neurology

The first great surge in the development of clinical neurology as an independent discipline occurred as a result of advances in epilepsy, which were made at the Harvard Neurological Unit of the Boston City Hospital in the 1930s. These advances were accomplished in two areas. The first was in the electroencephalographic (EEG) diagnosis of and research on epilepsy, and the second was in antiepileptic drug therapy.

ADVANCES IN EPILEPTIC DIAGNOSIS AND RESEARCH

The initial phase centered around the work of Dr. William Lennox, who was a most unusual figure in neurology inasmuch as his formal training in neurology was almost nil. Nevertheless, through persistent and single-minded effort, Lennox became the foremost epileptologist of his day, and his fascinating story must be recorded if one is to understand the early advances made in epilepsy.

WILLIAM G. LENNOX (1884-1960)

Born in Colorado Springs, where his father was a mine owner and rancher, Lennox graduated from Colorado College in 1909 and the Harvard Medical School in 1913. Following internship in Denver and at the Massachusetts General Hospital, he became a medical missionary in China at the Peking Union Medical College for 4 years. On his return to the United States in 1921, he obtained an M.A. degree at the University of Denver. In 1922, he started medical practice in Boston and became an assistant professor of medicine at the Harvard Medical School. More important, however, was the connection that he developed with Dr. Stanley Cobb as a fellow in neuropathology. Lennox followed when Cobb became chief of the neurology service at the Boston City Hospital and director of the Harvard Neurological Unit in 1925, supported by the Rockefeller Foundation grants, as discussed in Chapter 15. Cobb's primary interest in studying the mechanisms that produce neuropathology, rather than in the traditional end picture of neuropathology, suited Lennox well, and soon, they were involved in a review study of epilepsy (1). One of the leading theories for the cause of epilepsy at that time was based on the concept of cerebral anoxia produced by spasm of the cerebrovascular system. This led to studies of the cerebral circulation by Cobb and Harold Wolff.* Blood chemistry studies, for which Lennox developed the technique of obtaining blood samples, ruled out anoxia as a cause of seizures. Although carbon dioxide levels were found to vary with petit mal epilepsy in another study, this was not true for grand mal or psychomotor seizures.** In spite of still other theories, Lennox developed the opinion that seizures were a neuropathophysiological manifestation of disturbed cerebral neurochemistry.

Knowing about the brain wave studies on animals and the recent confirmation by Adrian (Professor of Physiology at Cambridge University) of Berger's studies on humans, Lennox and Frederic Gibbs consulted Halowell Davis, of the Department of Physiology at Harvard, as discussed in Chapter 5. This led to the development of EEG equipment by Albert Grass and the great breakthrough in the scientific diagnostic study of seizure types that soon followed (2,3). Electrophysiological studies with Frederic and Erna Gibbs also quickly followed that verified Lennox's theory of seizure activity, which established the inestimable value of this technique for neurophysiological research as well as for clinical EEG studies.

After the new Director of the Neurological Unit, Dr. Tracy Putnam, went to New York in 1939 and Dr. Denny-Brown was selected as his successor, the trio of Lennox and the Gibbses relocated at the Boston Psychopathic Hospital. I well remember that troubled period inasmuch as I worked with the Gibbses and Lennox and consulted with others at the Harvard Neurological Unit in early 1940 shortly before the move. Still later in 1944, Dr. Lennox was invited to establish the seizure unit at the Children's Medical Center. As chief of this unit, he introduced trimethadione, the first antiepileptic agent for petit mal epilepsy and developed the unit as a center for research and the clinical study of epilepsy.

In accordance with his missionary spirit and diverse background, Dr. Lennox's activities transcended his studies in the clinic and laboratory. He aided in the reorganization of the International League Against Epilepsy (1935), established its American branch, and served as president of both. In 1939, he organized the National Epilepsy League, a lay group to combat social discrimination against epileptic patients. This eventually led to the American Foundation of Epilepsy that, as a lay group, combats the fear and discrimination associated with epilepsy, aids in the educational and service aspects of this problem, and financially supports research. He also established the American Epilepsy Society and was the first editor of its journal, *Epilepsia*.

In addition to four books, Lennox wrote more than 240 articles on epilepsy. His studies, clinics, and laboratories were supported by the Rockefeller Foundation, the Markle

---

*Wolff was later Professor of Neurology at Cornell University School of Medicine and famous for his studies of headache.
**Early terminology for seizures later classified them as absence, generalized tonic-clonic, and complex partial seizures.

Foundation, the Association for Crippled Children and Adults, the National Institute of Neurology and Blindness (of the Public Health Service), and most frequently, patients and other friendly donors.

Lennox received a number of awards from societies such as the American League Against Epilepsy, the National Epilepsy League, and the American Pharmaceutical Manufacturers' Association. Colorado College and Boston University gave him honorary degrees, and he received the Lasker Award in 1951. He was honored by a dinner at the Harvard Club on the completion of his classic book *Epilepsy and Related Disorders*, which compiled his more important studies on epilepsy and migraine (4). Much to the consternation of all of us in attendance, Dr. Lennox collapsed near the end of the banquet and died 3 days later on July 21, 1960.

In his private life, Dr. Lennox was a quiet and retiring man. However, in his support of better teaching, practice, and research in epilepsy, he had no peer. He was a thoughtful and, in many ways, a saintly person in his selflessness and desire to help those whom he deemed might extend an understanding of epilepsy and of better care for epileptic patients. I spent many happy evenings in the Lennox home and, at a later date, was glad to initiate the William G. Lennox Trust (Boston), based on funds that he left to the American Epilepsy Society. His monumental book, *Epilepsy and Related Disorders*, well documents his clinical and research contributions and interests (4). The Gibbses dedicated their *Atlas of Encephalography* to Dr. Lennox, and, in his obituary, Frederic Gibbs paid him a fitting final tribute, "God grant that the human race will produce more men like William Lennox: men of wisdom, patience, kindness, and dedication" (5).

The Gibbses were so closely allied with Dr. Lennox that much of their story has been covered in the preceding account of Lennox. However, some additional points pertinent to the epilepsy story should be added. Mrs. Gibbs (née Erna Leonhardt, who emigrated from Germany) was the first to join the Lennox team. When Dr. Lennox was looking for a technician, Mrs. Lennox had suggested that he check the advertisements in the Boston papers. It was in this way that she was hired. Her unusual abilities soon became apparent, and she qualified as a collaborator from 1930 onward.

FREDERIC A. GIBBS (1903-1992)

The early life of Gibbs was spent in Baltimore, where he was born in 1903. He graduated from Yale in 1925 and from Johns Hopkins in medicine in 1929. He quickly joined the Cobb-Lennox team as an Assistant in Neuropathology at the Harvard Neurological Unit of the Boston City Hospital and, in 1930, was married to Erna. It was the Gibbses who developed the technique of measuring cerebral blood flow, which ruled out cerebrovascular spasm as the precipitating cause of seizures. Instead, they found that an increased flow of blood occurred during seizures. It had taken them 2 years to develop the technique of measuring cerebral blood flow while working at the Johnson Foundation of Medical Physics of the University of Pennsylvania School of Medicine.

When the Gibbses later moved to Chicago (1944), Frederic Gibbs became an associate professor of psychiatry, and from 1951 until his retirement in 1973, he was professor of neurology at the University of Illinois. He was the director of the Illinois consultation clinic for epilepsy, started in 1945, and was the founding editor of *Clinical EEG*, started in 1970. His contributions were in the teaching, service, and research aspects of epilepsy and electroencephalography. The Gibbses' *Atlas of Encephalography* was devoted to the normal EEG aspects of human development from birth on and to the diagnostic value of EEG in epilepsy and other neurological conditions (5). The Gibbses recognized the value of sleep as a seizure-inducing mechanism, and along with B. Fuster, a visiting research worker in clinical neurophysiology from South America, they were the first to describe the importance of temporal EEG foci in the EEG diagnosis of psychomotor epilepsy (later classified as complex partial epilepsy) (6,7). Their article on temporal foci in patients with temporal lobe epilepsy was indelibly printed on my mind, inasmuch as, in 1947, I was engaged in a 5-year review of our EEG localization, which showed a very high percentage of temporal foci in patients with temporal lobe epilepsy. Like many "firsts" in science, the lead is usually narrow and quickly supported by several other studies.

ADVANCES IN EPILEPTIC THERAPY

The second phase of the epilepsy account was initiated by Dr. Tracy J. Putnam shortly after he succeeded Stanley Cobb as director of the Harvard Neurological Unit at the Boston City Hospital in 1934.

TRACY PUTNAM (1894-1975)

In contradistinction to Lennox, but like Cobb, Putnam was a Boston patrician, who was educated at Harvard and graduated from the Harvard Medical School in 1920. Following training in surgery at the Massachusetts General Hospital, he trained in neurosurgery under Harvey Cushing and did research at the Peter Brent Brigham Hospital. He then worked with Cobb at the neurological unit. When Cobb turned to psychiatry in 1934 and moved to the Massachusetts General Hospital, Putnam became director of the Neurological Unit and was made professor of neurology at the Harvard Medical School. It was shortly after this that he conceived the idea that the phenyl derivatives of the various barbiturates accounted for the differences in their antiepileptic properties. A simple method for measuring electroconvulsive thresholds was developed, and a large series of barbiturates and related agents were tested (8).* The sodium salt of diphenylhydantoin stood out as a likely candidate for clinical trial (10). Houston Merritt led in the clinical evaluation of this agent, which later became known as phenytoin (11). The immediate success of phenytoin initiat-

---

*Although Dr. E. Spiegel had reported a more complicated method of measuring the convulsive threshold 1 year earlier, this was not generally used and, insofar as I know, was not the inspiration for the Putnam-Merritt technique (9). However, this again illustrates the close advances in scientific progress.

ed the modern era of antiepileptic drug therapy in epilepsy. Although Putnam's original thesis was proved to be incorrect, it does not detract from the great practical success of the study.

Perhaps even more significant than the discovery of the antiepileptic properties of phenytoin was the development of a method for testing antiepileptic agents. This technique was shortly adapted by pharmacologists and pharmaceutical manufacturers with the result that numerous other antiepileptic agents were developed over the next two to three decades.

In 1939, this remarkable development led to Putnam accepting the offer as the director of the Neurological Institute of New York and the appointment as professor of neurology and neurosurgery at the College of Physicians and Surgeons, Columbia University. As predicted by some of his Boston colleagues, this proved to be a grave mistake. Tracy's genius did not extend to administrative detail in a large and complex organization, nor could he cope with the intense political problems with which he was shortly confronted. He left New York in 1947 and worked for the rest of his life as the director of the neurological service at the Cedars of Lebanon Hospital in Los Angeles.

As Putnam's colleague, Dr. Houston Merritt, has written, "Tracy Putnam—a practical and wise counselor for me—was a unique and unusual person, understood by few, and really appreciated only by his colleagues in Boston" (12). That Putnam did extremely well in Boston and, for 5 years, was director of one of the most productive neurological units in history is in striking contrast to his fate in New York. As one who knew him in Boston, as well as later in New York and still later in California, it was my impression that the problem reflected more on the New York situation at that time than on Putnam.

In addition to his brilliant work on anticonvulsants, Putnam made significant studies on the physiology of the pituitary at the Harvard Medical School. He contributed to the surgical treatment of hydrocephalus and dyskinesias, invented several useful laboratory and neurosurgical instruments, and led in the development of the National Institute of Neurological Diseases.

H. HOUSTON MERRITT (1902-1978)

Merritt was one of my oldest acquaintances in neurology and became one of the brightest stars in the neurological firmament of the mid 20th century. Merritt primarily was a product of the Johns Hopkins Medical School and postgraduate training in Cobb's neurological unit at Boston City Hospital. He rose on the Harvard academic ladder to the level of associate professor and was associated with Putnam in the development of phenytoin, which as mentioned, revolutionized the treatment of epilepsy in 1937 (10). He went to New York in 1944 and, after 4 years as Chief of Service at Montefiore Hospital, became head of neurology at the New York Neurological Institute. Over the next 20 years, the Postgraduate Training Center at Columbia became one of the leading centers of neurology in the United States. Merritt's administrative abilities were almost more outstanding than his clinical abilities, and he rose to become Dean of the Faculty of Medicine and Vice

President in charge of Medical Affairs of Columbia University, positions he held from 1959 to 1970, when he finally retired. His excellent *Textbook of Neurology* (13) was published in six editions between 1953 and 1979. In addition to his classic book on cerebrospinal fluid with Fremont-Smith and another book, *Neurosyphilis*, he wrote over 200 articles and served for 9 years as Chief Editor of the *Archives of Neurology*. He was active in a number of neurological societies and was the recipient of many honors and awards.

My acquaintance with Merritt went back to early 1930, when he was a resident under Cobb in the neurological unit that Cobb had started at Boston City Hospital. He supervised my workups and the care of a number of patients, and I well recall his presentation of a clinical study of a series of patients with syringomyelia. Some 36 years later, I jokingly reminded him of this by asking if he still believed syringomyelia to be a common neurologic condition. Without hesitation, he seriously replied in the affirmative. My point in mentioning this, of course, was not to debate the relative incidence of syringomyelia (Merritt himself had written that syringomyelia was less common than spinal cord tumor or amyotrophic lateral sclerosis) but merely to point out Merritt's reaction, which I encountered on several other occasions. My conclusion was that it was not so much a lack of humor as a reflexive, defensive reaction. It made me wonder if he lived in an overly competitive climate that required this for survival.

Merritt did a fine job in holding things together at Boston City Hospital during the prolonged transition period from Cobb and Putnam to Denny-Brown. I was very sympathetic toward the remaining staff at Boston City Hospital, which was decimated following Denny-Brown's appointment; this staff included Lennox, the Gibbses, and Merritt. My sympathy was somewhat exaggerated by a suspicion of possible guilt. I had been consulted by one of the power brokers on the inside of the Harvard hierarchy at the time that Denny-Brown was being considered. I had approved of his choice without adequate thought as to its possible adverse effects on my friends. That my opinion had any real effect at that time is most unlikely. However, the individual mentioned did make a special trip out to the hospital in San Francisco to see me, a fact that left me wondering. Merritt's position for 3 years under Denny-Brown must have been very difficult; they were men of very different temperaments. It was a difficult situation, aggravated by wartime conditions. I have heard Merritt complain about many problems but never a word about the difficult problem he faced at Boston City Hospital.

I always believed that Putnam did well to draw Merritt to New York, but I thought that he should have worked him in as assistant director of the New York Neurological Institute in charge of operations. Merritt's practical sense and organizational genius might have saved the day for Putnam, considering how Merritt managed the same situation later. Putnam's brilliance, unfortunately, did not extend to administrative detail.

Following World War II, I had organized a symposium on epilepsy in San Francisco for the Western Institute on Epilepsy and invited both Putnam and Merritt as participants. This was my introduction to Putnam's reserve in extending credit to

Merritt for their development of phenytoin as an antiepileptic therapy. However, insofar as I had ever heard, Merritt made no claims with respect to the basic concept or early physiologic studies that were involved in this brilliant work. I happened to know about this because the laboratory testing of potential drugs was performed by a young woman whom I knew later as the wife of Robert Schwab, an old friend at Harvard. Merritt's part concerned the clinical trial of phenytoin, and I gained the impression that he was embarrassed by Putnam's defensive posture on this score. Perhaps other factors were involved as a result of Putnam's unfortunate experience in New York.

At later dates, Merritt participated at our center in a symposium on pain (1956) and as a visiting professor of neurology (1965). He was not a brilliant showman, like Macdonald Critchley or Henry Miller but, nevertheless, was extremely well organized and effective. His examinations of patients were thorough for the job at hand, and his analysis of clinical problems was excellent. He was not a Sir Charles Symonds, of course, but how many neurologists are?

I will never forget Merritt in Vienna, in September 1965, some 6 months after he had been our guest in San Francisco. While standing at an intersection in Vienna, a cab drew up directly in front of me and stopped because of the traffic. The rear window of the cab was down and there sat Merritt, 5 or 6 feet from me. He cut quite a figure, as I recall, in top hat, high collar with cravat, waistcoat, what I took to be a swallow-tailed coat, pin-striped trousers, spats, gloves, and cane.

My recall on the specific details mentioned may be faulty, but the general effect was striking and unmistakable. Impulsively, I cried, "Houston" What a resplendent sight! Now I have seen everything!''

I believe he was slightly appalled by this unexpected encounter, my outburst, and incredulous fixed gaze. However, Merritt was not one to be abashed for long and perhaps in another defensive reaction replied, "You yokels in the far West are too remote from the center of things.''

"But your costume, Houston! Where in the world could you be going in that array at this time of day?''

"`I'm on my way to see the committee that decides where the next International Congress is to be held, and I am making a plea for New York.''

As he said this, his cab pulled away, but I managed a wave and cried, "Good luck!''

As usual, Merritt was successful, and his organization of the International Congress in 1969 far surpassed the previous congresses that I had attended since 1949.

In my opinion, Merritt's *Textbook of Neurology* was the culminating glory of his brilliant career in neurology. His part in the development of phenytoin was that of an able clinical researcher. As an administrator, he was a genius. The fine group of academic "Merritt-orious'' professors that he developed probably equals or surpasses in value his book, but it is in the sound scholarly workmanship of his book and in its balanced practical presentations that his accomplishments are more apparent to most of us.

THE SURGICAL TREATMENT OF EPILEPSY
AND FURTHER RESEARCH

Other noteworthy advances in the study and therapy of epilepsy, which overlapped slightly with those advances made at the Harvard Neurological Unit, were developed by Dr. Wilder Penfield and his associates at the Montreal Neurological Institute. Starting in 1934, with generous Rockefeller Foundation support to McGill University, their studies reached a peak in the 1950s. Although the main impact of Penfield's studies was to delineate the role of neurological surgery in the treatment of epilepsy, his research also played a major role in the cerebral localization of clinical symptomatology and the underlying neurophysiology of the different seizure states. The story can largely be told in the career of Dr. Penfield.

WILDER G. PENFIELD (1891—1976)

Born in Spokane, Washington, the son and grandson of physicians, Penfield was educated in Wisconsin and at Princeton University. While obtaining his basic medical training at Johns Hopkins School of Medicine, he won a Rhodes scholarship. Further studies followed at Oxford where he did research on decerebrate rigidity with Sir Charles Sherrington. He worked with Gordon Holmes and Godwin Greenfield at the National Hospital, Queen Square, London; with Ramon y Cajal and del Rio-Hortega in Madrid; and with Otfrid Foerster in Breslau, Germany. In 1924, Penfield joined the Department of Surgery of the College of Physicians and Surgeons (Columbia) in New York City. Here he established a laboratory of neurocytology and wrote his book on neuropathology (14). In New York, he became acquainted with Alan Greg, later director of medical sciences and vice president of the Rockefeller Foundation. As in the case of Stanley Cobb, this explained their "magic carpet" of support for many years.

In 1928, Penfield was offered the support of the Rockefeller Foundation to start a neurological institute, and through the supportive efforts of Dr. Edward Archibald, Professor of Surgery at McGill, he finally settled on McGill University. He established the departments of neurology and neurosurgery at McGill with Dr. Collin Russell as chief of neurology and Dr. William Cone as chief of neurosurgery. This gave him a fine, supportive staff that freed him for his primary interests in research. However, it was not until 1934 that the new institute was finally completed.

Following the lead of Foerster, surgery on intractable epileptic patients became the main focus of his work. This involved careful initial neurological, psychological, and EEG studies, followed by his cortical stimulatory studies on conscious patients. This resulted in several classic reports on brain localization and function (15-17). Electrocorticography and neuropathological studies aided in the understanding of the underlying neuropathophysiology of symptomatic forms of epilepsy. His recruitment of Herbert Jasper from Brown University, Rhode Island, led, not only to thorough EEG studies before, during, and after surgery, but also to basic neurophysiological studies in the different forms of epileptic seizures (discussed subsequently). This comprehensive approach inevitably attracted a host of trainees in the clinical and preclinical specialties—many of whom went on to professorships in the United States, Canada, and other countries. He was the author of some 300 scientific publications, mainly concerned with the neurophysiology and neuropathology of epilepsy. In addition, he was the editor or author of seven monographs that summarize the studies of his group.

Penfield received many honors and wide acclaim as director of the Montreal Neurological Institute and as professor of both neurology and neurological Surgery at McGill. The large number and the variety of Penfield's awards, without question, made him one of the most honored physicians in the history of medicine.

Penfield always struck me as being somewhat of a saintly person; this went beyond his Bible reading on Sunday evenings. He was a thoughtful and kindly person in his relations with his patients and colleagues. At the same time, his critical mind demanded the best of himself and his staff in both his research and the operation of the institute. My contacts with Dr. Penfield extended over a period of 40 years and were always pleasant. I first met him in 1935 at a meeting of the American Neurological Association in Montreal and, later, at many more meetings of this society because both of us were regular attendants for over two decades. In addition, he served as a visiting professor of neurology at the University of California School of Medicine in 1960 (see account of Francis Walshe, discussed in Chapter 17), and in 1961, I attended one of the parties celebrating his 70th birthday. One episode may be worth recounting because it reflects the kind nature of Penfield.

I believe it was in 1947 that I presented the results of a study that correlated prolonged EEG abnormalities following cerebral concussion with an increased permeability of the cerebrovascular system, as determined by the spectrographic measurements of a tracer agent. These studies suggested that the perivascular pathology of cerebral concussion could be explained on this basis and, presumably, was related to the disruptive shearing forces of concussion between the soft cellular masses of the brain and their more rigid, supporting cerebrovascular tree (as I had found in earlier World War II studies) (18). In addition, both the EEG dysrhythmia and permeability changes were shown to be markedly reduced by a preceding series of injections of the supravital dye, trypan red, which in other studies, had been shown to reduce the permeability of the cerebrovascular system by some 30%.

Penfield, who was in the audience and who was aware of my previous articles on the protective effect of trypan red in experimental epilepsy, rose and asked why the dye's protective effect worked in other forms of epilepsy as well as against experimental convulsive agents. I was delighted with his question because the previous discussant had gone off on a tangent and, by twisting the subject to cite an article of his own, had obscured the point of my presentation. Penfield's question brought the subject back into focus and gave me an opportunity to relate convulsive susceptibility to the increased cerebrovascular permeability associated with cerebral pathology in symptomatic forms of epilepsy. My reply was that, with almost all forms of cerebral insult, the permeability of the cerebral blood vessels in the involved regions is abnormally increased, which alters the local homeostatic metabolic equilibrium.

Components of the blood stream escape into the parenchyma of the brain and disturb the normal extracellular exchange—its chemistry and physiology. Thus, abnormal brain wave activity is produced, and in seizure-susceptible patients, a convulsive diathesis might result. When the cerebrovascular permeability was lowered by the use of the supravital dye, this abnormal condition was controlled in some measure (19). In addition to the protective effect of the dye, the implication of this was that at least one form of abnormal brain wave could be caused by abnormally increased cerebrovascular permeability. This factor, of course, underlies differential staining techniques and the localization of central nervous system (CNS) lesions with radioactive isotopes. In other words, CNS stains and isotopes concentrate on pathological regions for the same reason that some abnormal brain waves have localizing potential—they all are secondary effects of focal impairments of the blood–brain barrier, as I and my colleagues were able to suggest in still a later study (20).

Dr. Penfield's question raised an important point, and I have always thought that, in asking his question, he was trying to help me by broadening the subject to an important related issue. Not only did Penfield's question reveal a kindly nature, but it also revealed his ability to bring the subject into focus, thereby emphasizing the subject's most important aspects.

In summary, Penfield's contributions to the field of epileptology were to define the potentialities and limitations of neurosurgery for epileptogenic foci in different areas of the cerebrum and to expand greatly the knowledge of the underlying neurophysiology of different seizure types. Although less important than the two phases of the diagnosis and treatment of epilepsy previously described (and coming much later), the surgical approach to epilepsy and the basic research accomplished at Montreal nevertheless contributed to several vital aspects of the epilepsy problem. Again, in the Penfield account, a noteworthy fact is that the studies on epilepsy, like the studies of Lennox, the Gibbses, Merritt, and Putnam in Boston, strikingly exemplify the dependence of modern neurology on the scientific advances achieved in the early decades of the 20th century.

The contributions of Herbert Jasper to the study of epilepsy should be mentioned because he was closely associated with Penfield for 27 years. Jasper was the main contributor to the neurophysiological studies at the Montreal Neurological Institute from 1933 to 1965.

HERBERT H. JASPER (1906-   )

Jasper was born in the Pacific Northwest at La Grande, Oregon. In rapid succession, he obtained a B.A. at Reed College in 1927, an M.A. at the University of Oregon in psychology and philosophy in 1929, a Ph.D. in psychology under Professor E. Trevis at the University of Iowa in 1931, and a D.duSc. in physiology under Professor Lapique at the University of Paris in 1935. He then obtained his medical degree, M.D.C.M., at McGill University under the stimulus of Penfield.

His first academic appointment was at Brown University where he served as an assistant professor of psychology and director of the neurophysiological laboratory for 5 years (1933 to 1938). In addition, he ran the EEG laboratory at the Bradley Home; it was there that I first met Jasper in early 1940. This apparently was in an overlapping period, inasmuch as Penfield had recruited Jasper as an associate professor at McGill University in 1938. He was then promoted to be a professor of experimental neurology at McGill in 1946 where he was the head of the neurophysiological laboratories of the Montreal Neurological Institute and in charge of graduate studies and research. He also was a consultant to the EEG and electromyography services of the five main hospitals in Montreal.

Five years after Penfield's retirement in 1960, Jasper transferred to the University of Montreal, when it became well supported by the Province of Quebec. From 1965 until his retirement in 1976, Jasper was a professor of neurophysiology, and from 1967 to 1976, he was the director of the medical research council group in the neurological sciences of the department of physiology. Following his retirement, he served as Honorary Consultant in Neuroscience for both the University of Montreal and the Montreal Neurological Institute of McGill University.

Jasper's early duties at the Montreal Neurological Institute primarily involved EEG studies. These included recording electrocorticographic studies during Penfield's operations and careful postoperative EEGs, which led to a collaboration with Penfield on the localization of symptoms produced by cortical stimulation and localization (17). In addition, he led in the neurophysiological studies of seizure states in animals, which have done much to establish the underlying pathophysiology of absence, temporal lobe epilepsy, and focal seizures.

I well remember Jasper's move to have his 10-20 system of EEG recording accepted as the international system. Several systems had been developed and were in use, among them my own,* based on a careful comparison of the electrical activity of all monopolar and bipolar recordings of one side with the other. This system followed the basic principle of the neurological examination and gave excellent results for purposes of localization as well as for more generalized EEG activity (21). The other systems, besides Jasper's and my own, seemed inadequate to me for the study of focal abnormalities because insufficient numbers of electrodes were used for localizations, yet at that time, one of these other systems threatened to become accepted as the standard. When Jasper agreed that other adequate localizing systems would be respected and articles based on such systems would be accepted by the *International Journal of EEG and Clinical Neurophysiology*, of which he was the editor and I was the associate editor, I voted for the international system. The "steamroller" tactics of the next generation, however, failed to uphold Jasper's point. Nevertheless, it served us well for nearly 30 years and was invaluable in certain research, such as a study of the spread of epileptic discharge from foci (22) and the discovery of an important depth sign (23).

Jasper extended his research to neurochemical mechanisms, including neurotransmitters and modulating substances, using microelectrode techniques for single cell activity under varying states of consciousness and cerebral activity. In addition to

* My system was also good as a teaching system. Criteria for significant localization were established, as opposed to stray variant recordings. For example, it did a better job of localization in the temporal regions than did the 10-20 system.

epilepsy, his studies ranged from head injuries to dyskinesias, sleep, anesthesia, coma, emotional excitement, and learning. Many of his studies involved the thalamocortical and thalamoreticular systems.

Jasper was an author or co-author of over 300 publications and served as editor or associate editor of seven journals. He was a member of over 30 professional associations. He received many honors and gave many invited lectures. Prizes have been established in his name, and two international neurophysiological symposiums were held in his honor.

Jasper greatly helped bridge the gaps between the basic techniques of neurophysiology, neurochemistry, and clinical neurology. Although he was one of the leaders in the field of epilepsy in the early phase of the flowering of neurology, his studies extended beyond epilepsy and beyond the flowering period.

A FEW LEADERS WHO FURTHER DEVELOPED THE FIELD OF EPILEPSY AND AIDED IN THE FLOWERING OF NEUROLOGY

Although the original stimulus to the clinical neurophysiological study of epilepsy and to its drug and surgical therapy developed (as noted in the previous sections), a host of related studies soon followed that extended the initial work. Because the expansion of the clinical studies was the first great impetus to establish neurology as an independent clinical discipline, a few careers involved in this important development will be used to illustrate it.

CAESAR LOMBROSO (1917-   )

It is difficult to understand the early, convoluted course of Dr. Lombroso's career without understanding his place of birth, family background, and the events leading to World War II. Born in Rome in 1917 into a distinguished family, he might have remained in Italy, except for the fascist movements of Hitler and Mussolini in the 1930s. His father was a professor of physiology who fled from Italy rather than pledge allegiance to Mussolini. An uncle and aunt were antifascist writers who were arrested and exiled from Italy. In his youth, Lombroso was a dedicated antifascist and a member of the Italian underground.

Following his graduation from the University of Genoa, Lombroso won a poetry contest that paid for a trip to the United States. He started medicine at Johns Hopkins University, but with the outbreak of World War II, he resumed his activities as an antifascist. Lombroso became involved with editing a journal, broadcasting to the Italian resistance movement, and working with various antifascist and anticommunist organizations. While attending the First World Youth Congress

---

* The charm and good wisdom of Eleanor Roosevelt is still one of my bright memories, and for this reason, I can understand the important impact of this meeting on Lombroso. In 1925, Mrs. Roosevelt was a guest in the Telluride House at Cornell University, and as one of the 18 members of this scholarship house, we came to know her quite well over the week she was with us. Furthermore, my mother, who was visiting at the same time, became a life-long friend of Mrs. Roosevelt.

sponsored by Eleanor Roosevelt* at the White House, Lombroso met his future wife Rysia, a Polish woman similarly engaged in antifascist work.

At the end of World War II, the Lombrosos returned to Italy. At the University of Genoa, Lombroso completed his medical studies, obtained a Ph.D. in physiology in 1956, and completed residency training in pediatrics. Having developed an interest in neurology, he next moved to Boston and worked with Dr. William Lennox at the Seizure Unit of the Children's Hospital. He received residency training in neurology and neuropathology with Raymond Adams at the Massachusetts General Hospital. Lombroso then returned to the Seizure Unit, and on Dr. Lennox's retirement in 1960, he was made his successor. Still later, he was appointed Director of the Division of Neurophysiology. Clinical and research fellowships were established for the unit and the laboratory. Lombroso next established the Family Service Team to better integrate and extend the activities of the Seizure Unit. This team included social service workers, psychologists, and psychiatrists, who worked closely with the neurological group in the Seizure Unit. Comprehensive studies with long-term follow-up were initiated, which became a model for other seizure units. Lombroso insisted on the integration of EEG and other laboratory studies with clinical work. I heartily cheered this especially notable action. It was to emphasize this integration that I joined the American EEG Society in 1947 and subsequently served as the first chair of the American Board of Qualification in Electroencephalography.

Lombroso published over 180 articles in addition to reviews and chapters in texts dealing with all aspects of epilepsy, including some new approaches. He won many honors and was elected to the top positions in the EEG and epilepsy societies. Like Aicardi, his counterpart in France (discussed in Chapter 9), Lombroso's work is a splendid example of the successful integration of the clinical and basic neurological sciences, which advanced modern neurology and established it as an independent discipline.

SAMUEL LIVINGSTON (1908-1984)

Most of those selected to illustrate the aspects of the field of epileptology had other interests and connections—not so Dr. Livingston. His *raison d'etre* was epilepsy, and he pursued it with tenacity and success. His primary objective was therapeutic improvement of the epileptic condition of his patients, but he also championed their social and legal rights.

Livingston was born in Philadelphia. He graduated from Georgetown University, magna cum laude, in 1928. He obtained an M.A. in chemistry at George Washington University and his M.D. at Vanderbilt University in 1934. His postgraduate training was in pediatrics at Johns Hopkins Hospital. He started private practice in 1936, but he continued to work in the Epilepsy Clinic at Johns Hopkins Hospital. Ten years later, he was made the director of the clinic. Using both his private and clinic groups of patients, he eventually accumulated over 30,000 epileptic patients for his studies.

His main clinical research involved the trial of almost all of the new antiepileptic agents as they became available. Equally notable was his study of seizure-inducing mechanisms and their effectiveness in the management of his patients. In this connection, his articles on the ketogenic diet and photogenic activation were particularly noteworthy. His emphasis on treating the patient as a whole was exemplary, which he emphasized in his text (24).

In his monograph, *Living with Epileptic Seizures*, Livingston describes measures to alleviate the social, emotional, and economic problems of epileptic patients (25). He showed that the driving safety record of epileptic patients was better than the driving record of the general population. He worked to reverse the American Medical Association's position against contact sports for epileptic patients. Livingston contributed to efforts to ease restrictions against the immigration of such patients, to obtain insurance privileges for them, and with the support of the United States Attorney General's office, to lessen legal bias. In addition to these major contributions, Livingston published over 300 articles, chapters, other texts, teaching brochures, and films. His was a dedicated life, and next to Dr. Lennox, Livingston probably did more to aid the cause of epileptic patients than did any other person.

HENRI GASTAUT (1915-   )

Another aspect of the broad development of the field of epilepsy is illustrated by the career of Henri Gastaut. His efforts were, not only in research, clinical diagnosis, care of epileptic patients, and teaching, but also in the international organization related to epilepsy, in the refinements of epileptic terminology, and in the classification of the epilepsies. No doubt much of this will change as research progresses, but his impact in the classification of a chaotic field was impressive.

The term *prima donna* has often been applied to Gastaut. This term suggests a distinguished performer but can also refer to an individual whose abilities are not in proportion to his or her temperamental and conceited manner. However, the term should be used with caution in the case of Gastaut. True, Gastaut was a performer and a very scintillating one, but he was also a teacher whose showmanship was in the best tradition of the old French school. Unlike the bombast and self-importance of the lesser German school, whose inflated performances had a pecuniary basis, Gastaut's teaching showmanship (sparkling and characterized by much wit, humor, and oratory) was sincere and effective. When I think of this aspect of Gastaut, I always think of the great spontaneity with which he conducted the clinical conferences at the Centre Hospitalier Universitaire "*La Timone*," which I attended in late 1957 as a Fulbright Research Scholar.

These conferences would start with Gastaut's precautionary remarks to the participating French physicians that they must speak clearly and in measured terms for my benefit. The French temperament, however, could not be so constrained for long. Like a locomotive slowly gaining speed, the conferences started very sedately. However, as interest in the patient's condition grew and debate advanced on uncertain aspects of the clinical problem, the tempo of the conferences accelerated and often culminated in excited exchanges with two or three of the participants talking simultaneously. At this point, my feeble ability to follow the tumultuous discourse rapidly waned. When Gastaut saw me lean back in relaxation, he would roar "*Attendez*," pound the conference table, and bring the conference to an abrupt halt. Once more, the conclave would take off with measured cadence but, inevitably, gain speed and momentum as the discussion waxed in intensity. I probably was little more than an ineffective and, perhaps, unwelcome brake to their spirited conferences. Nevertheless, except for Gastaut's thoughtfulness and command of the situation, I would have gained little from these fascinating clinical sessions. Also, I was fascinated with their ability to understand many of my English terms—lapses in the heat of the exchange—although the postwar ascendancy of English was officially not approved nor admitted in the 1950s. In quieter exchanges, it appeared that English was not understood.

That Gastaut was an orator at heart was clearly shown on his visit to San Francisco in 1955. He had arrived with three lectures written in English. Following his first lecture, which went perfectly well, he came to me and complained how "traumatique" it was to read the lecture. Reading slowed him down; his natural exuberant delivery was "crushed." He insisted that I read his second lecture, which he frequently interrupted. As a compromise, for his third lecture, he was to hold forth in French with an English interpreter translating each passage. Dr. Francis Schiller, a Czechoslovakian who spoke perfect French and English, served as the translator. Gastaut was on center stage, and Schiller sat at a side table. As Gastaut paused in his discourse, Schiller would translate but always with the close monitoring of Gastaut. On one occasion, a French term with two possible meanings was mistranslated by Schiller. Gastaut, with a resounding "*Non,*" bounded across the stage. Schiller, who had been facing the audience, cringed as he suddenly became aware of the unexpected and threatening advance of Gastaut toward him. The entire house was brought down by this amusing dramatic performance. For months afterward, people spoke to me of this final session—Gastaut holding forth with his sparkling eyes, animated gesticulations, and flow of beautiful French. Many flattered themselves on their ability to understand him, and all delighted in this third, concluding presentation.

Beyond all these more obvious aspects of Gastaut, he was a serious and sound scholar whose brilliance cannot be denied. This is best documented by his career and accomplishments.

Born in Monaco in 1915, his early training led to a *Licence de Sciences Naturelles* and then a medical doctorate. His interests in teaching and research led to advanced training in medicine and neurological sciences. Following World War II, he went to the Montreal Neurological Institute and studied electromyography with Jasper and with the distinguished group at the Institute in Epileptology. These subjects became his chief fields of interest and research. He developed an extensive laboratory at La Timone Hospital, which was the main teaching hospital of the University of Aix-Marseilles School of Medicine. This later was recognized by the World Health Organization (WHO) as a "center of excellence" for training and research in neurobiology. Basic neurophysiological studies were pursued to some extent in the research laboratories of the medical school. The main direction of Gastaut's interests, however, involved clinical studies that chiefly concerned electroencephalography and its activating techniques. On one notable occasion, I hit the jackpot in this connection. As a visiting lecturer in Sweden, I was asked to examine a man who had episodes of syncope and was suspected of having epilepsy. However, because all findings were normal, the problem was puzzling. On checking him and obtaining his story, I recalled a similar patient in La Timone. After obtaining permission from the patient and staff, I pressed on his orbits during EEG and EEG recordings and reproduced one of his episodes. The typical cardiac and EEG responses were obtained, much to everyone's delight.

In keeping with his clinical neurophysiological studies, Gastaut's other main interest was in epileptology following the well-established patterns in North America. Most noteworthy were his studies on complex partial seizures (temporal lobe epilepsy) and the EEG variant of epilepsy, which Dr. Lennox had reported long before in severe forms of childhood seizures associated with deep cerebral pathology. Because of Gastaut's many articles on this, the condition was later called the Lennox-Gastaut syndrome. His studies on the antiepileptic properties of diazepam and clonazepam (two of the benzodiazepines) were also notable.

Another episode illustrates Gastaut's enthusiasm and ability to overcome serious odds. At the time of Gastaut's visit to the University of California, San Francisco, in 1955, we discussed our mutual interest in temporal lobe epilepsy. For years, I had wondered about the bilateral asynchrony of temporal recordings as opposed to the normal bilateral synchrony of all other cortical areas. We had developed precise dual-beam cathode ray oscillographic recording techniques, and by clinical EEG correlation studies, I had hoped to explore this subject. When Gastaut stated that he had an oscillograph recording system adequate for the project, I decided to spend my forthcoming sabbatical leave (1957 to 1958) with him in Marseilles; I obtained a Fulbright Research Scholarship for this study abroad. Unfortunately, the equipment in Marseilles proved inadequate, and a substitute project with Mrs. Yvette Gastaut was conducted on posterior EEG rhythms (26).

I was amused by Gastaut's efforts to obtain the proper equipment. A German oscillograph capable of the task was well known but at that juncture could not be procured through the centrally controlled French system of university support; however, Gastaut was not to be stopped. He eventually succeeded in having a French scientific equipment company purchase the German oscillograph, and with proper adjustment of labels and paper nomenclature, the oscillograph was finally purchased for the University of Aix-Marseilles. The procedure was delayed, however; the equipment arrived just before I left.

Gastaut's publications number in the hundreds. Most significant was his ability to synthesize and summarize the vast background of his fields of interest. The most notable of these publications were *The Physiopathogenesis of the Epilepsies* (27), an international classification of epileptic seizures (in which he played a major role) (28) and the WHO *Dictionary of Epilepsy* (29).

In addition to his teaching and research, Gastaut organized many EEG conferences and international symposia. The Colloques de Marseilles was the most notable of these.

Alpine EEG ski meetings were held under his presidency for 20 years in France, Austria, Switzerland, Italy, and Germany. He was an enthusiastic skier.

Gastaut's enthusiasm extended into many fields of interest. He was an avid sailor, a collector of a number of ethnological treasures, a writer of several fascinating articles of the presumed medical conditions of prominent men of history, and as has been described by his friend and co-author Roger Broughton, a *"gastronome extraordinaire"* and a "connoisseur of painting and fine arts." That he was a bon vivant and fine connoisseur of wines, I can attest from many experiences, but one in particular serves to document the point. Mrs. Aird and I were invited to a Christmas party at his home when he lived on La Promenade de la Corniche. A select group of professors in the medical school and University of Aix-Marseilles had been invited. It was a lively and elegant party with excellent food and wine. Gastaut capped the occasion by introducing a rare wine in which each grape had been selected with care. The slope of the hill and location of the vineyard meant little to me, but obviously, this information was received with acclaim by his elite friends. My taste for fine wine had been developed to some extent by sampling California wines, but I quickly realized that the fine wine-tasting event of the Gastauts was far beyond the capability of my relatively unsophisticated taste buds. The wine was not wasted, of course, because it obviously was a fine wine. However, as I tasted the wine amid this select group and observed the sipping, the murmurs, and the expressions of delight, I realized that there must be subtleties of taste beyond my ability to discern.

Gastaut served with great distinction in several administrative posts. In addition to serving the International Federation of EEG and Clinical Neurophysiology, the International League Against Epilepsy, and the WHO, Gastaut was dean of the Faculty of Medicine of Marseilles for several years and, finally in 1971, was elevated to the presidency of the University of Aix-Marseilles.

As might be expected, many neurological, EEG, and epilepsy societies have honored Henri Gastaut. He has received honorary doctorate degrees from four universities and has been awarded several decorations in France and in other countries.

SUMMARY

The advances made in epilepsy, starting in the 1930s and extending through the flowering period of neurology, uniquely depended on neurophysiological techniques—EEG recordings, convulsive threshold measurements, and empirical neurophysiological research. The results, which greatly advanced our understanding of epilepsy and care of epileptic patients, were a great impetus to modern neurology because epilepsy continues to be one of the most common and important neurological disorders.

The diagnostic, therapeutic, and other aspects of these advances have been traced through the careers of those leaders who accomplished them. Starting in the Harvard neurological unit of the Boston City Hospital in the 1930s, the advances quickly spread to other centers. Significant surgical and research advances were later made at the Montreal Neurological Institute, and eventually the research on epilepsy, both clinical and basic, became international in its scope.

REFERENCES

1. Lennox, W.G., and Cobb, S. Epilepsy from the standpoint of physiology and treatment. *Medicine*, 7:105-290, 1928.
2. Gibbs, F.A., Davis, H., and Lennox W.G. The electro-encephalogram in epilepsy and in conditions of impaired consciousness. *Arch. Neurol. Psychiatry*, 34:1133-1148, 1935.
3. Gibbs, F.A., and Lennox, W.G. The electrical activity of the brain in epilepsy. *N. Engl. J. Med.*, 216:98-99, 1937.
4. Lennox, W.G., and Lennox, M.A. *Epilepsy and Related Disorders.* Boston, Little, Brown & Co., 1960.
5. Gibbs, F.A., and Gibbs, E.L. *Atlas of Encephalography.* vols. 1-3. Reading, MA, Addison-Wesley, 1950. revised 1964.
6. Gibbs, F.A., Gibbs, E.L., and Fuster, B. Anterior temporal localization of sleep-induced seizure discharges of psychomotor type. *Trans. Am. Neurol. Assoc.*, 72:180-182, 1947.
7. Fuster, B., Gibbs, E.L., and Gibbs, F.A. Pentothal sleep as an aid to the diagnosis and localization of seizure discharges of the psychomotor type. *Dis. Nerv. Syst.*, 8:199-203, 1948.
8. Putnam, T., and Merritt, H.H. Experimental determination of the anticonvulsant properties of some phenyl derivatives. *Science*, 85:525-526, 1937.
9. Spiegel, E.A. Quantitative determination of convulsive reactivity by electrical stimulation of brain with skull intact. *J. Lab. Clin. Med.*, 22:1274-1276, 1936.
10. Putnam, T., and Merritt, H.H. A new series of anticonvulsant drugs tested by experiments on animals. *Arch. Neurol. Psychiatry,* 39:1003-1015, 1938.
11. Merritt, H.H., and Putnam, T. Sodium diphenylhydantoinate in the treatment of convulsive disorders. *J.A.M.A.*, 111:1068-1073, 1938.
12. Merritt, H. and Putnam, T. *Trans. Am. Neurol. Assoc.*, 101:271-272, 1976.
13. Merritt, H.H. *Textbook of Neurology.* Philadelphia, Lea & Febiger, 1955.
14. Penfield, W.G. *Cytology and Cellular Pathology of the Nervous System.* New York, Hoeber, 1932.
15. Penfield, W.G., and Erickson, T.C. *Epilepsy and Cerebral Localization.* Springfield, IL, Charles C. Thomas, 1941.
16. Penfield, W.G., and Rasmussen, T. *The Cerebral Cortex of Man.* New York, MacMillan, 1951.
17. Penfield, W.G., and Jasper, H. *Epilepsy and the Functional Anatomy of the Human Brain.* Boston, Little, Brown & Co., 1954.
18. Aird, R.B., Strait, L.A., Zealear, D., and Hrenoff, M. Neurophysiological studies on cerebral conssion. *Trans. Am. Neurol. Assoc.*, 72:89-92, 1947.
19. Aird, R.B. Experimental studies on the origin of certain cerebral dysrhythmias of non-specific type. *IV* Congres Neurologique International, *Paris*, 5-10 Septembre 1949. *Communications.* vol. II. Paris, Masson, 1949, p. 129.
20. Sasaki, M., Aird, R.B., Kennedy, R., Kerber, C., Newton, T.H., and Powell, M. Correlative study of EEG and brain scintiphotography. *Trans. Am. Neurol. Assoc.*, 96:299-300, 1971.
21. Aird, R.B., and Bowditch, S. Cortical localization by electroencephalography: the value of quantitative and statistical analysis of homologous recordings obtained simultaneously. *J. Neurosurg.*, 3:407-420, 1946.
22. Aird, R.B., and Garoutte, B. Propagation of epileptic discharge, as revealed by activated electroencephalography. *Epilepsia*, 1:337-350, 1960.
23. Hasegawa, K., and Aird, R.B. An EEG study of deep-seated cerebral and subtentorial lesions in comparison with cortical lesions. *Electroencephalogr. Clin. Neurophysiol.*, 15:934-946, 1963.
24. Livingston, S. *The Diagnosis and Treatment of Convulsive Disorders of Children.* Springfield, IL, Charles C. Thomas, 1954.
25. Livingston, S. *Living With Epileptic Seizures.* Springfield, IL, Charles C. Thomas, 1963.
26. Aird, R.B., and Gastaut, Y. Occipital and posterior electroencephalographic rhythms. *Electroencephalogr.* Clin. Neurophysiol., 11:637-655, 1959.
27. Gastaut, H., Jasper, H., Bancaud, J., and Waltregny, A. *The Physiopathogenesis of the Epilepsies.* Springfield, IL, Charles C. Thomas, 1969.
28. Gastaut, H. Clinical and electroencephalographic classification of epileptic seizures. *Epilepsia*, 11:102-113, 1970.
29. Gastaut, H., and International Panel of Experts. *Dictionary of Epilepsy.* Part I: *Definitions.* Geneva, World Health Organization, 1973.

CHAPTER 3

Advances in
Clinical Neurological Diagnosis

IMPROVED NEUROLOGICAL HISTORY-TAKING AND EXAMINATION

It is a curious fact that, in tracing the many changes that culminated in the flowering of neurology as a clinical specialty, advances in clinical study have been among the most difficult to place in proper perspective and to validate. Certainly, William Gowers (1) in *A Manual of Diseases of the Nervous System* was one of the most successful early neurologists to systematize the existing knowledge. For years, this was considered the Bible of neurology (2). As history-taking became more precise and was routinely extended to include the patient's personal, family, and social history, many formerly hidden aspects of disease processes in their course of development were clarified. Genetic disorders and psychiatric conditions, in particular, were more clearly delineated. Thorough history-taking and comprehensive physical and neurological examinations, along with the later addition of many laboratory findings, have finally filled out the diagnostic aspects of medicine.

An amusing misconception of my early youth may be worthy of mention, inasmuch as it touches on the essential features of clinical diagnosis. Perhaps I misunderstood something that I had heard. In any case, I related the stories of detection developed by Sir Arthur Conan Doyle in the Sherlock Holmes mysteries to the evolution of clinical study. That his stories had any impact on sharpening medical diagnosis is most unlikely. Although this youthful misconception was corrected years before my own medical training started, it still served to heighten my interest in Doyle and his methods of detection as applied to clinical diagnosis.

My later knowledge of Doyle and his medical background was obtained from an introduction to Doyle's works in a family library book. Very briefly, I learned that he (1859-1930) was born and mainly educated in Edinburgh (M.B. in 1881 and M.D. in 1885) and had practiced medicine until 1891. While developing a practice, which in those days required years of effort, he found considerable time to write, and this proved to be more successful than his medical practice. Utilizing ingenious plots, Doyle applied the developing techniques of medical diagnosis to crime detec-

tion and highlighted these methods in the person of Sherlock Holmes whose prototype was Dr. Joseph Bell, one of Doyle's keenly observant professors at Edinburgh.
Starting with *A Study in Scarlet* in 1887, his stories, as related by Holmes' friend,
Dr. Watson, caught on and, ever since then, have been immortalized in plays,
motion pictures, radio, and television. Much of Doyle's success, no doubt, reflected
his keen insight, the web of mystery he achieved in his detective stories, and his
sense of the dramatic. He was knighted in 1902.

In spite of his great success with Sherlock Holmes, Doyle preferred historical subjects; his last Sherlock Holmes story was written in 1905. The later tragedy of the
death of his son in World War I considerably darkened his final years and probably
explained his late conversion to spiritualism. It was my interest in his earlier background, however, that made me eager to meet Doyle when the opportunity arose in
1925. However, it is necessary for me to first explain how this encounter occurred.

My father, Dr. John W. Aird, was a successful physician and surgeon. However, his
remarkable dedication to his profession, which involved intense and endless activity
day and night, seemed to me a questionable way to live. At a later date, as a result of
more advanced training and after wavering among architecture, history, and physics, I
finally realized that medicine might not be as bad a choice as I had imagined. It
became obvious that, no matter what career I selected, much in-depth training and critical thinking would be required. I greatly enjoyed college and discovered a scientific
bent, narrowing my career choice down to physics or medicine. It had reached the
point where I felt that I could not accept further scholarships without making a choice.
A decision was essential to meet the prerequisites for graduate school.

To decide the issue, I undertook a bicycle trip to Europe. While in Switzerland, I
finally decided on medicine. On returning to Paris, 2 weeks before my return to
America, I happened to hear that Sir Arthur Conan Doyle was to give a lecture in Paris
at Salle Wagrum. Although Doyle's subject was spiritualism, my enthusiasm for meeting him was not appreciably dampened. My interest, of course, was not in spiritualism,
and my reaction to this aspect of his talk was one of total disbelief. Although his slides,
which showed ectoplasm issuing forth from the mouths and ears of mediums could
easily have been faked, no one accused Doyle of deception insofar as I have ever
heard. However, his belief in a hereafter and his acceptance of spiritualism as evidence
of the hereafter probably fitted in with his desire to maintain contact with his son, tragically lost in World War I. This combination, of course, is one of the well-known attractions of spiritualism. On meeting him after the lecture, I mentioned that his application
of detailed study and deductive reasoning in crime stories may have been a factor that
led me to my decision on a medical career. The meeting, although brief, was stimulating in that he seemed interested in the idea that his detective stories had helped to influence my decision to go into medicine.

In retrospect, it is obvious that my thinking at that time involved a romantic conceptualization of medicine and its methods. Nevertheless, because the relationship
between detection and medical diagnosis seemed more than coincidental to me, the
thought of clinical work assumed thrilling proportions in my youthful mind.
Considering Doyle's preoccupation with spiritualism, my contact with him had an

effect that was entirely out of proportion to what might have been expected. Perhaps, this was due to the fact that my decision to pursue graduate study in medicine had been reached only 1 week before I met Doyle. In any case, this contact certainly served as a stimulus for me to undertake more thorough history-taking and examinations. Much later, as a consultant, who on average, was the fifth doctor to see referred patients, this paid rich dividends. Furthermore, I used this method in teaching by making neurological diagnosis a game of detection—a method whereby students might increase their acumen and improve their diagnostic yield.

Doyle's detective stories were a symptom of the striking changes that were developing in the medical world in the late 19th century. Physical examinations for other than deformities and wounds were essentially unknown before 1836 (3). By mid-century, however, thorough study was championed by the then-predominant French school, exemplified by such leaders as Trousseau, Charcot, and Duchenne. Keen observation and analysis were cherished features of Doyle's own student days (about 1880) in Edinburgh. However, if one can judge from the emphasis made by Gowers in his "manual" (1887 to 1888), the refinements of the neurological examination were still very much in an embryonic stage (Gowers, 1881). Gower's manual was called the "Bible" and was credited with being the source of a new, comprehensive order in neurology, which continued well beyond the turn of the century (2). It is interesting to note that Doyle's emphasis on precise observation and examination in his detective stories were written almost simultaneously (*Study in Scarlet,* 1887) with Gower's manual.

No doubt the clinicopathological correlations and new physiological studies of the 19th century had a healthy, stimulating influence on clinical diagnosis in the latter half of that century. It was a period of great change in which American medicine slowly emerged, and this included neurology following the American Civil War. In the case of neurology, Spillane, with particular reference to Gowers and the new British school, has designated this time as the "flowering of neurology" (3). There may have been a diagnostic flowering of sorts, but the true flowering of neurology, which included therapy, rehabilitation, and preventive measures, could not occur until the biomedical sciences of the early 20th century became available and vastly increased our understanding of neurological processes.

With the surge of more precise clinical observation, checked by clinicopathological correlations, neurology, nevertheless, made important gains in the post-Gowerian days. These advances, perhaps, can best be summarized in the careers of two colleagues, Robert Wartenberg and Macdonald Critchley. Having written three of the obituaries on Wartenberg and an article on Critchley for *Founders of Child Neurology,* I approach this task with some confidence (4).

DIAGNOSTIC TESTS IN NEUROLOGY AS ILLUSTRATED BY DR. ROBERT WARTENBERG

Diagnostic Tests in Neurology is the title to one of Professor Wartenberg's many writings on the subject of the neurological examination, a subject to which he devoted most of his life (5). As a good friend and colleague in the Department of Neurology at the University of California, San Francisco (UCSF), I worked closely with Dr. Wartenberg for 20 years. His story is a fascinating one and, in the context of the present subject of diagnostic testing, is particularly instructive (more about this colorful figure will be related in subsequent sections).

ROBERT WARTENBERG (1887-1956)

Born in Lithuania in the city of Grodno near the former German border, he pursued his medical training in Kiel, Munich, and Freiburg and received his medical degree magna cum laude from the University of Rostok in 1919. Postgraduate training with Cassirer (Berlin), Nonne (Hamburg), and Foerster (Breslau) followed, and in 1925, as a fellow of the Rockefeller Foundation, he visited the leading teaching centers of England, France, and the United States. He was made Physician-in-Chief of the Neurology Clinic at Freiburg in 1930 and was promoted to the equivalent of a German associate professor in 1931.

With the rise of Hitler in 1931 and the tightening of Nazi control in 1935, Wartenberg, along with many others, fled from Germany and started his second career at the UCSF School of Medicine in 1936 (as discussed under Sachs in Chapter 17). In spite of some early problems of adjustment (as discussed in Chapters 16 and 18), Dr. Wartenberg slowly won international recognition. Following the development of the UCSF Department of Neurology in 1947, his accomplishments as a neurological scholar and outstanding teacher soon won him promotion to Clinical Professor of Neurology. He became an honorary member of seven national neurological societies, and a Festschrift in his honor was published in December 1952 on the occasion of his 65th birthday. In 1954, he returned to Freiburg as a guest professor of neurology and, in 1955, was made honorary professor of neurology by the University of Freiburg.

His scholarly work was recognized worldwide. He was an associate editor of three journals, and his role as a critic, in his effort to raise the standards of neurology, was both internationally feared and admired. In addition to his 134 articles, he wrote four books. *The Examination of Reflexes,* which was translated into seven languages, was a classic and no doubt the most outstanding of his scholarly writings (5). It presents a simplification of an extraordinarily complicated body of literature and exemplified Wartenberg's scholarly capacity at its best. Wartenberg delighted in demonstrations of reflexes, signs, and tests, a few of which he was the first to describe, for example, the Wartenberg sign (thumb adduction with corticospinal lesions when fingers are flexed against resistance), the head retraction reflex, the head dropping test, and the pendulous leg test. He became a well-known and authoritative critic in this field. One of his final books, *Diagnostic Tests in Neurology*, summarized his contributions and the contributions of others; this book was translated into five languages (6). Of his 134 articles, 12 involved diagnostic signs, 18 concerned neurological tests, and about 15 were devoted to reflexes. Many other advances have been made, as will be recorded in these essays, but surprisingly little at Wartenberg's level of interest.

STILL OTHER EFFORTS

At one point, I thought that I might contribute to this field and was encouraged on this score by professor Wartenberg and other colleagues, such as Drs. Howard Naffziger and Ottiwell Jones. Because the test I developed is of potential value in selected patients, a brief description of it may be justified, considering the purpose of the present subject. The accentuation of signs and symptoms with coughing, sneezing, and straining, or again following pneumoencephalography and brain surgery, is not an uncommon observation in neurological practice and has been explained in terms of alterations of the intracranial pressure of space-consuming processes pressing on nerve roots or the central nervous system directly. Drs. Naffziger and Jones, for example, had used jugular compression as a test to differentiate radicular pain due to tumors or herniated discs from nonpressure-producing conditions. Digital neck pressure to produce jugular compression, however, is associated with widely variable results and, if enthusiastically applied, can cause compression of the internal carotid artery as well. Obvious dangers would be involved in the presence of subtentorial tumors and fragile, intracranial aneurysms or other cerebrovascular conditions.

Using the lengthwise folded cuff of an ordinary sphygmomanometer wrapped about the patient's neck and secured by a face towel, I was able approximately to double the cerebrospinal pressure with cuff pressures of 40 mm Hg. This level of pressure is well below arterial diastolic pressure and has no effect on blood pressure. This could be maintained for 10 or more minutes without discomfort to the patient while selected neurological tests might be repeated. Attention was focused on those findings that earlier examinations or the suspected condition suggested might be altered during the test. The intent was to standardize a safe procedure and clarify the diagnosis in questionable cases by accentuating their signs and symptoms (7). Its use, of course, was in that group of patients suspected of having space-consuming processes.

The results in a survey group were very encouraging, although a few false-positive and false-negative findings, based on the patient's subjective symptom reports, were encountered. The test was reported to the American Neurological Association, and the findings were confirmed by Professor James Ayer of Harvard and Tracy Putnam of Columbia. Dr. Wartenberg's enthusiasm for the test was considerably enhanced by the changes in the visual field of a patient who later was found to have a tumor of the left temporal lobe affecting the geniculocalcarine tract. However, the test required earlier studies to establish a base line and involved extra time, which was discouraging to many. Also, it may now be superseded by computed axial tomography and magnetic resonance imaging.

Another surprising observation was made in this study. Pressure on peripheral nerves had not been shown physiologically to stimulate them in 1940 when I presented the article, although considerable clinical evidence suggested it. This point had become an issue when I worked in the Johnson Foundation for Medical Physics at the University of Pennsylvania in 1939 to 1940. With Carl Pfaffmann, I was able to show that pressure along the length of nerves was indeed capable of stimulating nerve impulses (8).* I had envisioned this as a possible point of dispute when I presented my article on jugular compression and so was in a strong position to answer this point. Much to my surprise, the clinicians universally accepted this source of stimulation, and questions never arose, either at the meeting or in subsequent discussions.

HIGHER FUNCTIONS OF THE BRAIN
AS ILLUSTRATED BY DR. MACDONALD CRITCHLEY

Whereas Wartenberg's interests were primarily concerned with the signs and tests of the neurological examination and their clinical significance, Macdonald Critchley was interested in language, the symbols of communication, sensory perception, and the many disorders associated with such functions. His expertise on aphasia, developmental dyslexia, and the parietal lobe functions became world renowned, and he delighted in patient demonstrations in which sorting, drawing, and other psychological studies were required to establish the diagnosis. He was an actor at heart, and this, combined with his superb command of the English language, made him an outstanding teacher. His ability to explain esoteric concepts with apparent ease and great aplomb was phenomenal. In 1951, Critchley was a visiting professor of neurology at UCSF for 6 weeks. At first, the conferences had 18 or 20 persons in attendance, but by the end of Critchley's stay, the largest auditorium at that time (a capacity of 250) was inadequate to handle his audience.

To grasp fully the scope of his interests, his virtuosity, and his solid scholarly accomplishments, a few words about Critchley's background are necessary. Born in 1900 and raised in Bristol, he won a university place at the age of 15. Despite his service in both the Royal Air Force and Army in World War I, he won a first-class honors degree in medicine at the University of Bristol at the age of 23. Critchley did graduate training in London at the Great Ormond Street Hospital for Sick Children. He also trained in neurology at the Maida Vale Hospital and was at the National Hospital, Queen Square, for 3 years. His first medical article appeared in 1924, and by 1928, he was appointed as a consultant to the National Hospital and also as a consultant neurologist to King's College Hospital. His background plus his knowledge of French and German made him a popular lecturer and visiting neurologist in Europe before World War II.

Dr. Critchley served for nearly 7 years in the Royal Navy from 1939 to 1946 and, thus, was one of the few who served in all three military branches of Great Britain. Following World War II, he returned to the National Hospital where he remained until his retirement in 1965. However, he continued in private practice until 1984. Because of his outstanding ability as a lecturer and visiting neurologist, plus a peripatetic tendency developed in the navy, the whole world became his stage in this later period. In addition to his visit in 1951, he came to UCSF on five other occa-

---

*The late date on this published physiological study was due to further confirmatory testing by Pfaffman, his move to the Rockefeller Institute in New York, and also, according to Pfaffman, further delays in publication. The basic work, however, had been completed in early 1940.

sions. In 1965, Critchley was elected president of the World Federation of Neurology and served the maximum period of 8 years.

Critchley received many honors. He was president of numerous medical societies and an honorary member of about 33 national neurological societies, including the Royal Society of Medicine. He fulfilled 25 of the most outstanding lectureships of Great Britain and served as a *correspondent étranger* at the Academie Nationale de Medicine de France. In addition, Critchley was dean of the Institute of Neurology, Queen Square, and founder-editor of the *Journal of Neurological Sciences.*

His bibliography, which contains over 225 titles, clearly indicates his interest in the higher functions of the brain. His writings include such subjects as mirror writing, language of gestures, the parietal lobe, developmental dyslexia (four books), aphasiology, and silent language. His many essays in his well-known books, *The Divine Banquet of the Brain, The Citadel of the Senses,* and *The Ventricle of Memory,* deal with such subjects as aphasia, patholinguistics, dyslexia, visual and tactile perception, neuropsychology, psychopathology, mind blindness, visual disorientation, and phantom limb (9-11). When I last saw him (he was 91 years of age), he was retired at Nether Stowey in Somerset, and although nearly blind, his mind was still active, and he was continuing with his writing. Few neurologists, or authors of any type, can equal his highly productive record extending over 67 years.

The preceding, enthusiastic sketch of Critchley does not imply that he held a monopoly on either devising or using tests for the higher functions of the brain. This, in the main, has been the province of psychology. However, some psychologists in the past have promulgated bizarre claims about cerebral functioning based on either inadequate testing or lack of proper controls. Critchley, with his broad background in neurology, steered a conservative and yet enlightened course of evaluation that avoided such errors and helped to rectify the errors of others. His role was to evaluate carefully and to tie this exotic field in with the realities of neuroanatomy, neurophysiology, and neuropathology. On the other hand, he often advanced our understanding of the higher functions of the brain and, in the case of dyslexia, became a crusader for the study of a neglected condition (11).

A FEW OTHER OUTSTANDING NEUROLOGISTS WHOSE STUDIES HAVE ADVANCED CLINICAL NEUROLOGICAL DIAGNOSIS

Wartenberg and Critchley, although perhaps unique in their contributions to the clinical advancement of modern neurology, were far from being alone in this effort. Most contributions in this field were, in effect, a continuation of the descriptive phase of neurology from the period of the "founders" but were now being applied to the greatly expanded field during its "flowering" scientific period. Although it is neither practical nor necessary to review exhaustively this aspect of neurology, the contributions of a few other neurologists are included to illustrate the wide diversity of the contributions made in clinical neurological diagnosis.

KINNIER WILSON (1878-1937)

Although American born, Wilson was raised in Scotland and obtained his B.M. in 1902 and B.Sc. in physiology with honors in 1903 at Edinburgh. He was House Physician under Byron Bramwell in the Royal Edinburgh Infirmary and spent 1 year under Pierre Marie and Babinski in Paris. In 1904, he became a House Physician at the National Hospital, Queen Square, London, and spent the remainder of his career there and in related London institutions. His doctoral thesis in 1912 was "Progressive Lenticular Degeneration: A Familial Nervous Disease Associated with Cirrhosis of the Liver." This became known as Wilson's disease. The stories of his discounting the earlier observations of Westphal and Strumpell, essentially because they missed the liver origin, became apocryphal.

Wilson's clinical research involved a broad spectrum of neurological disorders, including epilepsy, epidemic encephalitis, tics, pathological laughing and crying, paralysis of emotional facial movements, and disorders of motility and muscle tone. In 1928, he published *Modern Problems in Neurology*, which well showed his broad neurological grasp and insight. When a group at Queen Square discussed the possibility of writing a modern text of neurology, Wilson announced that he was already doing it. However, his two-volume magnum opus, *Neurology,* was interrupted by his unexpected death in 1937 (13). His son-in-law, Ninian Bruce, completed the task. This text and his thesis in hepatolenticular degeneration constitute his main neurological legacy.

I had hoped to see Wilson, along with Holmes and others at Queen Square, in the 1930s, but this was not to be, because of the Great Depression and World War II. Webb Haymaker, however, has given a good description of Wilson, "His commanding physique, his rich voice, his keen, quick analysis of a situation, his ironical humor, and his skill at histrionics, made of him a figure of Olympic stature'' (14).

ROBERT FOSTER KENNEDY (1884-1952)

Foster Kennedy was born in Belfast where he obtained his early education. After graduation from Queen's College and the medical school of the Royal University of Ireland, he went to the National Hospital, Queen Square, London. He became a Fellow of the Royal Society of Edinburgh in 1910 and shortly thereafter migrated to New York. Following an initial connection with the New York Neurological Institute, he received the appointment of professor of neurology at the Cornell University School of Medicine and became the chief of the neurological department at Bellevue Hospital.

During World War I, he served with the British and French armies and made a special study of shell shock. For his services, he was awarded the English Military Cross and was made a Chevalier of the Legion of Honor of France.

On his return to New York, Kennedy developed many connections. In addition to his main teaching posts at Bellevue and Cornell, he was a consultant to many New

York hospitals, including the New York Hospital and Lennox Hill Hospital. He was a trustee of the Association for Research in Nervous and Mental Diseases and chair of the subcommittee of the National Research Council on Neurology. Kennedy received many honors, including an honorary doctorate of science from Queen's University, Belfast; membership in the Royal Society of Medicine, London, and the New York Academy of Medicine; and presidency of the American Neurological Association and the New York Neurological Society. He was an honorary member of five neurological societies, including the Parisian and Swedish societies.

His neurological contributions covered the whole field of neurology and also touched on psychiatry. Kennedy followed an *organic* approach to psychiatric disorders and strongly disapproved of the psychoanalytic school of thought. He published over 200 articles—the most notable of which dealt with the Foster Kennedy syndrome (homolateral papilledema and contralateral optic atrophy in frontal space-consuming lesions), the neurological complications of spinal anesthesia, and the neurological manifestations of allergy.

Above all, Kennedy was a teacher, and his ability in this respect was greatly enhanced by his quick wit, good humor, and his soft Irish brogue. Underlying this colorful approach to teaching was his keen observation and precise neurological testing. To his patients, Kennedy was a paragon; he exemplified the art of medicine. He was kind, thoughtful, and very supportive. He was equally popular with students, who cherished his delightful wit, kindly handling of patients, and sound neurological instruction. He also was a favorite among his colleagues, who highly respected his evaluations of the clinical problems encountered in his consultations. These same qualities, plus his cultured and scholarly background, made him a favorite speaker at meetings and an effective leader in his academic and medical associations. It was always a pleasure to see him in action. We had the pleasure of a visit with him in San Francisco in the late 1940s. His ability as a colorful raconteur was long to be remembered. He was the perfect host, and when the social tables were turned, he was the perfect guest.

LIDO VAN BOGAERT (1897-1989)

Of all the great neurologists of the modern period, Dr. Van Bogaert stands out as having reached the pinnacle of success without the usual academic background and support. He was born in Antwerp of Flemish descent, and it was in this city that his long career reached its ascendancy. His father was a successful physician. Van Bogaert once told me that he modeled his doctor-patient relationship and medical philosophy on his father's example.

His first 2 years of medicine were at the University of Utrecht, having fled Belgium at the time that it was overrun by the German army in World War I. His later service in the Belgian army ended when he was discharged because of a fractured spine and spinal concussion. Following World War I, he completed his medical training, summa cum laude, in 1922 at the Free University of Brussels. His training in neurology was in Paris with Pierre Marie and with Ivan Bertred in the German methods of neuropathology

He returned to Antwerp in 1923 as an assistant in medicine at St. Elizabeth Hospital and later was appointed staff physician at the Stuivenberg Hospital, where he started a pathological laboratory. In 1925, he successfully defended his doctoral thesis on amyotrophic lateral sclerosis at the Free University of Brussels. Van Bogaert was a prodigious worker; while completing his thesis, he produced 17 articles in 1924 and, during the next year, wrote 30. Although many of his articles were case reports and reviews, his overall literary production over the next 50 years has seldom been equaled. Over these early years, he also managed to visit the main neurological centers of England, Holland, Germany, and Austria.

In Belgium during the 1920s, neurology was still on a provincial level. There was only one department of neurology, at the University of Louvaine, in the country. Eventually, van Bogaert compensated for this by establishing an institute of neurology in Bunge under his directorship. He continued to serve in the department of medicine at the Stuivenberg Hospital until 1933 when the Institute of Bunge was established under his directorship (15). Joseph Rademecker joined the clinical staff, and Hans Scherer was made head of the neuropathological laboratory.

It was not until the end of World War II that the institute was able to add laboratories of electroencephalography, electromyography, biochemistry, and histochemistry. Van Bogaert's productivity also was accelerated, and many physicians from Europe and the Americas came for graduate training. The older International Congress of Neurology met in Brussels in 1957 and was reorganized as the World Federation of Neurology to foster the closer interaction of the many subspecialties of neurology. Van Bogaert was elected president, and several research groups were organized. It was in this capacity that he traveled widely, which included a memorable visit to the neurology department at UCSF.

With his international recognition in 1957, honors soon followed. He was made an honorary member of some 50 national societies of neurology and academies of science. He also received several honorary doctorate degrees.

It is difficult to evaluate all aspects of Van Bogaert and his career. That he was a prodigious worker and excelled in his clinical work—there can be no doubt. Essentially, no field of neurology escaped his attention, but encephalitis, metabolic disorders, degenerative diseases, inborn errors of metabolism, and extrapyramidal conditions were his main interests. His ability to add new insights and to lend perspective in these subjects was exceptional and highly regarded. In addition, Van Bogaert was wise enough to realize the limitations of pathology in studying the etiological factors involved in disease processes, and thus, in his later studies he invited the collaboration of neurochemists (16-19).

One exchange with Van Bogaert may be worth recording, inasmuch as it illustrates an important aspect of his background and medical philosophy. I had shown him an early patient with Alzheimer dementia, who still had some insight as to her progressive course. Van Bogaert handled her with the utmost tact, and when I complimented him on this afterward, he replied,

"I early learned the art of medicine from my father. Your patient retains some little insight, and it is important that we not leave her in a depressed mood by inept questions and handling. This may be difficult in a teaching demonstration with your students, but the art of teaching must not detract from the art of medicine. How to ask questions is as important as what to ask, and the teaching analysis is best done privately with the students following the examination, rather than in her presence. My aim was to conduct a thorough examination in a kindly and supportive fashion. This does not harm the patient and yet gives us the necessary data for the purposes of diagnostic analysis."

"It is precisely for those reasons that I made my comments," I rejoined. "My father was a wonderful person, too, but he was so dedicated, we in the family didn't see much of him. I grew up feeling that medicine was too demanding and that it was an unbalanced way to live."

"I know what you mean," he replied, "but it all depends upon one's sense of values. Did your father ever complain or resent the time he devoted to his patients?"

"On the contrary, he gloried in it. I was the one who complained, and it almost turned me away from medicine."

"Well, you seem to have done all right," he replied.

"In some respects, I am almost worse than my father, but I have taken pains to avoid neglecting my family."

"Yes," he replied, "The art of life is as important as the art of medicine and the art of teaching. It all depends upon the relative sense of values that one develops in life. Consideration of others is the basic precept that is involved, but to achieve this ideal in our handling of patients requires much thought, practice and experience."

No doubt we have all heard these sentiments before, but with Ludo Van Bogaert in the setting described, they assumed a vivid significance and sense of reality that is hard to convey. That Van Bogaert personified the ideals he expressed, there can be no doubt. As the leader in neurology from a small country that tried to remain neutral in the heyday of scientific nationalism, he exerted a great influence in developing a world community of neurology at a higher level (World Federation of Neurology). As an organizer and diplomat, he certainly was exceptional. He moved in all circles with ease. His career encompassed the old limited forms of neurology, with its syndromes and neuropathological correlations, and continued on into the diversified scientific basis of modern neurology. While recognizing the need of the new neurological subspecialties, he was anxious to maintain their cross-fertilization through research and joint meetings. As a person, Van Bogaert was simple, unpretentious, and unprejudiced, appearing to abhor class distinctions—academic as well as social and political. His warm, supportive relationship with patients was outstanding. His rapport with his colleagues was said to be excellent. He certainly was a highly cultured person with many interests beyond medicine. This description of him invites the tired phrase "Renaissance man." Certainly, as a neurologist and clinical research worker, he had few peers.

SUMMARY

Significant advances in neurological diagnosis were made in the latter half of the 19th century and achieved an early culmination in Sir William Gower's (1) A *Manual of Diseases of the Nervous System.* The detective aspects of Sir Arthur

Conan Doyle's stories were a symptom of these developments and, in my case, paid rich dividends in my later consulting and teaching work. However, these early clinical diagnostic advances did not constitute a true "flowering of neurology," as Spillane has postulated. As will be shown in subsequent chapters, the true flowering had to await the scientific advances of the early decades of the 20th century and the research and training support that did not materialize until after World War II.

The career of Robert Wartenberg was used to illustrate one aspect of the more recent advances of clinical diagnosis, while Macdonald Critchley's life well illustrated the diagnostic advances at the level of higher cerebral functions. A few examples of the careers of other leading neurologists were used to illustrate the wide scope of the clinical studies leading up to and during the flowering period of neurology.

REFERENCES

1. Gowers, W. *A Manual of Diseases of the Nervous System.* London, Churchill, 1886. revised 1888.
2. Kennedy, F. William Gowers. In: Haymaker. W., and Schiller, F., eds. *The Founders of Neurology.* Springfield, IL, Charles C. Thomas, 1970.
3. Spillane, J.D. *The Doctrine of the Nerves.* Oxford, Oxford University Press, 1981, p. 407.
4. Aird, R.B. Macdonald Critchley. In: Ashwal, S., ed. *The Founders of Child Neurology.* San Francisco, Norman Neuroscience Series No. 1, San Francisco, CA, Norman Publishing, 1990.
5. Wartenberg, R. *The Examination of the Reflexes.* Chicago, Year Book Publishers, 1945.
6. Wartenberg, R. *Diagnostic Tests in Neurology.* Chicago, Year Book Publishers, 1953.
7. Aird, R.B. Prolonged jugular compression: a diagnostic test of neurologic value. *Arch. Neurol. Psychiatry,* 45:633-648, 1941.
8. Aird, R.B., and Pfaffmann, C. Pressure stimulation of peripheral nerves. *Proc. Soc. Exper. Biol Med.,* 66:130-131, 1947.
9. Critchley, M. *The Divine Banquet of the Brain.* New York, Raven Press, 1979.
10. Critchley, M. *The Citadel of the Senses.* New York, Raven Press, 1986.
11. Critchley, M. *The Ventricle of Memory.* New York, Raven Press, 1990.
12. Critchley, M., and Critchley, E. *Dyslexia Defined.* London, W. Heinemann, 1978.
13. Wilson, S.A.K. *Neurology.* London, Arnold, 1940.
14. Haymaker, W. Kinnier Wilson. In: Haymaker, W., and Schiller, F., eds. *The Founders of Neurology.* Springfield, IL, Charles C. Thomas, 1970.
15. Institute Bunge. *Livre Jubilaire Hommage au Director Ludo van Bogaert.* vol. 15. Brussels, Les Editors Acta Medica Belgica, 1962, p. 24.
16. Van Bogaert, L., Cummings, J.N., and Lowenthal, A. Cerebral Lividosis: A Symposium, Basil. Oxford, Blackwell, 1957.
17. Van Bogaert, L. *Maladies Nerveuses Génétiques d'Order Metabolique.* Liege, Belgium, Revue Medicale de Liege, 1962.
18. Van Bogaert, L., and Bertrand, I. *Spongy Degeneration of the Brain in Infancy.* Amsterdam, North Holland, 1967.
19. Philippart, M., and Van Bogaert, L. Cholestandosis (cerebrotendinosis xanthomatosis). A follow-up study on the original family. *Arch. Neurol.* 21:603-610, 1969.

CHAPTER

4

Advances in
Neuroanatomy and Neuropathology

One may wonder at a joint consideration of neuroanatomy and neuropathology, usually considered as distinct disciplines and certainly taught as such in the orderly development of academic medical instruction. Anatomy is basic, always taught first, and is of special importance to surgery. Pathology is concerned with the end result of disease processes and is of special significance in the all-important subject of medical diagnosis. Nevertheless, both are related to a common structural base, their difference depending on abnormal function in the case of pathology as opposed to normal anatomical function. As physiological and other scientific techniques became available in the early decades of the 20th century, it was possible to relate function to anatomy in the complex structure of the central nervous system (CNS) and to understand abnormal function in the case of neuropathology. While pedagogical needs have maintained the departmental teaching distinctions between neuroanatomy and neuropathology, their modern research trends are difficult to distinguish. Neuroanatomy perhaps is more concerned with the developmental aspects of neurogenetics and the relation of CNS circuits to different transmitters.

My former professor, Stanley Cobb of the Harvard Medical School (as discussed in Chapter 15), was one of the first to branch off from the traditional emphasis on the end picture of neuropathology, a trend that now deals with the progressive stages of the abnormal functioning of structures secondary to the pathophysiological effects of disease processes. Although some new staining and fluorescent techniques have been added to the armamentarium of neuropathology, in the main, they have been refinements of the Spanish school of neuropathology, the Golgi stain, and other techniques developed by a past generation. Neurophysiological studies of function with stereotaxic recordings and neurosurgical techniques of ablation, neurohormonal studies, neurochemical studies of the neurotransmitters, radioactive isotope studies, tunneling microscopic studies at the molecular level, and other modern research techniques have almost entirely superseded the old research approaches of both neuroanatomy and neuropathology in the modern "flowering" period of neurology.

In some respects, the transition from the "founders" of neurology to the flowering period of neurology can be likened to the transition from the gold prospectors of 1849 to modern scientific methods of gold mining. As the "easy pickings" and "gold nuggets" of the founders became scarce and the association between clinical syndromes and neuropathology became difficult to find, it was inevitable that neuroanatomy and neuropathology would turn to research as the scientific techniques became available. This, after all, is the hope of the future, and as will be shown, the leading disciples of both disciplines followed this course with relatively little differentiation between the traditional distinctions of the two disciplines.

The shift from the old to the new schools of neuroanatomy and neuropathology is best illustrated by the careers of a few outstanding men from the transition period of the flowering of neurology when new scientific methods became available. To this end, I have chosen three students of that remarkable comparative anatomist, Professor J. B. Johnston of the University of Minnesota. James W. Papez, Andrew Rasmussen, and Stephen Ranson, who followed Johnston in the American tradition of comparative anatomy, of which Johnston was one of the founders.

JAMES W. PAPEZ (1883-1958)

Born and raised in Minnesota, Papez obtained his medical degree at the University of Minnesota School of Medicine where he came under the stimulating influence of Professor J. B. Johnston. Papez went on to teach in the Department of Anatomy at Emory University. In 1921, he transferred to Cornell at Ithaca where he taught and did research in neuroanatomy. It was there that he laid the groundwork for his celebrated study—the anatomical basis of emotion (1). At first, this had little effect, which in part was owing to his retiring nature and modesty as well as his neuroanatomical base. However, following the article by Kluver and Bucy (2) in 1939, it eventually became the stimulus for intensive research.

Although Papez was not one who used the new scientific techniques, like Rasmussen and Ranson, his career clearly overlapped into the modern era. This was because of his genius in relating function to structure, the factor that also made him a great teacher. Neuroanatomy, taught in the old traditional style, was a complicated and tedious ordeal, if not a threat to academic advancement. However, as Papez and other master neuroanatomists presented it, the subject sprang to life when related to function. In the case of Papez's later formulation of the function of the limbic system, neuroanatomy became fascinating (1).

I first met Dr. Papez at the Telluride House on the Cornell campus. The Telluride House was operated by a scholarship society, the Telluride Association, and entertained most of the guests of the university and many of the faculty.** Dr. Papez did

---

*Modern neuroanatomical teaching has further been extended to clinical demonstrations. The problems of patients are related to signs and symptoms, and the neuroanatomical basis of clinical diagnosis is emphasized. Here, again, the distinction between anatomy and pathology is blurred, and the two disciplines are joined to attain their common purpose more effectively. This still permits the presentation of explanatory slides and diagrams but, now, in a context that emphasizes their practical medical importance.

not object to my auditing his course, which was a stimulating supplement to my work in comparative anatomy. In retrospect, I believe this contact may have first stimulated my interest in the CNS. Certainly, it made me more aware of the central coordinating role of the CNS and its vital function in the brain–mind relationship. This was in the academic year 1925 to 1926, 11 years before Papez's famous article in *Archives of Neurology and Psychiatry* that described the CNS basis for emotional expression (1) and 13 years before the article of Kluver and Bucy (2). Papez was a quiet and unassuming person, but he was intense in his devotion to his work in neuroanatomy; he worked closely with his students in the laboratory. Because of his great knowledge and his correlation of function with anatomy, his individual instruction was a far cry from the flamboyant approach of Titchener and others who lectured in their full academic regalia to large audiences in the old-world style, as discussed in Chapter 15. Both methods have their place, of course, but in my estimation, the more formal lecture method of instruction, at least in medicine, does not hold a candle to the individual "bedside" teaching or the quiet and in-depth type of instruction characterized by Papez.

Because of his dynamic approach, his great knowledge, and his accommodating nature, Papez became an influential consultant to other professionals. Dr. William P. VanWagonen and I consulted with Papez' in 1932 and studied the CNS embryologic collections of the Department of Anatomy at Cornell Medical School in Ithaca. At the University of Rochester School of Medicine, we had made a collection of cases showing dilatations of the septum pellucidum and cavum vergae. One of the problems concerned how such dilatations developed. VanWagonen believed that stray embryonic rests of the pia arachnoid might be caught in the fusion of the anterior medial pallidal cells and that their formation of cerebrospinal fluid could account for the dilatations. Papez was most helpful, but we were not able to find convincing evidence for VanWagonen's thesis. Our Ithaca study was not mentioned in the final article that we published subsequently (3).

Apart from our embryological inquiry, I was astonished that Papez would remember me as a result of our limited contact 7 years earlier. I later wondered if this had been related to the help he offered me as I weighed my choices of medical schools,

---

** The association was endowed by Mr. L. L. Nunn, who first achieved the high voltage transmission of alternating current over long distances for the mines near Telluride City, Colorado, in 1891. He became the first hydroelectric magnate in the country and developed many power plants in the Rocky Mountains, as well as the first Niagara plant, and others. He had to improvise to obtain manpower to operate his plants since this was before the days that electrical engineers were trained. His improvisation involved recruiting young men raised in and inured to frontier conditions, but in obtaining the best young men, he had to provide for their education.

He was amazed by the influence of responsible work on the educational efforts of his young ``pinheads'' and, eventually, founded Deep Springs College in Inyo County, California to test whether half-time work in an academic setting (farm and cattle ranch of Deep Springs College) would produce similar results. Deep Springs has operated effectively for over 75 years. As director of the college for 6.5 years, I am convinced that some of our present educational problems could benefit by the techniques developed at Deep Springs. Student initiative and responsibility are potent peer influences.

The Telluride Association was established in 1911 as an outlet for the higher education of his more outstanding young men, which later included Deep Springs.

as well as to my unusual auditing of his course. In addition to Cornell Medical School, I had applied to Harvard and Johns Hopkins medical schools. Formerly, acceptance had been made on an irregular basis, and so I was accepted by Cornell at the end of my first semester in early 1926. I then wrote to both Harvard and Johns Hopkins to withdraw my application. One week later, I received a telegram from Harvard indicating my acceptance and requesting an answer within 1 month. Because it was still very early, Cornell graciously indicated that it would refund my registration fee if I accepted Harvard, inasmuch as they favored applicants whose first choice was Cornell. My many inquiries, which included my discussions with Papez, finally led me to choose Harvard. It was a difficult decision because of the circumstances and the respect that I had developed for Papez and a few others on the Cornell staff.

On one occasion, Paul Bucy expressed amazement at Papez's ability to deduce function on the basis of his neuroanatomical studies. In retrospect, however, this may not have been all that surprising, considering his great ability in comparative anatomy and his access to other data at the time. He knew of the "sham rage" described by Walter Cannon and the even earlier behavioral effects of decortication in the studies of Dusser de Barenne and Goltz and Rademaker. The inhibitory effect of the cortical association areas, as they developed with cerebral maturation, was also an old concept. However, I did not dispute Bucy's point, inasmuch as Papez's article did seem "far out" to all of us. As later studies verified and refined various aspects of the phenomenon of emotional expression, Papez's article of 1935 was perceived as establishing the necessary neuroanatomical substrate. This and the other studies mentioned gave rise to a whole new subdivision of neurology, as presented in Chapter 13 on behavioral neurology. When I audited Papez's course of comparative neuroanatomy in the mid-1920s, there was no inkling of this startling conceptual sortie. Because of the other developments mentioned, it is logical that Papez conceived it even after I saw him in 1932. Needless to say, I have followed this phase of neurology with great interest—especially since I was exposed to the fascinating theoretical formulations of Geschwind, as discussed in Chapter 13.

ANDREW T. RASMUSSEN (1883-1955)

In spite of the fact that Papez was one of the first anatomists with whom I had contact, when I think of neuroanatomists, the name of Andrew T. Rasmussen is the one that always comes to mind first. His father, also named Andrew, was a friend of my father, Dr. John W. Aird, when they were students at the University of Deseret, which later became the University of Utah in Salt Lake City. I still have the autographic signature of Andrew senior in my father's old student album, dated April 24, 1887. Andrew wrote in beautiful script, "A smooth sea never makes a skillful mariner," and signed it, "Your friend, Andrew Rasmussen." The future neuroanatomist, Andrew T. Rasmussen, was already 3.5 years old at that time.

In the early days of the West, students usually began college at an older age than they do today. Most of them worked and saved to go to college. My father, for example, was about 22 years old when he started at the University of Deseret and was about 24 when Andrew wrote in his album. As was the case for most students at the University of Deseret, the backgrounds of my father and Andrew Rasmussen were similar. Andrew came from the south central part of Utah (Spring City), and my father came from Heber, Utah, a town southeast of Salt Lake City in the Wasatch Mountains. It was a turbulent period of Mormon history when many of the young people were rebelling against the earlier fanaticism of the Mormon Church—its polygamy and theocratic manipulation of territorial government. I believe both families left the church. Certainly, my father's family left about the time that Andrew T. Rasmussen was born in 1863 when apostasy was dangerous (blood atonement) and later persecuted and when United States troops occupied the territory.

Because of this background, I was alert to Andrew T. Rasmussen when my father, as a physician in Provo, Utah, attended his family. Andrew graduated from the Brigham Young Academy (later it became a university in Provo). He married Gertrude Brown, the daughter of the dean of education at the academy, and 2 years after graduation, he was made head of its department of biology at the age of 28. Their first child, Theodore, was born in April 1910, and I recall seeing Theodore as a child playing in the yard on one occasion when I was driving with my father to visit them. This was before World War I and just before Andrew went East for graduate training. Later, I knew Theodore when he was with Dr. Wilder Penfield at the Montreal Neurological Institute (as discussed in Chapter 2) and still later when he was director of the institute.

I have always wondered if my father had helped Andrew with his graduate work. Andrew, as the bright and ambitious son of my father's old friend, would have been a logical choice for this. At that time, my father was making loans at low rates of interest to aid deserving young men in their graduate training. His interest in this stemmed from his own experience; he had struggled with large medical school debts at 12% interest for many years.

Regardless of this point, Andrew did graduate work in physiology under Sunderland Simpson at Cornell University and obtained his Ph.D. in 1916. He then accepted an instructorship in anatomy at the University of Minnesota and, 9 years later, succeeded Dr. J. B. Johnston as the head of neuroanatomy at Minnesota.

Rasmussen came to neuroanatomy with a rich background in biology and physiology and was known as a meticulous and perceptive teacher. His studies on the hypophysis, which paralleled the studies of Harvey Cushing (as discussed in Chapter 8), helped to establish a firmer basis for this important hormonal phase of medicine (4). I later became very conscious of this because I had done some research with Dr. Mary Montgomery in 1935 that disputed Cushing's concept of a central stimulation of paraventricular nuclei by intraventricularly injected pilocarpine or pituitary extract (5). It is now generally agreed that pituitary extracts are carried to the hypophysis by the portal vein and exert their effects through the cerebrovascular system. Rasmussen's studies on the hypothalamus were also basic neuroanatomical contributions (6).

Rasmussen's research on the long neuroanatomical pathways of the descending cerebellar and the secondary vestibular tracts were definitive studies (7). His great artistic ability was exemplified in the illustrative pictures of both this text and his *Outlines of Neuroanatomy* (8). He also did the sagittal series of CNS drawings in Villider's atlas. He was a dedicated teacher, and through his 15 graduate Ph.D. students and his research, he became one of the most influential neuroanatomists of the United States.

Following his retirement in 1952, he served as a visiting professor of neuroanatomy at the University of California, Los Angeles. His death in 1955 at the age of 72 was due to an unexpected heart attack.

STEPHEN RANSON (1880-1940)

Although included by Haymaker and Schiller in *Founders of Neurology*, Ranson is one of the few featured there who clearly overlaps into the modern era of neurology. His contributions extended over a period of 40 years. Initially, they involved anatomical studies and then gradually shifted to neurophysiological interests developed by relating function to neuroanatomical structures. He was so successful in these endeavors that a research institute was created for him by Northwestern University. This resulted in his training of many graduate students. One of his distinguished students, Dr. Horace Magoun of the University of California, Los Angeles, wrote Ranson's biographical sketch for the *Founders of Neurology*. His students have staffed several of our more prestigious institutions as teachers and research workers in the flowering period of neurology. His studies, which number well over 200, involved somatic and visceral reflexes concerned with spinal integration and the homeostasis of the body, water exchange, gonadotropic functions of the pituitary gland, and its hypothalamic innervation. Many other basic studies were undertaken, such as the emotional disturbance of and effect on body temperature by hypothalamic stereotaxic lesions (9). The anatomical basis of the Argyll Robertson pupil and the functional influence of the corpus striatum on the cortex were other notable studies.

The first issue of his classic text, *The Anatomy of the Nervous System,* appeared in 1920 but was modified in numerous editions over many years (10). Many honors came to Ranson in spite of his early death. Perhaps the greatest honor was the research institute of which he was the director. A volume of contributions on the hypothalamus was dedicated to him by the Association for Research in Nervous and Mental Diseases in 1940 (11). He was elected to the National Academy of Sciences and also the presidency of the American Association of Anatomists.

Unfortunately, I met Dr. Ranson only once and this but briefly in his laboratory. His unassuming and friendly bearing was obvious, as was his quiet dignity and obvious alert mind. I was informed that he had a charming family and that his family and laboratory were his two great loves, both of which had paid off handsomely in return for the time and care that he devoted to them. If true, Dr. Ranson would qualify as a selfless person, much as I found in the case of Dr. William Lennox, as discussed in Chapter 2. His monument was his laboratory and its accomplishments in research and training. His serenity of mind and happiness apparently were rooted in his personal integrity, his decency, and warm family ties.

PAUL YAKOLEV (1894-1983)

The career of Paul Yakolev is particularly noteworthy in illustrating the common bonds that exist between neuroanatomy, neuropathology, and clinical work. He slipped from neuroanatomy to neuropathology with the greatest of ease. On top of that, he was also a clinician. His whole-brain preparations constitute a valuable resource. They are now housed at the Armed Forces Institute of Pathology in Washington, D.C., and are available for special anatomical and pathological studies.

Although Yakolev was quietly making his sagittal brain preparations at Harvard while I was a student at the Harvard Medical School, I did not get to know him until I returned there for graduate study in 1940. This acquaintance grew from year to year in my contacts with him as a fellow member of the American Neurological Association. In Paris, in 1949, following a meeting of the International Association of Neurology, Yakolev took several of us on a walking tour of the Left Bank, where he had been a medical student following the Russian Revolution of 1919. The tour extended from the medical school area to the Panthéon, the Palais du Luxembourg, La Sorbonne (Faculty of Letters), and the Boulevard Saint Germain where it reaches the Seine River east of Ile de la Cité. Mrs. Aird and I continued on to Notre Dame and Saint Chapelle. I enjoyed revisiting sites I knew from a month-long stay in Paris in 1925, not long after Yakolev had completed his medical studies. It was a most interesting tour and gave me a much better insight into Yakolev and his unusual background.

Born in Touretz, Russia, into a military family, he moved to Wilno, Russia, after the early death of his parents, where he was raised by a maternal aunt. In 1914, he successfully applied to the Military Medical Academy in St. Petersburg. He became interested in the organic phase of neuropsychiatry through the influence of Vladimir Bekhterer, who Yakolev considered was the founder of Russian neurology. Pavlov lectured on conditioned reflexes in Yakolev's second year, and Alexander Maximow was one of his teachers in his third year. In 1917, however, the Russian Revolution and Communist takeover occurred. The population was confused, food was scarce, and typhoid was epidemic. Because of his family background, he felt that he would have no future in Russia after the Communist takeover. Maximow arranged for his early medical diploma ahead of time in late December 1919. With a friend, Yakolev took a train to Finland, but in anticipation of the approaching Red Army inspector and passport inspector, they moved from car to car and finally jumped off the slow-moving train into the snow while in a military zone short of the Finnish border. They then hiked to the Gulf of Finland, which was frozen over, and were able to cross the gulf. They escaped the Russian searchlights and dodged the border patrols that they occasionally encountered by covering themselves with sheets. After 2 nights and 3 days on the frozen Gulf, they finally reached the Finnish Border Patrol where Yakolev was recognized by one of the guards and allowed to enter Finland. After 2 months working on the docks of Helsinki, he obtained a visa to visit England. In London, he stumbled onto the British-Russian Brotherhood Society that aided him in earning enough to keep going for awhile by having him write his impressions of the Russian Revolution. Subsequently, his Bachelor of Medicine degree from the Military Medical Academy was accepted by the University of Paris, and during the following years, he proceeded to study for his M.D. Another year was spent with Pierre Marie at the Hospice de la Saltpétriere and another three years as a foreign assistant with J. F. F. Babinski at the Hôpital de la Pitié. He finally obtained his M.D. in early 1925. Through his former professor, Alexander Maximow, now at the University of Chicago, and C. Judson Herrick, Ph.D., he finally obtained an "extra quota" American passport on the basis of his special professional qualifications. After medical practice in Rhode Island for 6 months, he joined Stanley Cobb at the Neurological Unit at the Boston City Hospital to survey the foreign literature on epilepsy in preparation for a monograph by Drs. Lennox and Cobb, as discussed in Chapter 2. Between 1926 and 1936, he served as a neurologist at the Monson State Hospital in Monson, Massachusetts. A loan of $1,000 (secured by his salary of $37 per week) enabled Yakolev to spend 6 months in Zurich, Switzerland with Dr. M. A. Minkowski of the von Monakow's Hirnanatomisches Institute. However, he was careful to maintain his connection with the Harvard Neurological Unit at the Boston City Hospital. In 1932, he shifted from an assistant in neuropathology (1928 to 1932) to a research fellow in neuropathology (1933 to 1935) and then to research fellow in neurology (1935 to 1937) at the Harvard Medical School. He also was assistant visiting neurologist at the Boston City Hospital from 1934 through 1947.

Yakolev became Director of the Laboratory at the Metropolitan State Hospital in Waltham from 1936 through 1938. From 1938 to 1947, he was Clinical Director of Research at the Walter E. Fernald State School in Waltham. It was at this time that he had a large model of his Goddard microtome made, which was large enough for serial sections on the whole human brain. Numerous studies followed on epilepsy, mental retardation, neurocutaneous syndromes, frontal lobotomies, paraplegia in flexion, the limbic cortex, atlases of the human brain in sagittal section and also of the cerebellum, the development of the human brain, and many other studies on animal research (12,13). I was especially interested in his studies on schizencephalies with Dr. R. C. Wadsworth, who had been one of my dissecting partners in my first year of medical school in 1926; many of his studies were classic (14).

In 1955, Yakolev was promoted to Clinical Associate Professor of Neurology at Harvard and, in 1957, to Clinical Professor of Neuropathology. It was during this period, before retirement in 1961, when he was also curator of the Warren Museum of Harvard Medical School, when his collection reached its peak of expansion with 20 technicians at his command.

His great collection was housed for a period at the Walter E. Fernald State School but finally, in 1974, was relocated in the Armed Forces Institute of Pathology in Washington, D.C., as a National Resource of Histoanatomical Documentation in

Neurological Science. Yakolev spent his final years as the scientific advisor of his collection. During this period, he studied pyramidal tract decussation and prepared a detailed catalog for the collection.

I have always agreed with the description of Paul Yakolev by his colleague Dr. Thomas Kemper who wrote that Yakolev was "a kind, sensitive, gentle man . . . a man of uncompromising integrity, wisdom and devotion, a scholar who had knowledge beyond the narrow confines of neurology, and an open, keen and incisive mind'' (15). He well illustrated the rise of a refugee against great odds to the highest level of his field, his transcendence of the barriers between neuroanatomy and neuropathology, and the dependence of neurological advances on scientific techniques and research.

The careers of three additional men who were distinctively known as neuropathologists are added to this account to illustrate some of the changes that have occurred during the flowering period of modern neurology.

JOSEPH GODWIN GREENFIELD (1884-1958)

Neuropathology had taken a great leap forward with the silver staining of Ramon y Cajal in the late 19th century, but it remained for a retiring and modest Englishman, Godwin Greenfield, to lead the way between microscopic study and the keen clinical observations of the giants of neurology at the National Hospital, Queen Square, London. Greenfield's father was the professor of pathology and clinical medicine at the University of Edinburgh, and it was this bridge between the clinical findings and their end point in pathology that Dr. Greenfield was to pursue so successfully at the National Hospital.

Graduating in medicine from Edinburgh with first-class honors in 1908, Greenfield served as house physician to Sir Byron Bramwell and Alexander Bruce. The stimulus of neurology led him to Queen Square in 1910 where he served as house physician for 18 months. Following this, he accepted an appointment with Matthew Stewart, a distinguished morbid anatomist at the University of Leeds. However, he had to serve an assistantship in general practice to support himself.

In 1914, when Kinnier Wilson, as discussed in Chapter 3, forsook the post in pathology at the National Hospital, Greenfield successfully applied for it—a post he was to hold for the next 35 years. Previously, this position had been held by clinical neurologists with an emphasis on their more remunerative practice. With Greenfield, the emphasis was shifted to neuropathology, but always with a close bond to the clinical. This link was greatly strengthened by the training in neuropathology that he and his technical assistant provided for the endless chain of house officers of the National Hospital who rotated through his laboratory. Also, his summary comments on the pathologic findings in patients of exceptional interest were frequently sought.

In addition to his neuropathological duties, Greenfield was responsible for all the clinical pathology at the National Hospital. This included Wassermann reactions and the examination of the cerebrospinal fluid samples. The latter led to a book,

The Cerebrospinal Fluids in Clinical Diagnosis, with Dr. E. Arnold Carmichael in 1925 (16).

Greenfield's greatest contributions were to bring order to the early confusion of thought and findings on such subjects as encephalitis, spinocerebellar degenerative diseases, diffuse sclerosis, and the pathology of involuntary movements. In addition to a host of articles on a wide variety of subjects, he published two books on neuropathology. An early one with Sir Farquhar Buzzard was a simple review, and the second summarized the new knowledge that he and others had acquired over the years (17). This was a collaborative effort with his students Blackwood, McMenemey, Meyer, and Norman, but it was not published before his death in 1958.

Above all, Greenfield was a modest man who quietly kept at his work. Considering his limited quarters and staff for 35 years (as discussed in Medical Teaching in Great Britain in Chapter 15), which served the hospital routine in pathology and clinical pathology, his creative accomplishments and neuropathological training of the majority of neurologists of Great Britain can be appreciated in retrospect as outstanding. He befriended many. His door was always open, and he was a wise counselor to those in training, both those from the British Isles and those from abroad. He neither expected nor sought honors and relatively few came his way. Although he served as Dean of the Neurological Institute, the academic aspect of the National Hospital was not recognized by the University of London, and he was never provided with an academic chair. Only his own university, Edinburgh, gave him an honorary degree. He gave several lectureships and was the president of the Second International Congress of Neuropathology. Few men have lived, however, who were more revered for their humaneness and accomplishments. When I think of several acquaintances who have been excessively honored, considering their very modest accomplishments, the contrast with Godwin Greenfield makes one very suspicious of the "game" of honors. Because of the nature of the University of California, San Francisco, visiting professorship of neurology program, I could not invite him to come to San Francisco. His great modesty in his presentations, as well as his subject material, militated against this. He well understood this, and when he came on his own in the early 1960s, we went out of our way to take good care of him. His was an unpretentious, scholarly temperament that I have always admired.

JOSEPH H. GLOBUS (1885-1952)

Clinical pathological conferences are almost invariably characterized by clinicians who, on the basis of available clinical and laboratory data, discuss diagnostic possibilities, evaluate the evidence we hope correctly, and finally, arrive at a clinical diagnosis. With great composure, the pathologist sits on the side—ready with slides to pronounce the final judgment. This scenario, however, does not fit the picture of Dr. Globus. He was one of those rare pathologists who was also an accomplished neurologist and whose perspective encompassed both points of view.

I have always considered myself very fortunate to have had Dr. Globus as my examiner in neuropathology on the American Board examination in 1944. Earlier training and the influence of Stanley Cobb had made me aware of the importance of those pathophysiological and chemical factors that result in pathology; this was the approach of my neurological experimentation. Although I used pathology as a control and was well acquainted with the pathology of nerves, muscle, and brain tumors, I lacked a balanced, comprehensive mastery of neuropathology. Dr. Globus quickly sensed my situation and, after adroitly exploring my strengths and weaknesses, gave me a pass. In retrospect, I believe that I might have fared far worse in the hands of many traditional neuropathologists. Perhaps he had seen my article on the regenerative capacities of nerve and muscle, an experimental study of factors causing faulty recovery of the neuromuscular mechanism that had been published shortly before in the *Journal of the Mount Sinai Hospital*, of which he was the editor. He also may have known of my studies on experimental epilepsy that explained Stanley Cobb's results with brilliant vital red, or again, my showing in other parts of the American Board examinations may have weighed in my favor. In any case, I have always "thanked my lucky stars" for Dr. Globus. Many a neophyte has been tripped up on less.

Dr. Globus' background, no doubt, explained his broad perspective and pragmatic stance. Coming from Russia at the age of 20, he battled for years to obtain a Bachelor of Science degree at Columbia University. On going through the restored Immigration Center on Ellis Island recently, I was reminded that America was the land of hope for the immigrants of that period. Furthermore, education was the gateway to full self-development and success. I thought of Dr. Globus as I went through the various exhibits on Ellis Island. It was true in those days that superior youths could work their way through college on part-time jobs, but to do this while mastering a new language and to continue on through medical school required great sacrifices and much diligence and perseverance. One cannot go through such an experience without gaining considerable maturity and a broader perspective than that gained by American youths raised in well-established families with their more provincial outlook and less demanding circumstances. In thinking of Dr. Globus on Ellis Island, I began to feel somewhat guilty. My father was a very successful surgeon who had been among the founding members of the American College of Surgery. My mother was highly educated and was a member of our state legislature. I received scholarships for 10 years and, coming from the far West, had skipped through Cornell and then Harvard Medical School in luxurious circumstances. In the end, however, wasn't Joe Globus more successful? Furthermore, that he could deal with my situation on the American Board examination with such understanding and that he "bent over backward" to be fair struck me, once again, nearly half a century later, as I walked through the renovated Immigration Center on Ellis Island.

Globus' academic career started as a lecturer in anatomy at Cornell. He obtained his training in neuropathology at the Montefiore Hospital. Following his service in the U.S. Army Medical Corps in World War I, he returned to neuropathology at Mount Sinai Hospital in New York. From 1920 until his death 33 years later, he was director of the Department of Neuropathology at the hospital and became an associate professor of neurology and neuropathology at New York University. However, Dr. Globus also obtained clinical training in neurology, and in addition to serving on the wards at the Mount Sinai Hospital and being a consultant to several hospitals in Manhattan, Long Island, and in Connecticut, he was an associate professor of neurology at Columbia.

In spite of his busy schedule, Dr. Globus published over 100 articles on neuroanatomy and neuropathology. One of the main themes of his studies involved brain tumors. With Elsberg, he reviewed a large series of rapidly progressive brain tumors and with other colleagues reviewed 92 tumors of childhood (18,19). Altogether he published some 28 articles on the various types and aspects of brain tumor, one half of them between 1941 and 1946.

Another study that Globus did was of great interest to me. In 1943, he and his coworkers showed the perivascular pathology of electroshock therapy (EST) (20). This had been shown following human electrocution considerably earlier (study of O. R. Langworth, 1930), but that such changes might be significant in brief shocks of lesser degree was not known. With the introduction of EST for psychiatric conditions, as discussed under Cerletti in Chapter 13, this point assumed considerable importance. I found 11 reports written during the 1940s and early 1950s dealing with this subject, of which Globus' study was another.

In a series of studies with the supravital dye, trypan red, I and my colleagues were able to show that this agent uniquely stained the endothelial cells of the cerebrovascular system but did not extend beyond into the parenchyma of the brain per se. Such injections were found to reduce the permeability of the blood-brain barrier by as much as 30% and explained its protective effect in toxic forms of epilepsy and in preventing the cerebral electroencephalographic dysrhythmias of concussion and EST. Thus, an increased permeability of the cerebrovascular system could be correlated with electroencephalographic dysrhythmias and, presumably, with the perivascular neuropathology and clinical effects of EST (21). In other words, electroencephalographic dysrhythmias reflect abnormal function of the neural elements of the brain as produced by perivascular infiltrations and an altered homeostasis of the CNS secondary to an impairment of the blood-brain barrier. The fact that injections of the supravital dye could protect against such changes indicates that a high percentage of the electric current of EST is conducted and mainly restricted to the cerebrovascular tree (22,23).

At a later date, it was Dr. Globus who drew my attention to this experimental study of 1943. I suggested that he repeat his study after trypan red therapy, but I could never get him to do it. He considered my study as sufficiently definitive to prove the point.

Dr. Globus served as the editor of the *Journal of the Mount Sinai Hospital* and the *Journal of Neuropathology and Experimental Neurology*. He was active in neurological and neuropathological societies and was elected president of the American Association of Neuropathologists and the New York Neurological Society. He was the chair of the section of neurology and psychiatry of the New York Academy of Medicine. He had been elected to membership in the American Neurological Association in 1940 and became a senior member in 1950.

For an immigrant who had come to the United States at the age of 20, his was a great achievement over the subsequent 47 years that can only be explained in terms of his great ability, industry, and perseverance. On top of this, however, was an understanding man and a thoroughly pragmatic American of broad perspective. He was not our greatest neuropathologist, nor greatest neurologist, but he was unusual in that he mastered both fields and even more in that he triumphed over adversity.

WEBB EDWARD HAYMAKER (1902-1964)

Haymaker is another neuropathologist to be considered in this account. His contributions include the application of neuropathology to the more modern aspects of neurobiological research.

Haymaker had an early, colorful career—explained in his unpublished autobiography as due to "itching feet" (24). While attending the College of Charleston, he worked in the summers as a seaman. On one of his trips in 1924, he jumped ship at Bremerhaven and attended, for one semester each, the Universities of Wurzburg and Vienna, obtaining certificates in anatomy and physiology. He then went to the Medical College of the State of South Carolina and obtained his M.D. in 1928. He was a resident in pathology and then served a rotating clinical internship at the Pennsylvania Hospital in Philadelphia. His seafaring culminated in 1934 when he advanced to the position of helmsman on a four-masted schooner. His travels took him to Paris in 1932 where he served for 6 months as an intern at the American Hospital in Neuilly-sur-Seine and another 6 months at the Institute du Cancer.

In 1934, he became a fellow in neurology and neurosurgery at the Montreal Neurological Institute when it first opened. He described the experience as working in a small elevator shaft with makeshift experimental tools without supervision. Perhaps the most significant result of this experience was his meeting Dr. Evelyn Anderson, an endocrine physiologist from the University of California. She shared the elevator shaft with him, and later, they were married.

During 1935 and 1936, Haymaker worked as a clerk for Dr. E. A. Carmichael at the National Hospital, Queen Square, London, and also spent a few weeks with del Rio Hortega, a Spanish histologist and neuropathologist in Madrid. With thoughts of settling down, he pursued Dr. Anderson to the University of California where he obtained a post in neuroanatomy in Berkeley and attended the neurology clinic in San Francisco where he became a great devotee of Dr. Robert Wartenberg. It was at this time (1937) that I first met him. He was on the visiting staff as an assistant clinical professor of medicine in neurology and a neighbor of mine in San Francisco.

During the period when he was at the University of California (1937 to 1943), he was rather proud of his colorful earlier life, the details of which were usually glossed over with a humorous touch. On one occasion, he told me that his name "Haymaker," as used for a knockout blow in prize fighting, had its origin with one of his ancestors who was a pugilist and knocked out his opponents. Behind this colorful front, however, I became aware of a man of considerable ambition with scholarly interests and a prodigious capacity for work. His work as a seaman had not only paid for his travels but also allowed him considerable time for some of his early scholastic efforts (25).

In 1943, Haymaker was inducted into the United States Army as a First Lieutenant in the medical corps and was assigned to the Army Medical Museum in Washington, D.C., which later became the Armed Forces Institute of Pathology. When I visited him later in Washington, he had been made chief of the branch of neuropathology, a position he held throughout the war.

Following World War II, at the behest of Professor William Kerr (chair, Department of Medicine, University of California, San Francisco) and Dean Francis Scott Smyth, I made an effort to recruit Haymaker. Dr. Kerr's purpose was to enlist Haymaker's wife (Dr. Anderson), a brilliant endocrinologist. However, we could not compete with the war-time pay and retirement benefits of the Army.At that time, higher salaried full-time positions were still rare in American medical schools. It required another 15 years or so before this goal was achieved at the University of California, San Francisco and then only as an option to the previous limited private practice consultation plan. Although my letter had highlighted the benefits for his wife, his reply gave no consideration to this. On reviewing the correspondence, both Kerr and Smyth agreed that their purpose was to recruit Dr. Anderson and that Haymaker's terms were totally unrealistic. Although Haymaker would have been a good addition to neurology because of his neuropathological background, his clinical qualifications had not been helped by his years in the army. He had become an outstanding neuropathologist, and this had eclipsed his earlier clinical interests.

At a later date after the war, Haymaker was appointed assistant director for life sciences at the Ames Research Center for basic space research at Moffett Field near Sunnyvale, California. This involved his recruitment of a research staff, but he switched back to neuropathology in 1-year's time. As senior scientist (and ultimately Lieutenant Colonel), his work entailed sending animals into the stratosphere by balloon to determine whether or not cosmic rays would have destructive effects on the brains of astronauts. Haymaker was in the government services for the rest of his career; he served 18 years in the army and 18 years at the National Aeronautics and Space Administration.

Haymaker was a prodigious worker. His neuropathological articles dealt with many subjects, such as explosive decompression, altitude hypoxia, and the encephalitides. Later ones focused on the effects of irradiation on the CNS. At an earlier date, he co-authored, with Dr. Barnes Woodhall *Peripheral Nerve Injuries* and *The Hypothalamus* with his wife, Dr. Anderson, and Nauta (26,27). He also edited *The Founders of Neurology*, which had a second edition in 1970 with the co-editorship of Francis Schiller of our staff (28). His magnum opus, *Histology* and *Histopathology of the Nervous System*, however, was written with Raymond Adams (29).

Haymaker was elected president of the American Association of Neuropathologists in 1955 to 1956 and president of the Fourth International Congress of Neuropathologists in 1961. In addition, he received two honorary degrees. Not only did Haymaker achieve the highest levels of neuropathology, but he also utilized the most modern scientific techniques in his research and greatly contributed to the advances that mark the "flowering" period of modern neurology.

SUMMARY

Two transitional figures were included in this account to illustrate the beginning of the neurosciences in the early 20th century. The careers of Papez in neuroanatomy and Greenfield in neuropathology extended into the flowering period of neurology, and both made great contributions. Rasmussen and, particularly, Ranson became experimental neuroanatomists. Globus and Haymaker were experimental neuropathologists. However, Haymaker had taught neuroanatomy at the University of California, San Francisco, before going into the army (World War II). As the two disciplines utilized the modern scientific techniques of research, their differences began to fade. This was especially true in the cases of Globus and Yakolev, immigrants to America, who overcame great obstacles to become outstanding clinicians, as well as basic scientists (neuroanatomy/neuropathology) and research workers.

REFERENCES

1. Papez, J.W. A proposed mechanism of emotion. *Arch. Neurol. Psychiatry*, 38:725-743, 1937.
2. Kluver, H., and Bucy, P.C. Preliminary analysis of function of temporal lobes in monkeys. *Arch. Neurol. Psychiatry*, 42:979-1000, 1939.
3. Van Wagonen, W.P., and Aird, R.B. Dilatations of the cavity of the septum pellucidum and cavum vergae. *Am. J. Cancer*, 22:539-557, 1934.
4. Rasmussen, A.T. Innervation of the hypophysis. *Endocrinology*, 23:263-278, 1938.
5. Aird, R.B., and Montgomery, M. Studies upon the site of stimulation of salivation by intraventricularly injected pilocarpine in dogs. *J. Pharmacol. Exp. Ther.*, 56:290-306, 1936.
6. Rasmussen, A.T., Kabat, H., and Magoun, H.W. Autonomic responses obtained by electrical stimulation of the hypothalamus, preoptic region and septum. *Arch. Neurol. Psychiatry*, 33:467,1934.
7. Rasmussen, A.T. *The Principal Nervous Pathways.* New York, Macmillan, 1932. revised in 1941, 1945, and 1946.
8. Rasmussen, A.T. *Outlines of Neuroanatomy.* Dubuque, IA, William C. Brown, 1943.
9. Ranson, S.W. *The Hypothalamus: Its Significance for Visual Innervation and Emotional Expression.* In: Proceedings of the College of Physicians of Philadelphia. vol. II. 1935, p. 222.
10. Ranson, S. *The Anatomy of the Nervous System.* Philadelphia, WB Saunders, 1920 (and eight other editions to 1959).
11. Ranson, S.W. Regulation of body temperature. *Proc. Assoc. Res. Neurol. Ment. Dis.,* 20:342-399, 1940.
12. Yakolev, P., and Singer, M. *Human Brain in Sagittal Section.* Springfield, IL, Charles C. Thomas,1954.
13. Yakolev, P.L., Hamlin, H., and Sweet, W.H. Frontal lobotomy: neuroanatomical observations. J. *Neuropathol. Exp. Neurol.*, 9:250-285, 1950.
14. Yakolev, P.L., and Wadsworth, R. G.Schizencephalies: a study of the congenital clefts in cerebral mantle. *J. Neuropathol. Exp. Neurol.*, 5:116-130, 1946.
15. Kemper, T. Yakolev, Paul Ivan. *Arch. Neurol.*, 41:536-540, 1984.
16. Greenfield, J.G., and Carmichael, E.A. *The Cerebrospinal Fluids in Clinical Diagnosis.* London, Macmillan,1925.
17. Greenfield, J.G., Blackwood, W., McMenemy, W.H., Meyer, A., and Norman, R.M. *Neuropathology.* London, Edward Arnold, 1958.
18. Elsberg, C.A., and Globus, J.H. Tumors of the brain with acute onset and rapidly progressive course. *Arch. Neurol. Psychiatry*, 21:1044-1048, 1929.

19. Globus, J.H., Zucker, J.M., and Rubenstein, J.M. Tumors of brain in children and adolescence. *Am. J. Dis. Child.*, 65:604-663, 1942.
20. Globus, J.H., Harrer, A., and Wiersma, C.A.G. Influence of electric current application on structures of brain in dogs. *J. Neuropathol. Exp. Neurol.*, 2:263-276, 1943.
21. Aird, R.B. Neurophysiological effects of electroshock therapy. *Trans. Am Neurol. Assoc.*, 73:181-183, 1948.
22. Aird, R.B., Strait, L.A., Pace, J.W., Hrenoff, M.K., and Bowditch, S. Neurophysiologic effects of electrically induced convulsions. *Arch. Neurol. Psychiatry*, 75:371-378, 1956.
23. Aird, R.B., Strait, L.A., Pace, J.W., Hrenoff, M.K., and Bowditch, S. Current pathways and neurophysiologic effects of electrically induced convulsions. *J. Nerv. Ment. Dis.*, 123:505-512, 1956.
24. Vogel, F.S. In memoriam: Webb Haymaker. J. Neuropathol. Exp. Neurol., 44:220-223, 1985.
25. Haymaker, W. (ed.). *Bing's Local Diagnosis in Neurological Disease.* St. Louis, CV Mosby, 1940. revised in 1956 and 1969.
26. Haymaker, W., and Woodhall, B. *Peripheral Nerve Injuries.* 2nd ed. Philadelphia, WB Saunders, 1957.
27. Haymaker, W., Anderson, E., and Nauta, W.J.H. *The Hypothalamus.* Springfield, Charles C. Thomas, 1969.
28. Haymaker, W., and Schiller, F. (eds.). *The Founders of Neurology.* Springfield, Charles C. Thomas, 1970.
29. Adams, R., and Haymaker, W. (eds.). *Histology and Histopathology of the Nervous System.* Springfield, Charles C. Thomas, 1982.

CHAPTER 5

The Surge of Neurophysiology

Early neurophysiological observations had involved nerve–muscle preparations, the identification of motor and sensory roots of the spinal cord, the segmental innervation of muscle and cutaneous sensory areas, stimulation of the motor strips of the cortex, and many clinicopathological correlations. A good account of the background of neurophysiology in the 18th and 19th centuries can be found in Brazier's *Handbook of Physiology* (1). To bridge the gap between this older background and modern neurophysiology, I have chosen the career of Walter Cannon. Other notable neurophysiologists were in this transition period, but Cannon led the way in many different directions. His research constitutes much of the basis of modern neurophysiology.

WALTER BRADFORD CANNON (1871-1945)

Born in Prairie du Chien, Wisconsin, he was raised in St. Paul, Minnesota, and obtained his higher education at Harvard (B.A. in 1896, M.A. in 1897, and M.D. in 1900). Because Prairie du Chien was the site of Fort Crawford where William Beaumont in the 1820s had made his observation of gastric digestion on Alexis St. Martin, conjectures as to the influence of Beaumont's study on Cannon have been raised. While still a medical student and only 2 years after Roentgen's report on x-rays, as discussed in Chapter 7 on Neuroimaging, Cannon introduced the use of radiopaque agents for the x-ray study of gastrointestinal (GI) function (2).

In 1897, he observed that all GI activity ceased when a male cat became enraged. Other observations followed that clearly indicated the generality of the effect of excitement on GI activity. This observation drew Cannon's attention to the autonomic system and led to further physiological studies on "sham rage," as discussed in Chapter 13 on Behavioral Neurology.

Following his graduation in medicine, Cannon became an instructor in physiology. Within 6 years, he had advanced to the professorship and followed Henry P. Bowditch as chair of the department. Under his stimulating and wise guidance, the Department of Physiology greatly expanded over the next 20 years and became one of the recognized physiological research and teaching centers in the world. Usually regarded as the founder of modern physiology in America, he remained head of the department at Harvard until his retirement in 1942.

Starting in 1911, Cannon and his students explored the regulatory effects of stress via the sympathetic nervous system and the adrenal medulla (3). From these studies, Cannon developed the concepts of bodily adjustments to the emergency conditions leading to "fight or flight" as well as his thesis on homeostasis (4,5). This was dramatically verified in 1929 when he and his collaborators showed that cats from which the sympathetic ganglia chains had been removed could live normally under nonstressed circumstances but not under conditions of stress (6).

Further studies on the denervated heart led to the discovery of "sympathin" as a normal mediator of nerve conduction, which was an epinephrine-like substance that later was identified as norepinephrine (7). The sympathin hypothesis developed during the period when the electrical theory of nerve impulse transmission predominated, and it was one of the precursors of the chemical (electrolyte) nature of nerve and synaptic transmission, as discussed under Dale in Chapter 6.

In addition to these seminal studies, Cannon's suggestion and influence led to the introduction of the case method of study at the Harvard Medical School, an approach quickly adopted by others. During World War I, Cannon also drew attention to the important role of the circulatory system in what was then known as "shell shock." His role as a leader at the Harvard Medical School has been extolled by many, but he repeatedly turned down offers to be dean. Furthermore, his efforts to combat the early attempts of the antivivisectionists to halt animal research were also notable.

I was at Cornell University when I first heard of Dr. Cannon following the "Great Vosberg Hoax" that occurred shortly before I arrived. This amusing hoax illustrates the limitations of our knowledge in the early 1920s and the confused thinking of psychiatry and behavioral neurology at that time, as discussed in Chapter 13. The hoax was perpetrated by a graduate student in the College of Architecture, Charles Stotz, who in the guise of Dr. Herman Vosberg, a fictitious "psychoanalyst and pupil of Sigmund Freud," gave two lectures with slides on *The Freudian Theory as Modified by his Book Dreams and the Calculus.*" In a compound dialect of German and Jewish and in a suitably darkened lecture hall, Dr. Vosberg held forth to large audiences and even withstood the scrutiny of dinner and public receptions (8). A small inner coterie, which included the wife of the new president of the university, Livingston Farrand, helped in the masquerade. Indeed, the hoax was the inspiration of Mrs. Farrand, who later was described by Morris Bishop as "a great and vivid person, who imposed upon the community her robust vigor, humor, and charm." Daisy Farrand, in less than 3 weeks after her husband's inauguration, felt it highly desirable "to enliven the campus." Fortunately for Farrand, her role was kept a secret until her death 40-odd years later. Except for a small, discerning scientific group, Dr. Vosberg took in the masses, although the suspicions of some were later reinterpreted as disbelief. The hoax was a complete and hilarious success from the standpoint of the press and received worldwide publicity. A similar hoax was perpetrated at Cambridge University 3 months later.

In the early 20th century, relatively little was known about the biological effects of emotion. It was obvious, of course, that emotional reactions must be closely related to the central nervous system and must have an effect on the sympathetic nervous system. Various theories were advanced to cover the gap in knowledge during this confused period. The psychiatrists, following the lead of Freud, stressed that aberrations of thought and emotion could be corrected by mental processes. The absence of pathologic findings seemed to support this early line of thought. At that time, essentially nothing was known about abnormalities of neurophysiology and neurochemistry, either as the forerunners of neuropathology or as possible causes of limbic system dysfunction and psychiatric disorders.

Cannon's studies stuck directly into this nebulous area and, along with those of Pavlov on conditioned reflexes, had a profound effect in initiating much of the psychosomatic research of the past 50 to 60 years. Had Cannon been an aggressive self-promoter, as were some others of that period, I believe that he might have received a Nobel prize. A retrospective examination of the Nobel awards during the 1920s and 1930s indicates several recipients whose contributions were less distinguished and important than his were. Cannon's self-effacing modesty, however, was of no help in gaining honors.

I was first introduced to Dr. Cannon and his family when I was a first-year medical student in 1926. I was invited several times to the Cannon home in Cambridge, Massachusetts, and, on one unforgettable weekend, to their "farm" in Franklin, New Hampshire. This resulted in an acquaintance, not only with Cannon, but also with his remarkable wife, Cornelia; their son, Brad, who followed me in medical school; and the three younger Cannon children, Wilma, Marion, and Helen.*

My memory of Cannon involves his oft-repeated query, "What are the facts?" In my opinion, his inquiring mind and remarkable ability to obtain the facts most strikingly typified this remarkable man. These characteristics shone through, not only in his research, but also in his leadership role in the medical school faculty at Harvard, in the legal battles with the antivivisectionists to preserve the rights of research workers, and in many other ways, such as his report on Margery, the famous Boston medium of the 1920s (11). As previously indicated, he opened corridors that led to much of the modern neurosciences, which in turn led to the "flowering of neurology."

One other incident may be worth mentioning. When Dr. Cannon and his family visited my home in 1929, my father, Dr. John Aird, tried to treat Dr. Cannon's persistent skin itch with his "sure-fire" itch ointment. When this failed, father concluded that Cannon's itch must have had a central origin. Later developments suggested that this was probably true and resulted from Cannon's early exposure to x-rays. Lymphoma was diagnosed by 1930, and this no doubt hastened his death in 1945. However, in the interim, as Joseph Aub wrote, Cannon "did not let it interfere with his broad interests. His growth in stature paralleled his years. His wise and fair

---

*Marion has written an excellent account of the Cannon family life, although it does not do full justice to her father. However, a later report was much better (9,10).

judgment, and rare good humor, were attractive to friends of all ages. He remained the honest, simple, and devoted gentleman who was enthusiastic about the accomplishment of others, and modest about his own" (12).

In his later studies with Rosenbleuth, Cannon was using more modern technical equipment. This new technology was a key point in the advancement of neurophysiology. Modern neurophysiology really got underway when the technological advances of electronics made possible the development of electrical amplification and oscillographic recording.

ELECTRONICS

It may seem superfluous to review the background of electronics. We use the automobile and many modern devices without understanding the physics, electronics, and engineering that makes them possible. My object here is not to give a course in physics but to show how scientific advances established the basis for modern neurology. Perhaps even more important is that the evolution of a vital biomedical field depended on technological advances that were achieved step by step by many people and were all contingent on the application of basic scientific knowledge.

Fundamentally, electronics concerns the control of the flow of electricity through vacuum tubes, or the space lattices of transistors, by means of magnetic fields. Sir William Crooks initiated such studies in the late 19th century when he showed that electric currents transmitted through vacuum tubes consisted of particles, which were later identified by Robert A. Milliken as electrons. However, the application of electronics did not really get underway until 1904 when Lee DeForest added a third electrode to the tube (triode). The electromagnetic influence of the third electrode in the form of a grid controlled the flow of electrons in the vacuum tube. Small changes in the voltage of the grid produced large changes in the electron flow of the vacuum tube, and this current faithfully reflected variations of the grid current. Refinements of this basic phenomenon gave rise to amplifiers that could greatly amplify the minute electrical impulses of neurophysiological preparations in sufficient degree to enable their practical recording. The deflection and focusing of the electronic beam on a fluorescent screen inside the tube eventually made possible the photographic recording of high-speed variations of the minute electrical impulses of neurobiological phenomena.

The "spin-offs" of electronics have been almost endless and underlie much of our modern civilization, including radio, radar, television, tape recorders, industrial automation, photoelectric cells, electronic atom smashers, electronic microscopes, mass spectroscopy, and computers. With the development of transistors in 1948, the era of modern electronics was launched. In addition to the use of transistors and computers in neurobiology, they have found wide application in astronomy and all other fields of science—in industry, defense, and for many home uses. Concurrent advances in other fields, as well as in electronics, have tremendously extended our understanding of the nervous system. I am amazed that this has all occurred in my lifetime and that these advances catapulted neurology, after World War II, into its modern status as an independent, clinical discipline. In retrospect, it is well to remember that these developments, which are now referred to in a few deft terms and phrases that make them seem simple, involved years of slow improvement by H. D. Arnold, I. Langmuir, and many others.

THE APPLICATION OF ELECTRONICS TO NEUROPHYSIOLOGY

The selection of neurophysiologists to illustrate this section could be amplified many fold, and no doubt will be criticized by some. How can one ignore the contributions of Sherrington on reflex activity, inhibition, facilitation, reciprocal innervation, and postural reflexes or, again, the contributions of a host of other neurophysiologists such as Pavlov, Forbes, Bishop, Gerard, Magoun, and Jung? My object, however, is to illustrate how the new techniques of neurophysiology and their application to clinical problems established a firm foundation for modern neurology as an independent discipline.

The first major advance in modern neurophysiology occurred in the 1920s when Gasser and Erlanger used amplifiers and the cathode-ray oscillograph to study the transmission of nerve impulses in peripheral nerves. Although Gasser went on to an illustrious career, culminating in his presidency of the Rockefeller Institute, the story of Erlanger can best illustrate their seminal studies. In addition to nerve impulse conduction, the electronic techniques of amplification and oscillographic recording were soon applied to synaptic transmission, electroencephalography (EEG), electromyography, the study of cerebral centers and circuits, intracellular recording, and the study of cell membrane channels. These techniques were used in the work of Eccles in the case of synaptic transmission and in the work of Berger, Adrian, Lennox, Gibbs, Jasper, and O'Leary in the case of EEG. These and several others have been selected to illustrate the application of electronics to neurophysiology, but the early studies of Erlanger were particularly important in initiating this development.

JOSEPH ERLANGER (1874-1965)

I have chosen Dr. Erlanger to illustrate the first major application of electronics to neurophysiological studies because his adaptation of the cathode-ray oscilloscope for these studies led to the first precise measurement of nerve impulse conduction. He pursued and perfected this technique for some 20 years. This approach opened up the great surge of neurophysiology in the 1930s.

Erlanger was born in San Francisco and graduated from the University of California in 1895. He obtained his medical degree from the Johns Hopkins School of Medicine in 1899 and continued on there as an assistant in physiology. He had advanced to an assistant professorship of physiology by 1904 and, in 1906, accepted the position as professor of physiology and head of the department of physiology at the University of Wisconsin. His early research interest was on nervous stimulation of the heart, using a recording sphygmomanometer, which he had invented. In

1910, he was offered the corresponding position at Washington University, in St. Louis, where he became interested in the electrical activity of the nervous system. Herbert S. Gasser, a former student at Wisconsin, was invited to join him in these studies. With A. S. Newcomer, Gasser had used vacuum tube amplifiers for recording from the phrenic nerve.

Erlanger had conceived the idea of using the cathode-ray tube as an oscillograph. Deflection of the beam of the cathode-ray tube, however, required much higher voltages than those generated by nerve impulses. By utilizing Gasser's abilities in amplification, they finally achieved success, and they were able to make detailed studies on peripheral nerve impulses and their rates of conduction. The transmission characteristics were found to vary widely in individual nerve fibers, but conduction rates and fiber size could be correlated (13).

Their laboratory became a world center for neurophysiological research. Their joint studies continued until Gasser left in 1931 to become professor of physiology at the new Cornell University-New York Hospital Medical Center. In 1944, they were awarded the Nobel prize for their joint studies. George Bishop had joined their group in 1923, and he and Erlanger continued their studies on the mechanism of nerve impulse transmission and the nature of subthreshold stimuli. Erlanger retired in 1946 but lived on in St. Louis until his death in 1965.

The Erlanger-Gasser effort was certainly one of the first and most successful applications of the new electronic techniques to neurophysiological problems. Many others followed this lead, as had been my hope, in the early 1930s. Although I only met Erlanger once through my friend James O'Leary, I had made notes on essentially all of Erlanger's reports from the mid-1920s on. The idea had occurred to me that the application of the Gasser-Erlanger recording techniques on nerves might be of diagnostic value if applied more broadly to human problems. The concept involved recording from the vagus and other large nerves in the hope that abnormal patterns of sensory input from diseased organs and parts might be recorded and have diagnostic value. Assuming that the techniques could be developed, a study of the central nervous system (CNS) integration of body function conceivably might follow. The immediate goal, however, was to develop the necessary techniques, which involved shielded needle electrodes in addition to the amplifiers and oscillographic recording methods of the St. Louis group. These hopeful ideas were very stimulating to me and led to my accepting the position of research assistant at the University of California, San Francisco (UCSF), in 1932. Dr. Howard C. Naffziger, Professor of Surgery at UCSF, was in the process of developing a research laboratory there, and since I had always wanted to live in San Francisco, this appeared to be a good opportunity.

My youthful enthusiasm was soon tempered by the hard realities of the technical problems involved. Adequate amplifiers and recording oscillographic equipment were not available in UCSF during that period. Furthermore, the enlistment of the necessary electronic expertise (at that time still called electrical engineering) and progress on the equipment proceeded at what seemed to me to be a snail's pace. By working on other ideas and enlisting the research cooperation of staff men in different preclinical and clinical departments, I managed to survive, but this explains my intense and prolonged interest in Erlanger.

JOHN ECCLES (1902-   )

The career of John Eccles was an unusual one. Like the studies of Gasser and Erlanger on peripheral nerves, those of Eccles and his associates illustrate the unique dependence of scientific advances on the development and refinement of scientific techniques to record and measure electrophysiological activity. In his article, "Under the Spell of the Synapse," Eccles described the development of fine glass microelectrodes and technique of cellular fixation as vital to the studies on the mode of synaptic transmission and the excitatory and inhibitory forms of CNS neuronal activity (14).

Eccles also appreciated his indebtedness to his technical engineering associates who developed and maintained his equipment. In one article, he stated "electronics rapidly outstripped my understanding, but I always have maintained that the technical equipment must be the best. . . . My indebtedness to my associates is immeasurable" (15).

Born and raised in Melbourne, Australia, Eccles became fascinated with the puzzle of the mind–brain relationship as early as his teen-age years, and he later attributed his attraction to neurophysiology to this early interest. Following his training at the University of Melbourne (M.S. and B. S.), he won a Rhodes scholarship and went to Oxford in 1925 where he earned an M.A. and finally a Ph.D. (physiology) in 1929. He worked with Sherrington for 3 years (1928 to 1930) and served as a university lecturer at Magdalen College, Oxford, from 1934 to 1937.

Eccles returned to Australia to become the director of the Kanematsu Memorial Institute and the director of medical science in the Sydney Hospital. Associated there with B. Katz and S. W. Kuffler, he worked on neuromuscular transmission. They showed that nerve impulses to the muscle endplate were successful in stimulating muscle contraction only when the endplate potential reached a critical level.

Eccles was offered and accepted the position of professor of physiology at the school of medicine of Otaga University in Dunedin, New Zealand, in 1944. Over the next 8 years, he worked on the monosynaptic knee jerk reflex, and during this time, he developed the technique of extracellular fine glass microelectrode recording (16). This made possible the recording of inhibitory postsynaptic potentials that disproved the electrical hypothesis of synaptic transmission and confirmed Dale's theory of neuromuscular transmission, as discussed in Chapter 6 (17).

Eccles had accepted the appointment to the professorship of physiology at the Australian National University at Canberra, but his laboratories were not ready until 1953. In further studies on inhibitory synaptic transmission, he noted changes in the recording that were explained by the diffusion of chlorine ions from the intracellular microelectrodes placed in the cell. This led to the technique of intracellular ionic injections and studies of cell membrane tonic gates. Further studies on the inhibitory action of Renshaw cells and newly discovered inhibitory interneurons led to the theory that the CNS primarily involves two types of neurons: excitatory and inhibitory. This has led to many studies that suggest exceptions to this generalization in invertebrate nervous systems but not in mammalian nervous systems. These findings were summarized in his Herter lectures at Johns Hopkins and in his book *The Physiology of the Nerve Cells* (18). His studies on synaptic action were summarized in his book The Physiology of Synapses (19). Other studies on the inhibitory action of the basket cells of the hippocampus and cerebellum greatly added to our knowledge of the physiological activity of these structures (20).

Eccles's mandatory retirement in 1966 ended his 13 years in Canberra. This led to two appointments in the United States, as director of the Institute for Biomedical Research in Chicago and as distinguished professor of physiology at the State University of New York in Buffalo. It was in the latter position that models for the mode of operation of the cerebellar cortex were formulated. Here again the studies depended on advances in instrumentation. Eccles's active scientific life ended in 1975 with his retirement from the University of Buffalo. He retired to Switzerland, absorbed with his original fascination of the mind-brain problem.

I had learned a great deal about Dr. Eccles as the result of two visits to his laboratory in Canberra. In 1962, I had been invited to participate in the first Asian and Oceanic Neurologic Congress in Tokyo. A loop flight on the early jet planes was made to New Zealand, Australia, Indonesia, Thailand, and Japan. While in Canberra, I visited the physiological laboratories and also the aboriginal collection in the Department of Anatomy. I had heard a considerable amount about Eccles and his work before this time, but the visit to his laboratory gave me more detailed knowledge of his neurophysiological studies.

A second trip to Australia developed as the result of an invitation from Dr. Graeme Robertson to attend the second Asian and Oceanic Congress scheduled for Melbourne in 1967. On this trip, we again visited the neurophysiological laboratory of the National University in Canberra. It was then called the John Curtain School of Research. Eccles was not there, but Professor David Curtis was most hospitable in showing us the setup and describing the continuing work.

Between these two trips, Eccles visited us in San Francisco in November 1964. He had just completed his book on synaptic action, and we obtained a wonderful review of this (19).

I saw Eccles once again in London when we both participated in the 1968 centennial celebration of the birth of Gordon Holmes. Lady Eccles urged me to join them in retirement in Switzerland. Perhaps this merely reflected the graciousness of Lady Eccles in dinner conversation, but she did go into considerable detail as to how this might be accomplished on the Swiss end. Because of my great love of Switzerland, this was tempting, but it did not make sense from the standpoint of my work and family.

One additional aspect of Eccles's career should be noted. He well illustrates the importance of imaginative creative powers to develop hypotheses that are consistent with past factual knowledge and to extend them into a generalization or principle. Only when the problem is clearly defined can critical experiments be designed to prove or disprove the theory. Eccles attributed much of his success in this respect to Karl Popper, a philosopher of science (21).

In summary, the career of Eccles illustrates an important advance in the transmission of nerve impulses with vital implications for CNS function as well as peripheral nerve physiology. In addition, Eccles's methods exemplify the adaptation of new scientific techniques to the study of cellular function.

EDGAR DOUGLAS ADRIAN (1890-1977)

Adrian, one of Great Britain's most distinguished neurophysiologists, has been selected because of his pivotal role in initiating the study of brain waves and evoked cortical potentials as commonly practiced today in EEG. I first met Adrian in 1953 when he came to Boston for an International Congress of EEG and Clinical Neurophysiology. This was combined with the annual meeting of the American EEG Society of which I was president. I was also chair of a committee on EEG training in the international society. Thus, between the two meetings, my presidential address, committee report, and a talk with Norbert Wiener (on the side) about Fournier analysis of brain waves, I was extremely busy. The situation was further complicated by my plans to attend the International Congress of Neurology in Lisbon where I was to present an article. In spite of all this organizational turmoil, I managed two pleasant meetings with Professor Adrian and had dinner with him at the banquet of the international society. When I saw him in 1953, he was at the peak of his illustrious career, and yet he remained a simple, unaffected man, who impressed me by his modesty and friendly manner.

The events leading to Adrian's study of brain waves can only be understood in the context of his research activities and background. Adrian was born and raised in London. He attended Cambridge University and as a student worked with Keith Lucas in experiments that proved Lucas's "all-or-none" law of nerve impulse conduction. Following Lucas's death in an airplane accident in 1916, Adrian completed the final chapters of Lucas's monograph, "The Conduction of Nervous Impulse" (22).

Adrian trained in neurology at the National Hospital, Queen Square, during World War I and served in various assignments in military hospitals. Following the war, he became a fellow and lecturer in physiology at Cambridge University and pursued neurophysiological research the rest of his life. His earlier student work with Lucas was the determining factor of his career.

His research involved all aspects of nerve conduction, the recording of afferent impulses from sensory end organs, including the rod and cone responses of the optic nerve, and the rhythmical activity of motor units. Adrian's work on inhibition was also noteworthy. He and Alexander Forbes at Harvard favored an interference of impulses by other impulses, as proposed by Wedensky, but this was later explained in terms of synaptic activity, as discussed previously and under Dale in Chapter 6.

Perhaps, most importantly, he confirmed the report of a little-known German neuropsychiatrist who had reported the recording of brain waves* Hans Berger had secretly recorded the electrical activity from the cortex of animals and finally humans and, in 1924, had succeeded in obtaining the EEG on a brain-injured human, which thus established the basis for human EEG. However, it was not until he recorded brain waves from the scalp with intact craniums that he finally began to publish in 1929 (23). It was this background and the series of articles that followed that finally attracted the attention of Adrian. Because Berger's results were of questionable quality and published in a relatively obscure psychiatric journal, no attention was paid to them until Adrian and B. H. C. Mathess finally confirmed them in articles published between 1934 and 1936 (24). As indicated in Chapter 2, it was their reports that finally initiated the further clinical research on EEG, epilepsy, and additional neurophysiological studies on the brain. Adrian and Sherrington shared the Nobel prize in 1932.

Adrian's first article was written as a student while working with Keith Lucas at Cambridge in 1912; his last was in written 1977. Aside from his many lectures, books, and reviews, his bibliography shows some 113 scientific publications. The majority of his studies were done on his own, but he collaborated with a number of other physiologists from 1912 to 1947. I knew four of the physiologists who collaborated with him, including Bronk, Olmstead, and Forbes, mentioned in these essays.

In his later life, Adrian received many honors in recognition of his contributions. From his appointment as chair of physiology at Cambridge in 1937, it was not until 1951 that he was made master of Trinity College at Cambridge. Other appointments soon developed. He became vice chancellor of Cambridge in 1952 and finally chancellor in 1959. He was elected president of the Royal Society (1950-1955) and was made a baron, which carried the title of Lord Adrian in 1955. Numerous prizes, honorary degrees, and lectureships followed. Except for the great surge of clinical neurophysiology, which followed his confirmation of the work of Berger (as discussed in Chapter 2), and winning the Nobel prize in 1932, it is not likely that this very unassuming man would have been deluged with so many later honors. I have always believed that he well deserved all the honors he received to which his position at Cambridge and long life no doubt contributed.

JAMES LEE O'LEARY (1904-1975)

The career of James O'Leary was unusual in that it demonstrated the close bonding of the basic neurosciences with EEG and clinical neurology. Starting as a neuroanatomist with Heinbecker and Bishop, O'Leary became a neurophysiologist. Later, he became interested in EEG and clinical neurology and, eventually, started an independent department of neurology at the University of Washington, St. Louis.

His story is an interesting one. O'Leary's mother, Nancy, had operated the family business in Iowa and supported three children after the death of her first husband. She

---

* Others had reported the electrical activity of the brain in animals earlier, for example, Catron in 1875, Beck in 1891, and Pravdich Nominsky in 1912, who for the first time, obtained a record of this activity.

later married James O'Leary and gave birth to James O'Leary III in Tomahawk, Wisconsin, where his father had gone to practice law after obtaining a law degree at the University of Wisconsin. After James's birth, Nancy O'Leary developed a pulmonary infection. To obtain a better climate, the family moved to San Antonio, Texas, where James III grew up. His father died when he was 11 years old. His mother again rose to the occasion by developing a real estate business to support her family.

James did brilliantly in school and was encouraged to study medicine at the University of Chicago. Robert R. Bensley in the Department of Anatomy became his mentor, and with a scholarship in anatomy, he obtained a Ph.D. in this field. In anatomy, he worked with G. W. Bartelmez and C. J. Herrick. He accepted an assistant professorship of anatomy at Washington, in St. Louis, following obtaining his Ph.D. in 1928. However, he also managed to obtain his M.D. degree by doing summer clinical work in the joint program offered by the University of Chicago, which he completed in 1931.

Following the pioneering neurophysiological studies of Gasser and Erlanger on the peripheral nerve, Bishop and Heinbecker undertook a project to relate fiber size and physiological activity with nerve function. This required correlative studies with peripheral nerve stained sections; O'Leary, as a young neuroanatomist, joined them in this research. This collaborative effort quickly resulted in all of them becoming interdisciplinary experts, and O'Leary's neurophysiological expertise grew as their research work was extended into other areas. O'Leary extended his nerve staining technique by learning the Golgi technique under the auspices of Raphael Lorente de No, who had been a student of Ramon y Cajal, the great Spanish neuroanatomist. O'Leary in particular was proud of his histologic analysis of the lateral geniculate nucleus and visual cortex as related to evoked electrical potentials (25).

In 1941, O'Leary undertook clinical neurological instruction under Irwin Levy, a certified neurologist on the staff of the Barnes Hospital, the teaching hospital for Washington University in St. Louis. At this time, he became an assistant professor of anatomy. World War II intervened in 1942, and O'Leary was assigned to the Army School of Neuropsychiatry at the Mason General Hospital. There he established standards of EEG and became the head of the EEG department at the Mason Hospital; secondarily, he gained experience in psychiatry.

Following his return to Washington University in 1946, he worked again with Bishop on evoked potentials of the brain and undertook research in experimental epilepsy, which involved EEG control studies. Several other studies followed, such as the one with Sidney Goldring, in which they analyzed the slow voltage changes of the brain (26).

With Levy and a few other part-time neurologists on the staff of the Barnes Hospital, O'Leary established a training program in neurology; his role was concerned with EEG and electrophysiology. His daily EEG review and teaching conferences became a focus for clinical neurophysiology in which the residents of both neurology and neurosurgery participated. In 1963, an independent Department of

Neurology was established during his time as chair.

O'Leary's public service involved several committees of the National Institutes of Health in its developmental period and later with the National Multiple Sclerosis Society. He served on the editorial boards of several neurological journals and aided me in establishing the Certification Board of the American EEG Society. He later was president of the American EEG Society and received the W. G. Lennox Award. Still later, he was elected president of the American Neurological Association and received its Jacoby Award in 1971. Shortly before his death, O'Leary was given the Doctor of Science Honorary Degree by Washington University. Following his retirement in 1970, O'Leary continued full time in research and research training. His final book, *Science in Epilepsy*: Neuroscience Gains in Epilepsy Research, came out following his death (27).

For many years, O'Leary and I were very friendly because of our common interests in EEG and clinical neurophysiological research. He followed me as chair of the Certification Board of the American EEG Society and also as chair of the William G. Lennox Trust Fund of the American Epilepsy Society. At the time, the American Neurological Association was bearing down on the certification of non-M.D.'s by the Certification Board of the American EEG Association (1962). I was the one, as a member of the nomination committee of the American Neurological Association, to suggest his nomination as president of the association. This was important in relieving the pressure on the American EEG Society and gaining O'Leary's support in changing the rules of the EEG certification board. O'Leary reviewed some of my material for one of my books on epilepsy, and on two to three occasions, he participated with me in the UCSF visiting professor program.

Our friendship extended over that exciting time (1946 to 1975) when there was a cross-fertilization of backgrounds from neurology, psychiatry, psychology, physiology, and even, electrical engineering and physics. I was more the clinical neurologist, and he was more the neurophysiologist—but with these interests overlapping with EEG and epilepsy. The previous comments of Dr. Thomas Kemper on Dr. Paul Yakolev (discussed in Chapter 4) could equally well be applied to James O'Leary. Certainly, he was a kindly man, a scholar, and a man devoted to his research. In addition, he was a loyal friend and a man of uncompromising integrity.

WALTER R. HESS (1881-1973)

The career of Walter Hess, a Swiss Nobel prize winner in 1949, was unusual in two respects. His early career was in the practice of ophthalmology, and because his later career in neurophysiology climaxed during World War II, his work was not well known in the Western English-speaking world. I visited him in his laboratory at the University of Zurich in early September 1949 and later became acquainted with his son, Dr. Ruedi Hess (of EEG fame). Through these connections, I gained some insight into Professor Hess's background and contributions.

Hess was born and grew up in Fauenfeld where he attended the local *gymnasium*. His father was a college teacher of physics, and he early acquired a good grounding in this field. His other main interest in early life was in nature, both fauna and flora. He was attracted to medicine through the family doctor who took care of him when he developed pleurisy due to tuberculosis. His medical studies extended from 1900 to 1905 at the Universities of Lausanne, Bern, Berlin, Kiel, and finally, Zurich. Postgraduate work followed as an assistant in the departments of surgery and ophthalmology from 1905 to 1908 in Zurich. During this period, Hess qualified for the M.D. degree at Zurich (1906). Over the subsequent period of 4 years, he practiced as an ophthalmologist and married in 1909. In 1913, he obtained the position of assistant and lecturer in physiology at the University of Zurich and also at Bonn, Germany. In 1971, he was made professor of physiology and director of the physiology department at Zurich, a position he held until his retirement in 1951.

During his medical studies, he developed an interest in the vascular system and problems of hemodynamics. He was attracted to ophthalmology in the hope that it would provide a good income and still allow time for research. This led to developing techniques for analyzing oculomotor disturbances and stereoscopic vision. His medical practice, however, took so much time that it crowded out his research. The conflict between his practice, which involved a sense of duty to his growing family, and his desire to do research finally reached a climax in 1912 when the position in physiology became available. Physiology won out in spite of a considerable loss of income. He became a *privatdozent*, which combined teaching and research. This was interrupted by World War I, following which he did graduate work with Max Verworn at the University of Bonn. His research involved the regulation of regional blood flow. Further military service plus teaching duties interrupted his research, and in 1916, on the retirement of his ailing chief, he became the acting head in charge of lectures and laboratories. He managed so well that, in the following year, he was offered the chair of physiology at the University of Zurich. To improve the teaching and research at Zurich, he traveled to England, saw the laboratories of Starling, Langley, and Sherrington, and attended many international physiological congresses.

His research on the circulatory system was followed by studies on the respiratory system (28,29). The close relationship and synergistic functioning of these systems led him to central integrative control mechanisms of the vegetative nervous system at the higher level of the diencephalon. This project involved technical advances in stereotaxic needle insertions, checked by pathological control studies. A stimulatory technique, which allowed local stimulation, but without spread, and determination of the physiological effects so produced involved a meticulous study, the technical aspects of which were described in a monograph published in 1932 (30). These studies extended from 1925 to 1950, but the great mass of data warranted the publication of two monographs in 1948 and 1949 (31,32). It was these publications that won him the Nobel prize in 1949 for his "discovery of the functional organization of the diencephalon and its role in the coordination of the functions of the inner organs." Switzerland was closed off during World War II. This and his publications in German resulted in the obfuscation of his work among the allied nations of that period.

His son, Dr. Ruedi Hess, has repeatedly stressed that his father's studies went beyond the diencephalon and were particularly important with respect to the organization of the motor system, studies which predated those of Granit (see subsequent section) and the cybernetics of Wiener (see section of Adrian and the discussion on McCulloch in Chapter 17) (33-35).

In addition to his physiological studies, Professor Hess was involved in the high altitude research center at the 11,000-foot level on the Jungfraujoch and served as its director for 5 years. He also aided in a time-consuming movement against a lay proposal to ban all animal research and initiated the establishment of the Swiss Physiological Society and its journal, *Helvetica Physiologica et Pharmacologica Acta*. He was particularly proud of his efforts in starting the interdisciplinary Commission for Brain Research, which finally culminated in the Brain Research Institute.

The saga of a medical practitioner with research interests slowly evolving into a Nobel prize neurophysiologist is a fascinating story and is well related in Hess's "From Medical Practice to Theoretical Medicine: An Autobiographical Sketch," Perspectives in Biology and Medicine (36).

JOHN FARQUHAR FULTON (1899-1960)

John Fulton was one of the most distinguished neurophysiologists of the 20th century. He was a dynamic person whose interests went well beyond physiology. As a bibliophile, his enthusiasm succeeded in convincing Harvey Cushing and Arnold Klebs to contribute their libraries on the history of medical sciences, along with his own, to found the great collection at Yale University. As an editor, he founded the *Journal of Neurophysiology* (1938) and, later, the *Journal of the History of Medicine and Allied Sciences* (1946). He also played a leading role in the founding of the *Journal of Neurosurgery* (1951). As a teacher, he served in two roles at Yale University: as Sterling Professor of Physiology (1929 to 1951) and as Sterling Professor of the History of Medicine (1951 to 1960). His infectious enthusiasm stimulated many projects, including a harrowing one for myself. Fulton knew of my studies on epilepsy, electroshock therapy, and cerebral concussion using supravital dyes to determine changes in the permeability of the cerebrovascular system, as discussed in Chapter 2. Thus, in early 1940, when I was on sabbatical leave in the East, Fulton enticed me (perhaps "collared" would be a more accurate term) against my better judgment to give a lecture on the clinical effects of blood–brain barrier impairment at his neurophysiological institute. Had I had time to prepare it, I could easily have put on a good show, but the lecture involved much data that would be difficult to present because I did not have the proper slides with me. The result was a very questionable presentation from my standpoint but apparently satisfactory to his group at the Neurophysiological Institute of Yale.

Because I had many contacts with Fulton over the years and his accomplishments touch on several aspects of this book, a fuller account of his background and contributions is justified. He was the son of an ophthalmologist in St. Paul and attended the University of Minnesota from 1917 to 1918. He transferred to Harvard and obtained his B.A. degree in 1921. He won a Rhodes scholarship, undertook an honors course in physiology, and obtained another B.A. from Magdalen College,

Oxford University. This led to a fellowship with Sherrington and Laidell, which initiated his interest in neurophysiology. His work resulted in a M.A. degree in 1925 and, finally, his Ph.D. in 1927. His thesis was published later in an expanded form as a monograph, "Muscular Contraction and the Reflex Control of Movement" (37). He then returned to Harvard and obtained his M.D. in 1927 at the medical school where I first knew him. In the following year, he served as an assistant in neurosurgery under Harvey Cushing at the Peter Brigham Hospital. It was in a laboratory provided by Harvard, and while working with J. Pisuner, that they made the classic distinction between muscle spindles *in parallel* as opposed to the *in-series* position of tendon organs concerned with muscle stretch and contraction. Except for Pisuner, I doubt if he could have covered both assignments simultaneously. However, it may be that Cushing allowed him considerable leeway. They had discovered their common interest as bibliophiles and especially their fascination with the Osler Medical Library at Oxford. This background, no doubt, was important in Cushing's later Pulitzer Prize-winning biography of William Osler, Fulton's later Pulitzer Prize-winning biography of Harvey Cushing, and the founding of the great Yale Library of Medical History, as previously mentioned (38,39). In 1929, he was appointed professor of physiology at Yale. However, he had already agreed to return to Sherrington's laboratory, which meant that his duties at Yale did not really begin until 1931.

His chief contributions to neurophysiology can be summarized as follows:

1. He organized the first primate laboratory in America and undertook a series of ablation studies of apes to understand human neurological disorders better. One of these studies with Carlyle Jacobsen showed striking behavioral changes when the anterior association areas of the frontal lobes were extirpated (40). They gave a report on this at the Second International Congress of Neurology in London. As recounted in the chapter on behavioral neurology (Chapter 13), Egas Moniz, after hearing their presentation, conceived the idea of frontal lobotomy for which he won the Nobel prize in medicine in 1949. Fulton's primate studies quickly led to similar work in many other institutions, and although some of his early reports were criticized, his lead unquestionably resulted in a tremendous advance in our understanding of cerebral and cerebellar physiology.
2. His classic studies on muscle tone and contraction are considered by some to be his most outstanding contributions.
3. His training program in neurophysiology attracted a fine group, who later became leaders at other institutions.
4. In addition to his training program, his book *The Physiology of the Nervous System* gave a great impetus to neurophysiology (41). Fulton's editorial work and his accomplishments in the field of medical history have been mentioned previously.

His later years were troubled by ill health, and it was for this reason that Fulton switched from physiology to his historical post. Another contact will illustrate a complication of his diabetic condition. Following the International Congress of Neurology in Lisbon in 1953, Mrs. Aird and I went to Madrid to attend a special meeting of the Spanish Neurological Society to dedicate a new auditorium at the University of Madrid in honor of Ramon y Cajal. The program was long and involved, aside from a good address in English by Russell Brain. Fulton gave a talk in French that later both the French and Spaniards said they could not understand. Fulton was sweating profusely (I believe that he was on the edge of an hypoglycemic attack, probably induced by insufficient food and the stress of the occasion). I felt keenly for him, but there was nothing one could do. Fortunately, his talk, like that of Brain's, was reasonably brief. As the rest of the program of Latin language speakers droned on, dusk fell, and lamps were brought in to allow the speakers light for the reading of their endless articles. At that time, Madrid electricity was rationed and did not come on until 9 p.m. As the auditorium darkened, muffled snoring could be heard as many dozed off in the comfortable new seats. Promptly at 9 p.m., the lights burst forth in dazzling intensity. The somnolent audience was slumped in their seats to a person. The effect of bright light under such circumstances was wondrous to behold. As each person shuffled to sit fully erect, they looked about with disdain at others who were a mite slower and, in some cases, sluggards. Within 30 seconds or so, the room appeared quite prim and proper. The considerable commotion appeared to have no effect on Professor Trelles from Lima, Peru, who was the one reading at that point.

Finally, at the end of the addresses, a delightful symphonic piece was broadcast. Several officials rushed out. Eventually, the music was subdued, and we heard the words of Cajal. The program was a success, however, inasmuch as it was concluded by a reception that featured the tasting of the finest Spanish sherries.

The elaborate social events of the old neurological congresses helped to make up for the limitations of their scientific programs. This was highlighted by the inability of the Southern European and Latin American delegates to keep to a schedule, with the result that it was impossible to go from room to room to hear anticipated talks. Nevertheless, the congresses provided a wonderful opportunity to see old acquaintances and to visit teaching and research units abroad. In this relaxed atmosphere, Fulton's difficulties were glossed over, if noted at all. One has to understand his stimulating enthusiasms, his endless interests, and his tremendous energy in his younger days to appreciate fully his impact on a whole generation at the peak of the flowering of neurology.

Still another neurophysiologist, Ragner Granit, deserves consideration for his efforts to elucidate visual sensation and motor activity at higher cerebral levels. It has been said that only psychologists with organic leanings would undertake such complex studies in their attempts to interrelate the mind–brain puzzle. In any case, this pattern occurred with several neurophysiologists, such as Trevis, Jasper, and Granit.

RAGNER ARTHUR GRANIT (1900-   )

Granit was born of Swedish parents in Helsingfors (Helsinki), Finland. Before graduation from the University of Helsingfors, he engaged in Finland's war of liberation from Russia and won the Finnish Cross of Freedom. Returning to the university, he combined the humanities and chemistry to obtain a major degree in philosophy (1923). He continued in medicine and obtained his M.D. degree in 1927. He studied in the field of experimental psychology and adapted physiological approaches to the problems of vision. He was an assistant in the Physiological Institute of Helsingfors and, by 1929, became a "docent."

Granit's horizons, however, had greatly expanded in 1928 when he spent half a year (1928) in the Oxford laboratory of Sir Charles Sherrington. In 1929, Ragner married the Baroness Marguerita Emma Brunn, the daughter of the Swedish State Councillor, Baron Theodor Brunn. From 1929 to 1931, he was a fellow in medical physics under Detlov Bronk, as discussed in Chapter 16, at the Eldridge R. Johnson Foundation at the University of Pennsylvania. From 1932 to 1933, he worked in Sherrington's laboratory at Oxford. In 1935, he was appointed deputy professor of physiology at the University of Helsingfors, and 2 years later, he was formally appointed to the chair.

In 1940, Granit accepted the professorship of physiology at the Royal Caroline Institute of Stockholm. His setup there was supported by a special grant of the Nobel Foundation plus Rockefeller Foundation funds. Five years later, the Caroline Institute made his neurophysiological laboratory a department of the Medical Nobel Institute, and in 1946, Granit received a personal research chair in neurophysiology from the Swedish Ministry of Education. The new Nobel Institute building was opened in 1947, and Granit continued in this position until he retired 20 years later. However, he also served as a visiting professor at several institutions from 1955 to 1978, including Rockefeller University, Oxford, and the Smith-Kettlewell Institute in San Francisco. He aided the trustees of the Nobel Foundation for several years and was awarded the Nobel prize himself in 1967. His early studies on vision and later studies on motor control and cerebral integration, as discussed subsequently, were the basis for this prestigious award. His many other awards, lectureships, honorary memberships, medals, and other honors were worldwide and too numerous to add.

How Granit managed to accomplish so much good research in his bustling life is a mystery. However, his early start on problems of vision and his concentration on this and the higher aspects of locomotion probably account for it. Beginning with psychophysics in 1920 and electrophysiology in 1930, his main research centered on the retina. His analysis of the electroretinograms and discovery that very slight amounts of visual purple were capable of suppressing the electroretinograms were notable. Microelectrode studies on the responses of single-fiber retinal nerves of frogs to spectral light were of two types—either they were broad or narrow bands of sensitivity, the latter affecting three specific regions: red, green, and violet. This work was extended to many other species and led to the conclusion that sensitivity to visual wave lengths was sharpened and improved by neural interaction (42). Similar narrow bands of wave length sensitivity have been found by others in the geniculate bodies and cortex of monkeys.

Granit's later studies on motor control were initiated with Berger Kaada of Norway in 1947. They demonstrated that the thin gamma fibers of spinal motor neurons could be activated or inhibited from sites in the cerebrum, cerebellum, and basal regions of the brain. Because the gamma fibers were known to act only on the intrafusal fibers of muscle spindles and the brain centers were known to have a corresponding effect on the extrafusal fibers of muscle contraction, the concept of central control systems for muscle action developed (43). Muscle contractions by control systems in the brain that could be demonstrated by cathode-ray spiking from single neurons or sense organs became a popular approach that soon extended to other laboratories.

Granit also differentiated tonic motor neurons from phasic motor neurons. Only the tonic neurons sustained prolonged discharge when activated by the stimulus of repeated stretch (44). In his last studies, Granit showed (by means of intracellular recording) that cellular firing and inhibition were summarized algebraically and, quantitatively, were equivalent to reflex stimulation at corresponding rates of discharge (45).

Granit's interest in the integrated action of the nervous system had been stimulated by Sherrington, and it was in this area that he enunciated two general principles (46). The first postulated that higher degrees of sensory discrimination, finer degrees of motor manipulation, and greater levels of perceptiveness and "consciousness" required greater numbers of brain cells in proportion to their "elaboration." On the motor side, he noted the expanded areas of the motor cortex for thumb and finger control and, on the sensory side, the great cortical expansion for the small fovea of the retina in contrast to the rest of it.

The second general principle postulates that the greater the need for cortical expansion in terms of "motor contact points to facilitate the extensive combinations of data required for exclusion and anticipation" is, the greater the number of sites in the brain engaged in mediating such functions. He pointed to the large number of sites widely separated that are engaged in a motor act as defined by anatomical, clinical, and physiological studies. Another example concerned the numbers of visual centers, "a number of nine at the moment" (47). He pointed out that these biological concepts dealt with the purposeful responses of living organisms to their environment, which thus placed them in the teleological aspects of physiology (48).

A neurophysiological friend once expressed the opinion that Granit's success was considerably enhanced by his aristocratic marriage and his close association with the trustees of the Nobel Foundation. Although human interactions are difficult to evaluate, I have always thought that this was not fair to Granit. He had achieved considerable success before his marriage. Furthermore, Sweden is highly socialistic, a democracy, and favors to aristocracy are sharply limited, as shown in the account under Wohlfart in Chapter 15. The main point, however, turns on the quality and impact of his research, which cannot be denied in Granit's case. His studies on vision and cerebral motor control, including their higher cerebral integration, constituted a significant contribution to the flowering of neurology.

SUMMARY

The careers of several neurophysiologists have been used to illustrate the striking advances that have been made in this field, extending from the seminal studies of Walter Cannon, which probably were the earliest biomedical research with x-rays, to the integrated balance of body chemistry controlled by the nervous and endocrine systems, which he termed *homeostasis*, and to other studies that have helped to open the fields of the neurotransmitters, psychosomatic medicine, and behavioral neurology.

Because of Erlanger's early adaptation of the cathode-ray tube to oscillographic recording, precise neurophysiological studies became possible and were quickly used for recording nerve impulse transmission and both research and clinical studies on the central nervous system. Eccles extended such studies to the synapse and confirmed its electrolyte basis. Adrian and O'Leary illustrated different aspects of EEG and other neurophysiological studies on the CNS.

Still others illustrated the use of stereotaxic stimulation (Hess), primate neurophysiology, muscle tone and contraction (Fulton), and vision, motor control, and nervous system integration at higher levels (Granit).

Four of these investigators won Nobel prizes, and at least two of the others might well have qualified. Although those selected for this account by no means illustrate all aspects of the progress made in neurophysiology, they indicate some of its main facets, show how scientific advances are adapted to neuromedical research, and document the dependence of modern neurology on such research.

REFERENCES

1. Brazier, M. *Handbook of Physiology.* vol. 1. Cambridge, American Physiological Society, 1959, pp. 1-58.
2. Cannon, W.B. *The Mechanical Factors of Digestion.* London, Arnold, 1911.
3. Cannon, W.B. *Bodily Changes in Pain, Hunger, Fear and Rage.* New York, Appleton, 1915.
4. Cannon, W.B. *Autonomic Neuro-Effector Systems.* New York, Macmillan, 1937.
5. Cannon, W.B. *The Wisdom of the Body.* New York, Norton, 1932. revised 1939.
6. Cannon, W.B., Newton, H.F., Bright, E.M., Menkin, V., and Moore, R.M. Some aspects of the physiology of animals surviving complete exclusion of sympathetic nerve impulses. *Am. J. Physiol.,* 89:84-107, 1929.
7. Cannon, W.B., and Rosenblueth. *The Supersensitivity of Denervated Structures. A Law of Denervation.* New York, Macmillan, 1929.
8. Stoz, C.M. The Vosberg Hoax. *Cornell Alumni News,* 12:7-11, 1964.
9. Schlesinger, M.C. *Snatched from Oblivion.* Boston, Little, Brown & Co., 1979.
10. Schlesinger, M.C. The Way of Walter B. Cannon. Harvard Med. Alumni Bull., 59:47-51, 1985.
11. Russell, F. *The Witch of Beacon Hill.* New York, American Heritage Publishing, 1952.
12. Aub, J. *Harvard Medical School Perspectives: Passing the Torch.* Cambridge, MA, Harvard University Press, 1991, p. 2.
13. Gasser, H., and Erlanger, J. The role played by the size of the constituent fibers of a nerve trunk in determining the form of its action potential wave. *Am. J. Physiol.,* 80:522-547, 1927.
14. Eccles, J.C. Under the spell of the synapse. In: Worden, F.G., Swazey, J.P., and Adelman, G. (eds.). *Paths of Discovery.* Cambridge, MA, MIT Press, 1975.
15. Eccles, J.C. My scientific Odyssey. *Am. Rev. Physiol.,* 39:1-18, 1977.
16. Brock, L.G., Coombs, J.S., and Eccles, J.C. The recording of potentials from motor neurons with an intracellular electrode. *J. Physiol.,* 117:431-460, 1952.
17. Coombs, J.S., Eccles, J.C., and Fatt, P. The specific ionic conductances and the ionic movements across the motor neural membrane that produce the inhibitory post-synaptic potential. *J. Physiol.,* 130:326–373, 1955.
18. Eccles, J.C. *The Physiology of the Nerve Cells.* Baltimore, Johns Hopkins Press, 1957.
19. Eccles, J.C. *The Physiology of Synapses.* Berlin, Springer-Verlag, 1964.
20. Eccles, J.C., Ito, M., and Szenta Geitha, J. *The Cerebellum as a Neuronal Machine.* Berlin, Springer-Verlag, 1967.
21. Popper, K.R., Eccles, J.C. *The Self and Its Brain.* New York, Springer-Verlag, 1977.

22. Lucas, K. *The Conduction of Nervous Impulse.* New York, Longmans, 1918.
23. Berger, H. Uber das Elektrenkephalogrnsm des Menschen. *Arch. fur Psychiatry,* 87:527-570, 1929.
24. Adrian, E., and Matthess, B.H.C. Interpretation of potential waves in cortex. *J. Physiol.,* 81:440-471, 1934.
25. Bishop, G.H., and O'Leary, J. Electrical activity of the lateral geniculate of cats following optic nerve stimuli. *J. Neurophysiol.,* 3:308-322, 1940.
26. O'Leary, J., Goldring, S., Ulett, G.A., and Greditzer, A. Initial survey of slow potential changes obtained under resting conditions and incident to convulsive therapy. *J. Electroencephalogr. Clin. Neurophysiol.,* 2:297-308, 1950.
27. O'Leary, J. *Science in Epilepsy: Neuroscience Gains in Epilepsy Research.* New York, Raven Press, 1976.
28. Hess, W. *Die Regulierung des Blutkreislaufes.* Leipzig, Georg Thieme, 1930.
29. Hess, W. *Die Regulierung der Atmung.* Leipzig, Georg Thieme, 1931.
30. Hess, W., Thieme, G. *Die Methodik der localisierten Reizung und Ausschaltung Subkortikaler Hirnabschnitte.* Leipzig, Georg Thieme, 1932.
31. Hess, W. *Das Funktionelle Organisation des Vegetative Nervensystems.* Basel, Schwabe, 1948.
32. Hess, W. *Das Zwischenhirn, Syndrome, Lokalisationen, Funktionen.* Basel, Schwabe, 1949.
33. Hess, W. Biomotorik als Organisationsproblem: Parts I and II. In: *Die Naturwissenschaften.* vol. 30 Berlin, Springer-Verlag, 1942, pp. 441-448, 537–541.
34. Hess, W. Cerebrale Organization somatomotorischer leistungen. Part I. vol. 207. *Arch Psychiat Nervenkr* 1966, pp. 33-44.
35. Hess, W. Cerebrale Organization somatomotorischer leistungen. Part II. vol. 208. *Arch Psychiat Nervenkr* 1966, pp. 209-233.
36. Hess, W. From Medical Practice to Theoretical Medicine: An Autobiographical Sketch. *Perspectives in Biology and Medicine.* 1963, pp. 400-423.
37. Fulton, J. *Muscular Contraction and the Reflex Control of Movement.* Baltimore, Williams & Wilkins, 1926.
38. Cushing, H. *Life of Sir William Osler.* Oxford, Clarendon, 1926.
39. Fulton, J. *Harvey Cushing,* A Biography. Springfield, Charles C. Thomas, 1946.
40. Fulton, J.F., and Jacobson, C.F. Functions of the frontal lobes of the brain, a comparative study of lower apes, chimpanzees and man. *Fiziol Zhur* 19:359-370, 1935.
41. Fulton, J., and Kellar, A.D. *The Physiology of the Nervous System.* 3rd ed. New York, Oxford University Press, 1945.
42. Granit, R.A. *Receptors and Sensory Perception, Silliman Lectures.* New Haven, CT, Yale University Press, 1955.
43. Granit, R.A., and Kaada, B.R. Influence of stimulation of central nervous structures on muscle spindles in the cat. *Acta Physiol. Scand.,* 27:130–160, 1952.
44. Granit, R.A., Henatsch, H.D., and Steg, G. Tonic and phasic ventral horn cells differentiated by post-tetanic potentiation in cat extensors. *Acta Physiol. Scand.,* 37:114–126, 1956.
45. Granit, R., and Strom, G. Autogenic modulation of excitability of single ventral horn cells. *J. Neurophysiol.,* 14:113-132, 1951.
46. Granit, R.A. *Basis of Motor Control.* London, Academic, 1970.
47. Granit, R.A. *Half a Century with Neurosciences*: Personal Comments on Choices and Decisions. Stockholm, Nobel Institute for Neurophysiology, Karolinska Institute, 1969.
48. Granit, R.A. In defense of teleology. In: Karczmar, A. G., and Eccles, J. C. (eds.). *Brain and Human Behavior.* Berlin, Springer-Verlag, 1972, pp. 400–408.

CHAPTER 6

Advances in Neurochemistry
and Neuropharmacology

Scientific advances develop slowly in a stepwise fashion and in a highly interdependent and even interdisciplinary fashion. The emergence of science in the late decades of the 19th century and, particularly, in the early decades of the 20th century made possible the development of the neurosciences and, finally, the clinical disciplines of neurology and its related fields. As in the case of neurology, neurochemistry did not become a recognized and independent neuroscience until after World War II (1). Nevertheless, because of its obvious great importance, the origins of neurochemistry date back into the 18th century and even earlier, when the pseudoscience of alchemy held sway.

Liebig and his contemporaries developed organic chemistry in the early 19th century. Biochemistry came later with the studies of Bernard, Pasteur, Pfluger, and a host of others in the late 19th century. The earliest serious studies of the brain were undertaken by Thudichum, a student of Liebig (2). However, it was an isolated effort and not directly related to brain disorders or clinical problems. This background finally set the stage for modern neurochemistry. This involved studies on tissue oxidation, glycolysis, and vitamins; on the role of iodine in goiter and of insulin in diabetes; and on many other developments. The recognition by Garrod of the inborn errors of metabolism and of the biochemical basis of genetics was especially notable, as discussed in Chapter 12 (3). Biographical sketches of some of the leaders of these early advances, Hensing, Vauquelin, and Thudichum, have been provided by Tower (4).

Early metabolic studies involved carotid artery-jugular vein differences for many agents in the early 20th century, as well as in the *in vitro* studies of Winterstein and others (5). The investigations of Szent-Gyorgyi, Quastel, Krebs, and Meyerhof led to the modern era of neurometabolism. The studies of Peters on vitamin B deficiency were notable, as was his concept of the biochemical lesion (6). Another important advance occurred when Cannon discovered his "sympathin" (7). This was an epinephrine-like substance, which was later identified as norepinephrine. In the same year (1921), Otto Loewi recalled a forgotten technique to prove the electrolyte transmission of nerve impulses, which later won him a Nobel prize. With stimulation of the vagus nerve of a frog preparation, he obtained a perfusate, which decreased the cardiac action of a separate frog heart preparation, thus demonstrating that his "vagusstoff" was a neuromuscular transmitter (8). This effect could be blocked by atropine, and Dale eventually identified the "vagusstoff" as acetylcholine (see later section on Dale).

Liebig had originally proposed the intracellular-extracellular concentration of potassium and sodium, but it was not until the studies of Hodgkin and Huxley that this was demonstrated on the squid giant axon, which led to the modern concept of electrolytes as the basis for action potentials and axonal conduction (9).

In spite of their late developments, the fields of neurochemistry and neuropharmacology are so vast that only illustrative examples to highlight some of their principal aspects can be included. In other chapters, consideration has been given to the pioneering studies of cerebral blood flow by Lennox and Gibbs, the synaptic studies of Eccles, and the investigations of Walter Cannon, which led to the latter's concept of homeostasis. Ehrlich's discovery of the blood-brain barrier and Cannon's concept of homeostasis involve neurochemical balances for optimal metabolic functioning of the central nervous system. Also, because of the revolutionary advances that are taking place in the delayed infectious processes of the central nervous system, neurogenetics, and behavioral neurology, separate chapters have been devoted to these subjects in the next section.

JUDAH H. QUASTEL (1889-1987)

K. A. C. Elliott has written that "Q (a reference used by Quastel's friends) was the first modern biochemist to work extensively in the field of brain metabolism, and he remained one of the leaders of it" (10). Because of his remarkable studies with brain slices and homogenates, Quastel well illustrates the field of cerebral metabolism. However, it is a complicated field, and Quastel is one of the few people featured in these essays that I did not know personally. Luckily, I have an extensive communication on him from his son, David M. J. Quastel, Professor, Department of Pharmacology and Therapeutics, of the University of British Columbia (personal communication, 1992). This and the excellent biographical sketch of the Royal Society, in addition to still other background data, was of great help (11).

His story is a very unusual one, and it would appear that his roots went far to explain his brilliant pioneer work in brain metabolism and his persistent endeavors, which extended for a period of over 40 years in this field. There were at least three phases that appear to be crucial to Quastel's development and career. Born in Sheffield, England, of orthodox Jewish parents from the old Austrian Hungarian empire, he became a "lone wolf" as a youngster in the traditional environment of Victorian England. Thanks to his discovery of the Sheffield Public Reference Library, he tells us that he read "all the forbidden literature," including "growth, genetics, reproduction, about sex...textbooks of chemistry, physics and mathematics, and of the great creative artists...and writers...that I had missed in all my formal education at school." As a result, he slowly threw off the old orthodoxy and became a "free thinker" (11).

At the age of 9, he aspired to a career in chemistry, and by dint of much hard work, at the age of 17, he won a scholarship to Imperial College, London. However, this was postponed because of his anticipated induction into the army within 1 year. During this interval, he worked as a volunteer in the laboratory of the Sheffield public analyst, which began the second phase of his development. It was in this laboratory that he learned many of the basic scientific techniques, including the use of the microscope. After his induction into the military, the sergeant in charge of his company on one occasion unexpectedly yelled, "Anybody 'ere who can use a microscope? If so, one step forward, march." Quastel's fellow conscripts looked at the sergeant as though he had lost his senses, but Quastel stepped forward. He later wrote, "To me, this step forward turned out to be every bit as important as the first step of the famous astronaut on the moon's surface" (11). His transfer to the pathological laboratory of the local military hospital completely transformed his life in the military. Here he learned much about bacteriological media, vaccines, microbiological techniques, and postmortem examinations. Here, also, he made several good friends and learned of professor F. G. Hopkins of Cambridge University.

On discharge from the army in early 1919, with the aid of his scholarship and an ex-service grant, Quastel attended Imperial College, where he majored in chemistry and graduated in 1921. Before graduation, he learned of a scholarship in Trinity College, Cambridge, which involved graduate studies in biochemistry under professor Hopkins. Since this was what he now aspired to do, he successfully applied, and so began his graduate training in biological chemistry and studies on bacterial metabolism. Using bacterial suspensions, he discovered a number of basic biochemical mechanisms, and working with bacterial dehydrogenases, he obtained evidence, which permitted him to postulate the principle of competitive inhibition of enzymes by their analogues. Malonate was the classic example of this process, being a competitive inhibitor of succinic dehydrogenase.

Quastel obtained his Ph.D. at Cambridge in 1924 but continued in his research there until 1930, when he was offered the post of director of research at the Cardiff City Mental Hospital, Wales. It was here, at the age of 41, that his career in the biochemistry of the brain started, a third phase that he brilliantly pursued for the next 41 years. In 1947, he accepted the professorship of biochemistry at McGill University in Montreal, Canada, and was director of the Montreal General Hospital's new research institute. Following mandatory retirement from McGill, he was appointed professor of neurochemistry at the University of British Columbia, Vancouver, in 1966 and carried on with his research until 1979.

Quastel's contributions to brain metabolism have been so numerous that many pages would be required to present them. For the purpose of this account, his contributions are listed with references to a few of the more important ones.

SOME OF QUASTEL'S NEUROCHEMICAL ACHIEVEMENTS

1. First to demonstrate the unique role of glucose in supporting the respiration of brain *in vitro*. He also showed for the first time that glutamate is effective in suporting brain respiration and is a source of brain energy (12).

2. First to demonstrate that the cerebral oxidation of glucose proceeds through pyruvate and not through lactate (13).

3. First to demonstrate the existence of amine oxidase in the brain, that a variety of amines (aliphatic or derived from amine acids) play a metabolic role in brain, and that amphetamine blocks the activity of amine oxidase (14).

4. Discovered that the synthesis of acetylcholine takes place in the brain as a normal metabolic process and demonstrated its linkage with cerebral carbohydrate metabolism (15). He showed the presence of a bound form of acetylcholine in the brain, which could be released by potassium ions, phospholipase A, and others (16). This work, all details of which have been amply confirmed, was the first demonstration of a biological acetylation *in vitro*, and it initiated all later work on choline acetylase and on acetylcholine localization on brain cells.

5. First to study fatty acid oxidation (17).

6. First to describe the effects of nicotinamide on brain metabolism (18).

7. First to demonstrate the specific inhibitory effects of fluoroacetate (at low concentrations) on ammonia metabolism in the brain *in vitro* and glutamine biosynthesis, observations that have led to new views on the site of action of fluoroacetate in the brain (19).

8. First to demonstrate the quantitative importance of acetoacetate in the general metabolism of infant brain (20).

9. First to demonstrate the effects of barbiturates and other anesthetic agents on brain metabolism, to specify the site of action of barbiturates in respiration (a conclusion that has been fully confirmed), and to describe the effects of ouabain, tetrodotoxin, and others (21).

10. Discovered that active (energy-assisted) transport of glucose across intestinal membranes required sodium ions (22). This was a forerunner of many studies showing the requirement of sodium ions on other energy-assisted transport systems.

11. First to demonstrate the glutamate-glutamine cycle in the brain. The glutamate was released by stimulation of neurons and converted to glutamine in the glia and reformed to glutamate when taken up again by the neurons (23).

12. First to demonstrate the active transport of vitamins (thiamine and ascorbic acid) into the brain *in vitro* and the dependence of acetic acid oxidation on vitamin B1 (24).

S. C. Sung has reviewed Quastel's contributions in more detail and includes 16 more basic contributions than the 12 listed here (25). This list also corresponds fairly well with the account given by Macintosh and Sourkes in the memoirs of the Royal Society (11). The lists of both his son and the Royal Society credit Quastel with many more firsts. This amazing number of fundamental discoveries and observations is partly explained by Quastel's pioneering role in neurochemistry but obviously would not have been possible except for his brilliance and great industry. Small wonder that he was made honorary president of the XIth International Congress of Biochemistry in 1979. Twenty-five other honors were listed in the Royal Society memoirs, including two honorary academic degrees and two visiting professor lectureships.

Quastel's son, David, has described him as "perhaps the typical over-achieving product of (then) poor immigrant parents 'turned on' to science by his studies in the Sheffield Public Reference Library and working with the public analyst of Sheffield." His Royal Society memoirs describe him as "never aggressive...and even kindly in argument" (11). He was cheerful and optimistic in temperament. In spite of his early orthodox Jewish origin, he greatly cherished his many friendships with "nonracial" Gentiles. He was an effective teacher and in his later years and never lacked graduate students, who held him in great respect.

RUDOLPH ALBERT PETERS (1889-1982)

I first heard of Peters through Dr. J. M. Walshe, the son of Sir Francis Walshe, as discussed in Chapter 17. My contacts with Sir Francis Walshe had always been most cordial, and it probably was this background that led to his son's visit in 1966. Dr. J. M. Walshe had just completed studies with Peters on the toxicity of copper for brain tissue. On the side, I wondered if he had been drawn to this subject by the hope that his expertise in the detoxifying use of BAL might be applied to copper in early cases of Wilson's disease. Regardless of this point, he was enthusiastic about his copper studies, his setup at Cambridge, and collaboration with Peters. Because I kept up on the research of one of my postgraduate students (Dr. Sean O'Reiley, later a professor of neurology at George Washington School of Medicine, Washington, D.C.) who worked extensively in this same field, I was able to follow Walshe's discussion. This paid rich dividends in extending my knowledge of both Walshe and Peters.

The broad training of Peters in medicine, physiology, and biochemistry was probably an important factor in explaining his pioneering efforts in deficiency disorders and in being the first to show the function of vitamins. Peters came from a distinguished Danish and English family background. His father was a physician, and his mother was a musician who encouraged his violin playing (26). His early hobby was science; excellent contacts and training in his preparatory schools extended this enthusiasm.

At Cambridge (1908 to 1914), he developed contacts with such distinguished professors as Joseph Barcroft, A. V. Hill, J. N. Langley, and others. His studies in physiology included physiological chemistry, and in this field, he did a study of the iron-oxygen relationship in hemoglobin. He especially enjoyed his contacts with A. V. Hill and studied heat and lactic acid production of muscle, which helped to disprove the Meyerhof lactic acid theory of muscle contraction.

With the outbreak of World War I, he trained in medicine at his father's school, St. Bartholomew, in London. He qualified in 1915 and joined the Royal Army

Medical Corp. After various assignments in France, which won him the Military Cross, he was recruited for studies on the chemical warfare that had been initiated by Germany in 1916. He served for the rest of the war under Barcroft, who had been made head of the physiological laboratory. This background greatly influenced his later career in biochemistry and his studies of toxic agents (26).

In 1918, Peters returned to Cambridge where he taught in physiology and did research in biochemistry under Gowland Hopkins. He continued with studies on the mechanisms of action of toxic agents and the effect of phosgene and other war gases on the alveolar epithelium of the lung. It was his toxic agent studies that led him on to studies of vitamin B extracts of yeast, the latter being used in the media for the growth of protozoans and paramecia.

In 1922, at the age of 34, he was invited to assume the Whitley Chair of Biochemistry at Oxford. The biochemical setup at Oxford was closely associated with the physiological department under Sir Charles Sherrington. Sir Archibald Garrod, of "inborn errors of metabolism" fame, also encouraged his appointment, and shortly thereafter, the Rockefeller Foundation considerably expanded the biochemical laboratory.

Peters pursued his studies on vitamin B at Oxford. Because it was then unknown that vitamin B was a complex of essential nutritional factors, Peters centered his studies on the "anti-neuritic" factor of yeast and the mediation of its effects. His first investigations involved the extraction and purification of the antineuritic factor of yeast, using the head retraction of pigeons fed on polished rice as a gauge of its concentration (27). Previously, vitamin B1 had been shown to have a predominantly peripheral polyneuropathic effect. Peters, however, pursued its central effect, based on his belief that the head retraction of pigeons fed on polished rice had a central origin. This concept was encouraged by his observation that glucose temporarily cured the head retraction and that the excess of lactic acid found in the brains of his affected pigeons disappeared after treatment with thiamine (B1). His basic study on the oxidative effect of B1 on the pigeon brain followed. By 1936, Peters and his collaborators showed that B1 was essential to the oxidative removal of pyruvic acid, a degradation product of carbohydrate metabolism (28). Thus, for the first time, the mode of action of a vitamin was demonstrated.

With the onset of World War II, Peters headed another research group involved in studies to protect against chemical warfare; one aspect of this concerned thermal burns. His group showed that high dietary protein significantly reduced the tissue wasting and urinary loss of nitrogen. Other contributions concerned his studies of nutritional factors on vitamin B, vitamin C, calcium, and others. He was chairman of the Accessory Food Factors Committee of the Medical Research Council from 1943 to 1954, as well as chairing several of its subcommittees.

Following the war, Peters studied the toxic actions of fluoroacetate and eventually showed that it was enzymatically converted to fluorocitrate, which competitively inhibits aconitase and blocks the metabolism of citrate in the tricarboxylic acid cycle (29).

After retirement at Oxford in 1954 at the age of 65, Peters accepted an invitation to head the biochemistry department of a new institute of animal research at

Babraham, 6 miles south of Cambridge. With several of his team from Oxford, he studied the toxicity of plants found in livestock pastures. This mainly involved studies on the toxicology and biochemistry of various fluorine-substituted metabolites. Fluorooleic acid, extracted from the seeds of *Dichapetalum toxicarium* and used by the witch doctors of Sierra Leone for trials by ordeal, was shown to be extremely toxic.

When Peters retired from Babraham, he accepted the invitation of Sir Frank Young to continue work in the University's Department of Biochemistry at Cambridge. Here, he continued his research on the pharmacology and biochemistry of fluorine-containing compounds of plants. Other studies, however, were pursued with various collaborators, including Dr. J. M. Walshe, as previously mentioned (30).

Peters was an unusual man in several respects. He was a kindly person who encouraged young investigators. In the case of R. W. Wakelin, a laboratory assistant whose technical skill greatly contributed to Peter's research at Oxford, Peters included him as a co-author on ten papers, a very unusual practice in England at that time. He always gave full credit to his co-workers. Of his 218 publications, over 60% were joint efforts with his students and colleagues. His friendly and supportive interest was reciprocated many fold through the loyalty of his colleagues, which in part explains his selection to important posts.

Although a man of high intellect and great shrewdness, he sometimes appeared vague and confused in his speech. His diversion of thought, however, was a foil to gain time for further consideration when important decisions were involved. Clear thinking and appropriate decisions were announced hours or days later. Like many scientists, his writing was not lucid, although he coined many popular terms, such as "biochemical lesion" and "lethal synthesis."

His breadth of training and interests have already been mentioned and account for his insistence on the close association of biochemistry with physiology. No doubt the cross-fertilization of ideas by means of contacts with members of other disciplines paid rich dividends. The extension of the biochemical to the lesion and its medical effects account for his most important studies.

Peters maintained his interests in music and his violin throughout life and greatly enjoyed playing in chamber music groups. He was on the Faculty Board of Music at Oxford and was chair of the Caius Musical Society at Cambridge.

In the field of nutrition and vitamins, Peters well illustrates the importance of the role of biochemistry in the neurosciences and of the step-by-step approach in scientific advances. His innovativeness, which introduced ultracentrifugation to English science, was noteworthy, as was his early utilization of quantitative methods of microchemical analysis.

As with most other subjects of these essays, Peters was deluged with honors (15), honorary degrees (8), medals, prizes, named lectureships (18), and honorary memberships in distinguished societies (13). He was elected to membership in the Royal Society in 1935 and was knighted in 1952.

CHOH HAO LI (1913-1987)

Born and educated in Canton (Guangchou), China, Li obtained his B.S. degree in chemistry in 1933 at the University of Nanking. His first scientific article, published in 1935, led to his being accepted as a postgraduate student at the University of California. Three years later, he received his Ph.D. and was recruited by Herbert Evans in the Institute of Experimental Biology, University of California, Berkeley (UCB), as discussed in Chapter 16.

I have always felt very grateful to Dr. Li for providing his early extracts of the anterior pituitary to me.* Evans had organized a group of chemists and biologists in his Institute of Experimental Biology to extract, purify, and test the anterior pituitary hormones, but they had not been fully successful prior to Dr. Li's recruitment. Li personally constructed for the institute the first Tiselius apparatus that was used for obtaining the electrophoretic patterns of these agents. However, I was informed by Evans that the earlier extracts supplied for my studies on exophthalmos in 1939 (discussed under Evans in Chapter 16) were reasonably pure, and this was corroborated by my studies. It was the thyrotropic extract that produced the exophthalmos—not the gonadotropic, mammotropic, or growth extracts used as controls.

When Li started his research at the university in 1938, none of the six anterior pituitary hormones known at that time had been identified chemically. In the next 49 years, Li was in the forefront of pituitary endocrine research. He identified and synthesized a variety of peptides, in addition to the six originally known pituitary hormones, that now are known to mediate a variety of physiological functions. Li's other contributions on α-adrenocorticotropin (ACTH), ß-endorphin, and the human growth hormone made him preeminent in this field.

By the mid-1940s, Li had isolated a protein that possessed high ACTH activity. His evidence suggested that this was a carrier or precursor of smaller peptides with ACTH properties. By 1954, he identified the smaller molecule, α-ACTH, that was a very potent stimulator to the adrenal cortex and, in addition, was a fat mobilizer and melanocytic (MSH) stimulator. Li identified this molecule as a 39-amino acid peptide and later synthesized the portion of the molecule that had potent ACTH activity (31).

In later studies, Li and his collaborators isolated two new substances that were different from ACTH and MSH but had lipolytic and MSH activity. The larger molecule was named ß-lipotrophin (ß-LPH). When two pentapeptides were later found that competed with morphine for central nervous system binding sites, the amino acid sequence of one of them, methionine-enkephalin, was noted to be part of the sequence of ß-LPH and Li's other 31-amino acid peptide. The latter was shown to have pain-relieving properties several times greater than morphine and was named ß-endorphin, which was shown to be present in many animals (32). The primary molecular structure is highly retained in evolutionary species. To a great extent,

---

*This followed my earlier studies on exophthalmos, and because the studies with Li's extracts were limited and did not alter my earlier conclusions (as discussed under Evans in Chapter 17), they were never reported.

Li's studies on the various peptides have led to the current hypothesis that the pituitary produces a large molecule, propiomelancortin, that breaks down into many smaller peptides with various endocrine properties.

Li's studies on growth hormone started in the early 1940s, and his preparation was known to be the most potent growth hormone in the world. However, it was shown that humans do not respond to growth hormones from mammals below the high primate level. Thus, it was a major advance when Li isolated human growth hormone in 1956 and later determined its structure (33). This led to the synthesis of human growth hormone by both chemical and recombinant DNA means. Still other studies involved the thyrotropic and the two gonadotropic hormones of the anterior pituitary. Li was able to show that all of these were glycoproteins and had a comparable structure (34).

In 1950, Li established his own laboratory in Berkeley, the Hormone Research Laboratory. He was director of this until his retirement in 1983. Following retirement, he established still another laboratory at the University of California, San Francisco (UCSF), the Laboratory of Molecular Endocrinology, where he remained active until weeks before his death in 1987.

Li's honorary degrees (10) other honors (28) visiting professorships, and lectureships (17) are too numerous to recite, but they include the highest international awards in the field of endocrinology. He served on many advisory boards and was honorary president of the Eighth International Congress of Endocrinology. Li published over 1,000 scientific papers and served as editor on many journals and neurochemical books.

One anecdote may be worth recording, inasmuch as it suggests Li's breadth of knowledge and his care in writing. Following his Faculty Research Lecture at UCSF, I happened to encounter him in one of the elevators of the Medical Sciences Building. I congratulated him on his lecture and added that he must have taken great pains in writing it and that, in spite of its scholarly subject, it was delightful. His reply surprised me. Quoting Voltaire, he said "Every kind of writing is good save that which bores." How he happened to come up with that one, I have no idea. It was new to me, but I looked it up later, and sure enough, he was right. I suspect that Annie Lu, his wife, had a hand in his lecture. For years, she had worked on the introductions and conclusions of his articles, and she had considerable ability as a lucid writer.

Li was generous to a fault in providing hormone preparations, which may well have started with myself but later reached worldwide proportions. In addition, he was generous to his laboratory colleagues, who over the years exceeded 200 people; they were like a large family, and when technicians contributed significantly to the work, Li included them as co-authors.

Li was a leader in an unparalleled period of endocrine research on anterior pituitary proteins and peptide hormones. His legacy of scientific accomplishments in this important field is enormous. It is a pleasure to include Dr. Li, a friendly, unassuming, and generous person, in these essays.

RADIOACTIVE ISOTOPES AND ERNEST LAWRENCE

A major advance in neurochemistry was initiated before World War II with the development of radioactive isotopes. This was accomplished by Ernest Lawrence when he created the cyclotron at the University of California in 1932. The use of the isotopes in biology and medicine has been well established and especially in clinical scintiphotography and positron emission tomography for research and for purposes of clinical radiation therapy.

A brief sketch of Ernest Lawrence's career is justified, not only because of his great perceptiveness of the value of the isotopes for medical research, but also for his extraordinary generosity in supplying the isotopes for such research, dating back to his original cyclotron. The story is an interesting one and important because isotopes have assumed a vital role in neurochemistry. Furthermore, it concerns an excellent illustration of how scientific advances have been used to greatly extend and support the development of modern neurology.

ERNEST LAWRENCE (1901-1956)

Born and raised in South Dakota, his advance education was at the Universities of Minnesota, Chicago, and Yale, where he obtained his Ph.D. in 1925. In 1928, he transferred to UCB, where his first cyclotron was built. This involved the acceleration of destabilized atoms, energized by an alternating current to extremely high speeds and energy levels, and held in a circular course by its strong, 80-ton magnet.

Radioactivity was discovered by Henri Becquerel in 1896 and Georg Hevesy used thorium B, a radioactive isotope of lead, in studies on plant metabolism in 1923. However, it was not until Ernest Lawrence produced isotopes with his cyclotron in the 1930s that their practical use in biomedical research became possible.

As in the case of the chapter on neurophysiology, where a short section was devoted to electronics, so, in the case of neurochemistry, the subject of radioactive isotopes must be mentioned. Radioactively labeled ions and molecules can be detected and quantified for neurochemical study of metabolism, as well as for purposes of clinical diagnosis and therapy. In effect, this is another manner in which the electrical activity of biomedical phenomena can be followed quantitatively. In view of the fact that the interaction of electrolytes, with respect to cell membranes and synaptic activity, constitutes the basis of all living organisms, the potentialities of isotopes can be seen to be enormous.

In the mid-1930s, Ernest brought his younger brother, John, to UCB, who was instrumental in establishing the Donner Laboratory as a division of medical physics in the radiation laboratory. Through John Lawrence, a classmate of mine at Harvard Medical School, I came to know Ernest. John Lawrence had a brilliant career of his own in the Donner Laboratory and in the early use of the isotopes. Later, he was made a regent of the University of California. Through John Lawrence's influence and Ernest Lawrence's marriage to Molly Blumer, the daughter of the professor of medicine at Yale, Ernest's interest in the medical application of isotopes was kindled.

I can vouch personally for Lawrence's generosity in supplying isotopes for medical research. In 1937, Dr. David Greenberg and I obtained isotopes for a study that concerned the blood and spinal fluid levels of magnesium and calcium in epilepsy and convulsive states (35). This was one of the first radioactive isotope studies in neurology, using isotopes produced by the original cyclotron. Products of the later and larger cyclotrons were employed in several other isotope studies over the next three decades.

The neurological and other biomedical applications of isotope research, which were started in the mid-1930s, were quickly expanded by many workers. For example, as a result of my research showing increased permeability of the blood–brain barrier in electroshock therapy, cerebral concussion, and lesions of the brain, I was well aware of the diagnostic potential of the isotopes. It was obvious that isotopes that could be detected by brain scans would concentrate in the regions of increased permeability. The trick was to find isotopes of sufficient radioactivity that were biologically nontoxic. While I was testing the possible therapeutic value of reducing the blood–brain barrier permeability clinically, others exploited the diagnostic potential of the isotopes. A host of better agents for brain and bone scans soon followed. That electroencephalographic (EEG) localization depended on the same underlying altered blood–brain barrier permeability produced by pathological cerebral processes was later suggested by a close comparison of EEG and brain scintiphotography using technetium pertechnetate performed simultaneously on the same patients (36).

The therapeutic use of radiation therapy, using Ernest Lawrence's second cyclotron, as I remember, was initiated by Dr. Robert Stone, chief of the x-ray division at the UCSF at that time, as discussed in Chapter 7. I well recall how horrified Dr. Stone was over the earlier lack of protective measures in the Berkeley Radiation Laboratory. His initial therapeutic studies in Berkeley and his later evaluation in San Francisco of the fast neutrons (synchrotron) for the treatment of malignancy are presented in Chapter 7.

Ernest Lawrence's later career was greatly influenced by the World War II effort. He was associated with Arthur H. Compton and Harold C. Urey in the production of plutonium for the first atomic bomb. The huge cyclotron of 1942, developed with the aid of the theoretical physicist Robert Oppenheimer, was converted for this purpose. In 1946, Ernest Lawrence completed the synchrocyclotron, which energized particles up to 400,000,000 electron volts. From 1947 to 1948, he produced the first human-made mesons (unstable particles responsible for the forces acting between the electrons and neutrons in the nuclei of atoms) with the synchrocyclotron. He also was involved in the development of the first bevatron, a particle accelerator that obtained an energy level of 7 billion electron volts.

Endless accounts have been written about the atom smashers, the development of the atom bomb, and the security disqualification of Oppenheimer during World War II. I knew Oppenheimer in the late 1930s and followed the subsequent careers of both him and Ernest Lawrence with great interest. In spite of the many arguments that have raged over the years, it always seemed to me that Oppenheimer's disqualification in the super-security appointments of World War II was inevitable based on his earlier associations with ultraleft contacts. It also was my impression that the later sensational reports of the disrupted personal relationships that were involved were greatly exaggerated. A good book on Lawrence and Oppenheimer written by N. P. Davis is available for interested readers (37).

Ernest Lawrence won many awards, such as the Hughes Medal of the Royal Society in 1932, the Comstock Prize in 1937, the Enrico Fermi award of the Atomic Energy Commission in 1957, and the Nobel prize in 1939. A great career was tragically ended with his postoperative death in 1958.

DONALD TOWER (1919-   )

Tower played basic roles in the advancement of neurochemistry during the flowering period of neurology. This involved both his research and administrative services in the National Institutes of Health, Public Health Service. His interests in history have also helped to clarify the abstruse background of neurochemistry.

Born in Orange, New Jersey, in 1919, his early life conformed to the traditional pattern of bright students in "upper crust" families—Philip Exeter Academy, Harvard College, and Harvard Medical School. He discovered his scientific bent early, majored in chemistry, and graduated cum laude from Harvard in 1941. World War II had its effect on Tower, as it did on all young men of that period. A series of assignments in the Navy (mainly in the Philippine Islands from 1945 to 1947) followed postgraduate training in surgery at the University of Minnesota (1944 to 1945).

Following the war, Tower obtained further training in neurochemistry and neurosurgery in the Montreal Neurological Institute and McGill University and received B.Sc. and Ph.D. degrees. This background and the focus of his studies on epilepsy at the Montreal Neurological Institute explain his neurochemical approach to this subject.

Tower next served as an intern under Dr. E. A. Carmichael at the National Hospital, Queen Square, London, for 5 months. Thus, in addition to extensive postgraduate training in neurochemistry, Tower obtained excellent clinical training in surgery, neurosurgery, and neurology, as well as in public health and general medical experience in the Navy.

From 1951 on, his career was devoted to neurochemistry. Returning to the Montreal Neurological Institute, he served as an assistant neurochemist for 2 years and then rose from an instructorship in epilepsy and neurology to an assistant professorship at McGill University.

The National Institute of Neurological Diseases and Blindness (NIND&B) had been inaugurated in 1951, and its intramural program was expanded rapidly over the next few years. Along with several others from the Montreal Neurological Institute, Tower joined the Bethesda setup in 1953 as chief of the section of clinical neurochemistry at NIND&B. Various administrative titles followed over the next 20 years, and by 1974, he was made director of the National Institute of

Neurological Diseases and Stroke. He served in this important post for 7 years, retiring in 1981. Tower's main contribution was to delineate the neurochemical basis of epilepsy. As recounted in Chapters 5 and 6, it was known that electrolytes constituted the basis of bioelectric action potentials (9). It was this background that led Tower to his studies and his summary of the neurochemical basis of seizures (38). Table 1 summarizes his 23-page review.

Table 1. *Neurochemical basis of epileptogenesis*

Mechanism	System Involved	Cause	Result
Acetylcholine and its choline esterase	Acetylcholine transmitter	Organophosphorous poisoning and other derangements of the acetylcholine transmitter system	Excessive stimulation of postsynaptic enzyme effector motor units
B6 γ-aminobuteric acid	γ-aminobuteric acid, the transmitter for post-synaptic inhibitory systems of CNS	Derangements of transmitter system (glutamic carboxylase). Hydrazides or other inhibitors of pyridoxyl kinase	Reduction of inhibitory neuronal activity of CNS
Deprivation of cerebral oxidation and supply of glucose	Transport of sodium and potassium across neuronal membranes	CNS anoxia or deprivation of glucose	Edema and depolarization of cerebral neurons
Adinosine triphosphatase	Transport of sodium and potassium across neuronal membranes	Ouabain-inhibition of Na & K transport Mobilization of CA ions and mitochondrial uptake of CA	Depletion of neuronal K and failure of Na pump resulting in depolarization of cerebral neurons

Tower emphasized that the common denominator of these four known mechanisms of epileptogenesis probably involved the excitability of neuronal membranes necessary to support the response of the neurons for incoming impulses. Mechanisms 1 and 2 concerned excitatory (acetylcholine) and inhibitory (aminobutyric acid) transmitters in explanation of the postsynaptic effector action. Mechanism 3 concerned the cerebral oxidative mechanism necessary to maintain the cation transport system of neuronal membranes and their normal neurophysiological functions. Mechanism 4 more directly implicated derangements of the cation transport across neuronal membranes and the central role of this mechanism to epileptogenesis.

Following the publication of his article, I inquired as to the regional differences that might fit in with the neurophysiological studies on temporal lobe epilepsy (complex partial seizures) and absence seizures (corticoreticular system), but such studies had not been done. At that time, the International Classification of the epilepsies did not recognize these types of seizures as regional forms, which seemed to me and my co-authors to produce a somewhat muddled and confusing situation.

Although many investigators have been involved in these studies, Tower's own research has been important to mechanisms 1, 2, and 4 of the table. Tower is a clear and interesting writer, and readers would be well advised to consult his review articles (39,40). In addition to his articles on acetylcholine, γ-aminobutyric acid, and glutamic acid, his articles on cerebral compartmentation, brain edema, glia, and astrocytes are also notable and testify to the breadth of his studies (41-43).

Tower's interest in history was well known and led to his appointment in 1984 as the historian of the American Society for Neurochemistry. He has written about 20 articles dealing with the historical development of neurochemistry and several of the early leaders in this field. Interestingly enough, his own memoirs and a genealogical study of his family are included in his bibliography. His story is unusual mainly in his devotion to developing neurochemistry as an important facet of the Public Health Service and in his service in other government roles. Tower's honors and awards have included several important lectureships, the Distinguished Service Medal of the Public Health Service, and an honorary degree from McGill University.

In summary, Tower's career bridged the gap between neurochemistry and clinical neurology. He was particularly conscious of the advances in neurochemical instrumentation and techniques, utilizing them all in his governmental posts. In addition, he served in important governmental administrative posts, both in the Public Health Service and the Navy but, especially, in the Public Health Service where he was the director of the National Institute of Neurological Diseases, Communicative Diseases, and Blindness (NINDCDB, later stroke) for 10 years. By taking advantage of the great impetus of support of the NINDCDB, he played a major role in the development of neurochemistry in the flowering period of neurology.

HENRY DALE (1875-1968)

Henry Dale is one of the few neuroscientists included in these essays that I did not know, although I heard a great deal about him through Chauncy Leake. In this account of neurochemistry and neuropharmacology, however, he cannot be neglected. His studies on synaptic transmission and his advocacy of a neurochemical basis for nerve and synaptic transmission won him the Nobel prize, and he brilliantly bridged the gap between neurochemistry and neuropharmacology.

Born and raised in London, he attended Trinity College, Cambridge University, where he worked under Langley. He completed his medical training at St. Bartholomew's Hospital and Medical School, London, in 1903. He obtained a student fellowship the next year and worked with Ernest Henry Starling on his physiological studies of the heart. One year later, he was made director of the Wellcome Physiological Research Laboratory. Dale became a prototype for those engaged in industrial pharmacological research, which has become so widespread and important in more recent years. However, he did not fit into prescribed lines of research dictated by the pharmaceutical company. He was an original thinker and did much basic research, spanning the gap between neurochemistry, neuropharmacology, and neurophysiology.

In his studies on ergot, he isolated ergotoxine and discovered its effect in reversing the pressor action of epinephrine. Posterior pituitary extracts were used as controls, which led to his discovery of the contracting action of ergot on uterine muscles and their use in obstetrics (44). Another early study concerned the sympathomimetic action of the amines. His co-worker, George Bayer, a chemist, synthesized many amines, and their pharmacological studies resulted in the introduction of several important drugs into clinical practice.

In 1914, he was made director of the National Institute for Medical Research (Great Britain), where he conducted his studies on histamine and its effect on anaphylaxis, as well as developed his studies of synaptic transmission. Dale was aware of Sherrington's earlier studies showing long-lasting effects on central summation and inhibition, which suggested the accumulation of excitatory and inhibitory "substances" at the synaptic junction. A chance observation of a muscarine-like action of an atypical ergot extract on cardiac function reminded him of a report of my former professor of pharmacology, Reid Hunt, given 8 years earlier on the intense vagomimetic action of acetylcholine. Dale then confirmed the fact that the muscarine-like ergot extract was acetylcholine. Still later, he found that acetylcholine also had nicotinic effects. Although it has been pointed out how close Dale came to discovering the chemical transmission of acetylcholine in 1914, it was not until some 19 years later that he proved it to be the transmitter for the autonomic nervous system (45). As indicated in the introduction above, Loewi had demonstrated that his vagostuff was a chemical transmitter in 1920. Dale's breakthrough was quickly extended to the voluntary neuromuscular system (46). The studies of Dale were basic in identifying the synaptic "substance" and in showing different types of neurotransmitters. Dale and Loewi shared the Nobel prize in 1937.

Several other important drug effects were discovered during Dale's period of research at the National Institute of Medical Research. The use of curarine derivatives in some of his experiments led to their clinical use as muscle-relaxing agents in surgery, as discussed under Laborit in Chapter 13. Drugs that block the synaptic destruction of acetylcholine, such as physostigmine, were useful in myasthenia gravis.

Dale's experimental studies ended in 1938 when he became president of the Medical Research Council. With the onset of World War II, his administrative duties were further expanded. He proved to be as excellent in the field of administration as he had been in the experimental field. When he retired from the council in 1942, he carried on in many administrative posts, including the Royal Society and Wellcome Trust.

His bibliography of 295 articles, as listed in the memoirs of the Royal Society, is incomplete in the sense of the many articles he inspired among his staff and co-workers. At his research peak, he produced 54 articles for each of two decades and an overall average of almost 5 per year for 38 years. Over the next 25 years, after retiring from research, his output remained almost as high but changed to administrative reports, review articles, introductions to meetings, historical articles, and obituaries.

Henry Dale undoubtedly is one of the most honored men of neuroscience. He received 16 of the highest honors internationally, won 21 prizes and medals, including the Nobel prize, and was awarded 25 honorary degrees. He was made an honorary member of 37 national societies and fulfilled a great many lectureships.

Dale was knighted in 1932, was president of the Royal Society from 1942 to 1945, and was the Fullerian professor and director of the Davy-Faraday Laboratory of the Royal Institution from 1942 to 1946. He became the chairman of the Wellcome Trust in 1938 and guided the growth of the Wellcome Medical History Museum and Laboratory until 1960. No doubt his early success in research and later his long and illustrious life account for his honors, but it is still an astounding record.

Chauncy Leake has described Dale as a kindly, cheerful, and most hospitable person, who at the same time was a brilliant and witty speaker (47). Others have described his sense of humor and his abilities as a raconteur. Certainly few have equaled his brilliance in both research and administration.

LOUIS S. GOODMAN (1906-   )

As one of the most distinguished pharmacologists of the past generation, when neurology was in its flowering stage, Louis S. Goodman well deserves inclusion in this account. His textbook of pharmacology, *The Pharmacological Basis of Therapeutics*, with Dr. A. Gilman was perhaps his most acclaimed achievement (48), but his ability to establish an outstanding department of pharmacology and to develop a world-recognized program in the pharmacology of antiepileptic drugs and basic studies on epileptogenesis made him an acknowledged leader in the field of neuropharmacology. Like so many included in these essays, Goodman's background of training and development was thorough and excellent.

Born and raised in Portland, Oregon, his early education was at Reed College (B.A., 1928) and the University of Oregon (M.D. and M.A., 1932). He interned at Johns Hopkins and then obtained a National Research Council Fellowship in Medicine at Yale in 1934. He was appointed an instructor in pharmacology at Yale in 1935 and was promoted to the assistant professorship in 1937. In 1943, Goodman moved to Vermont to be professor and chair of the Department of Pharmacology and Physiology at the University of Vermont College of Medicine. This was quickly followed by a move to Salt Lake City in 1944, where he became professor and chair of the Department of Pharmacology at the University of Utah College of Medicine, remaining there until his retirement in 1971.

Goodman's "magic carpet" to recognition and success came after writing his outstanding text of pharmacology with Dr. Gilman (48). This was started when they worked together in the department of pharmacology of the Yale School of Medicine. Published first in 1941, it had immediate success, and over 200,000 copies were sold within the next 30 years. It became known at the "Blue Bible" of medicine and pharmacology. The original 900,000 words were extended to 1,500,000 in the 1955 edition. This encyclopedic effort at first seems at variance with Goodman's own admonition that "if you can't organize your subject within ten pages, forget it." His "escape hatch" on this, of course, was that his textbook involved thousands of subjects. As research progressed and the field of pharmacology expanded, it was inevitable that the Goodman and Gilman text would enlarge. As pharmacological subdivisions have grown, other collaborators have participated in newer editions. Its quality and practical usefulness, however, have been maintained by the critical editorship of Goodman and Gilman.

Starting with two associates and limited facilities in the newly expanded Utah School of Medicine, his department had achieved national recognition by the early 1950s when, with funding by the National Institutes of Health, considerable expansion was made possible. I served on a progress site visit of the NIND&B in 1968 that awarded the department excellent funding for its research and training programs. There was no question of the high caliber of the people and work, which became nationally and internationally recognized. Goodman's ability to select superior associates and to organize a highly productive teaching, research, and graduate training program was outstanding.

In addition to his book and departmental commitments, Goodman fulfilled many public service roles. At different times, he was a member of six prestigious national committees and councils, two international assignments to Russia, and the American representative to the International Union of Physiological Sciences. He was a member of many national boards, associations, and foundations. In addition, he was chief editor of Pharmacological Reviews and president of the American Society of Pharmacology and Experimental Therapeutics in 1959.

Goodman was the author or co-author of 200 articles and reviews in the field of pharmacology and experimental therapeutics (49). These dealt with a broad variety of subjects but, in particular, with neuropharmacology and anticonvulsants. With E. A. Swinyard, E. P. Toman, and others, he co-authored some 42 articles on the physiology and pharmacological aspects of experimental epilepsy. Techniques of studying the electroconvulsive threshold were evaluated, and the convulsive action of a dozen agents were tested. The modes of action of anticonvulsant drugs were studied. The broad approach employed by Goodman and his associates to the study of brain excitability and the mechanisms that modify convulsive threshold is impressive. Many of his articles dealt with this approach, perhaps best exemplified by his early effort with Toman (50). His laboratory became a world center. An outstanding group was attracted to his department, among whom were E. A. Swinyard, E. P. Toman, J. Gordon Millichap, and Dixon Woodbury. Of the first 15 John Jacob Abel awards presented by the Society of Pharmacology and Experimental Therapeutics, 5 were from Goodman's department. Two members won the research award in pharmacodynamics of the American Pharmaceutical Association Foundation.

In addition to his many offices and assignments, Goodman was a member of the National Academy of Science and received honorary Doctor of Science degrees from the Universities of Manitoba and Utah.

As a teacher, stimulator of research, and administrator, Goodman had few equals. When I was chair of a National Institutes of Health committee on "Orphan Drugs," it was inevitable that he would be assigned to the committee. Our problem concerned the unavailability of drugs for rare medical conditions. Years before the government took action to deal with this difficult problem, their limited sales did not justify the tremendous expense of their development and marketing by pharmaceutical manufacturing companies.

During one of our contacts, Goodman and I exchanged experiences on our respective trips to Russia. He had gone in 1958 as a representative of the Departments of State and Health, Education, and Welfare on a neuroscience mission, while I had led a neurological group on Russia's invitation in 1965. The isolation and doctrinaire atmosphere of Russia at that time made it difficult for its scientific community with their crowded living conditions, poor remuneration, and limitations on visiting or attending meetings in foreign countries. The few who managed visits in the United States could not believe that the standards of living were so high and suspected that they were being manipulated (as indeed Russia attempted to do for others in its Exhibition of Economic Achievements). Our highways, crowded with cars, and our privately owned homes constituted a world beyond their wildest dreams. Goodman informed me that, when he entertained a group of Russians in his lovely Salt Lake City home, they were stunned and suspicious of another "American trick."

Dr. Goodman has been described as looking like the typical absent-minded professor, but he certainly never appeared that way to me. It is true that he is a quiet and unpretentious person, but his brilliance and wisdom quickly became evident in committee, departmental, or other group activities. He was the acme of consideration and support for his staff, a reaction richly returned by their loyalty. The words of his first graduate student and early associate, Dr. E. Swinyard, come to mind in this connection. When he asked Goodman how he could ever repay him for his help and understanding, Louis answered that it was easy—all Swinyard had to do was to treat his graduate students in the same way. In this fashion, his efforts to develop young people would be expanded and carried on. He added that this should be done without regard to the color or creed of his students (51). Goodman was more than a teacher, research worker, and administrator—he is a superior man of vision whose abilities catapulted him into the highest levels of his field.

DIXON M. WOODBURY (1921-1991)

To include Dr. Woodbury, who was a member of Dr. Goodman's department, in these essays may seem redundant, following the account devoted to Louis Goodman. However, the two were quite different. Goodman was more the pharmacologist whose background enabled him to relate pharmacology to the needs of medicine. Woodbury, on the other hand, was primarily a research worker whose broad background in neurochemistry and neurophysiology, plus his inquiring mind, made him an outstanding investigator. He was in charge of the postgraduate training program under Goodman and led in much of the department research. The two complemented each other in their interests; they made a remarkable team. Goodman was the wise administrator, author, and able representative of pharmacology. Woodbury was in the front line as an investigator and, because of the many advances he achieved, well illustrates this aspect of neuropharmacology in the flowering period of neurology.

Although Woodbury was born and spent his first few years in St. George and the southwestern corner of Utah, his family moved to Salt Lake City when his father, Angus Woodbury, was made assistant professor of zoology in 1927 at the University of Utah. It was a family of unusual scholarly attainment.

Woodbury's college training was at the University of Utah where he majored in zoology in 1942. In addition, he obtained a M.S. degree in herpetology. Fortunately for the neurosciences, his interests turned to medicine, and after 3 years of this, he went into graduate study at UCB in physicochemical biology and cellular physiology. While writing his thesis for his Ph.D. (1948), he served as a research instructor in pharmacology at the University of Utah School of Medicine and obtained further graduate training in the Department of Pharmacology. He was advanced to an assistant research professorship of pharmacology and from 1953 to 1958 served as an assistant professor of pharmacology. In 1958, he also was made Scientist of the National Neurological Research Foundation and, in 1961, was promoted to the full professorship of pharmacology.

Professor Goodman had become his mentor from 1947 on and influenced his interests and research on cerebral excitability, pharmacological methods of modifying this, brain metabolism, the changes occurring with cerebral maturation, and especially, the mode of action of antiepileptic drugs. Many other interests were interwoven, such as basic neurophysiological and neurochemical studies on the effects of various pharmacological agents and hormones (desoxycortisone acetate and thyroid) as well as studies on the blood–brain barrier. His bibliography contains 159 scientific articles, another 127 preliminary reports and abstracts, and 33 invited lectures, 12 of which were in foreign centers. In addition, he wrote chapters or was a co-author of 62 books. Although the bulk of his research, either directly or indirectly, concerned epilepsy, there was a solid base of physicochemical biology and pharmacology in both his teaching and research. It was Woodbury who wrote the chapter on "General Principles" for the Goodman and Gilman text, as well as other chapters, such as "Analgesics and Antipyretics" and "Parathyroid" (48). Again, "Physiology and Biophysics" he wrote the chapters on "Physiology of the Body Fluids" and "Blood-CSF-Brain Fluid Relations."(49)

Woodbury obtained research career awards from the National Institutes of Health from 1962 on and also received honors for his teaching. He was the director of the graduate training program in pharmacology from 1966 to 1971 and served as head of the Department of Pharmacology at the University of Utah from 1971 to 1980. His research, writing, and consulting work became so involved with epilepsy that a special division of neuropharmacology and epileptology was created for him; he served as head of this for his last 11 years. Near the end of his life, he was involved in an exciting study of the anticonvulsive effect of vagus nerve stimulation.

My first contact with Woodbury was in 1952 or 1953. He came to San Francisco to explore the possibility of a research connection in the neurology department. Unfortunately, it was well before our new research towers were built, and space was a hopeless problem. I knew of Woodbury through my mother, who as a former trustee of the University of Utah, had developed a high opinion of Professor Angus Woodbury, his father. I never did discover the precise reasons for Woodbury's approach at that time, but it probably was related to his earlier postgraduate contacts in Berkeley and his continuing research work with Professor Paola Timaris in Physiology at Berkeley. Woodbury knew of my early research on desoxycorticosterone acetate in epilepsy (52). In the late 1940s, he had published eight or nine articles on this subject and was to continue with it in four reports with Timaris and others over the next decade. He may also have been attracted by my research interests in epilepsy and the blood–brain barrier.

While on a project site visit for the National Institutes of Health in 1968 to pass on a large grant request from the Department of Physiology at the College of Medicine, University of Utah, the possibility occurred to me of collaborating with Woodbury on a book dealing with the subject of epilepsy. I had begun the book with the aim of summarizing the tremendous research literature on epilepsy that had been compiled from two international symposiums (53,54). Although the articles were published in book form, a practical summary for the clinical neurologist, faced with the problems of the management of epilepsy, was lacking, and I had turned my attention to this objective. However, I quickly realized that I could benefit from the cooperation of someone steeped in the neurochemical and neurophysiological aspects of this subject. Woodbury had almost finished medical school training before changing to his postgraduate Ph.D. studies, had become one of the leaders in research on the underlying mechanisms of epilepsy and antiepileptic drugs, and in addition, was a pleasant person to work with. He was receptive to the idea, and out of this, grew our book *The Management of Epilepsy*, which finally was published in 1974 (55). I had emphasized the need of a comprehensive approach to the clinical management of epileptic patients, with special attention to the control of the underlying seizure-inducing mechanisms in each patient. Woodbury saw the importance of this at once, which led to chapters on the basic seizure-inducing mechanisms and their control, insofar as possible, in the clinical setting. From this contact, several articles developed, such as the role of the blood–brain barrier in epilepsy and a proposed modification of the classification of the epilepsies (56,57).

Two other episodes in my many contacts with Woodbury may be worthy of mention. The first was notable because it established a closer bond between us and aided in the subsequent rapport of our several ventures of co-authorship. In 1970, Woodbury complained of left shoulder pain, and subsequently, he was studied for a suspected heart condition and, then, scheduled for a catheter study of his heart. Further inquiry revealed that his pain had no connection with effort or fatigue, which with his description of his pain and of its distribution sounded to me to be atypical for referred cardiac pain. I then examined him and discovered tenderness over the left trapezius muscle at its lateral edge below the posterior shoulder level, probably involving the spina scapulae. Pressure on this elicited his pain. After questioning him about accidents and injuries, he recalled a fall about 1 year before that had injured his left shoulder and caused pain. This had improved, and so he had not related his present pain with the fall. His present pain had developed over the previous few months during which heavy lifting may have caused a recrudescence of his earlier pain.

Woodbury was fascinated with my explanation of a possible neurological referred basis for his pain problem and was convinced when I could reproduce his pain with pressure on his tender spot. I advised him to discuss my evaluation with his cardiologist but to proceed with the planned study if the cardiologist still believed it to be indicated. I heard a few days later that the catheter study had been done and the findings were negative. Woodbury was greatly reassured and was most grateful for my examination and advice, which finally led to appropriate treatment.

The second episode occurred while working on our second book * (58). Because of our many contacts, which extended over several years, he had learned of a trip that I had taken to Southeastern Utah in 1923, when he was still a baby. He knew about the Posey Indian War near Blanding, Utah, and was amazed that I and a friend had "bumped" into this situation on a pack trip to the natural bridges some 57 miles west of Blanding by way of the old Indian trails. Because I had been asked to write an account of the trip by the widow of my companion, my plan was to motor to this same area for research purposes and illustrative color photography for a written account of the trip. Dr. and Mrs. Woodbury became fascinated with the story and insisted that they be included in the expedition. Later, they requested a copy of the book" ** (59).Although we had spent a great deal of time in close association working on the two books for more than 10 years, I believe this trip and story did more to cement our friendship than anything else.

Woodbury was a very scholarly man, who at the same time was a master experimentalist. His broad background in neurochemistry, neurophysiology, neuropharmacology, neurobiology, and medicine equipped him well for the many basic studies previously mentioned. Initially, his abilities to write well were somewhat limited. However, his teaching taught him to summarize the essentials, and his writing improved tremendously over the years (60). These factors plus his pleasant personality and solid integrity made him the obvious choice as director of the Graduate Training Program under Goodman and finally Goodman's replacement as chair of the department on Goodman's retirement in 1971. Whereas Goodman was a schol-

---

*This new book was undertaken with Richard L. Masland, M.D., as well as with Woodbury, and its purpose was to emphasize the clinical problems arising from the confusion of inaccurate diagnosis and classification of epilepsy as well as the limitations of treatment, when seizure-inducing mechanisms were not included in the overall management of epilepsy.

**Bound copies were also supplied to the Utah State Historical Society and the Library of the State Historical Monument (The Edge of the Cedars at Blanding) at their request.

arly and practical man of great vision, Woodbury was a superb research worker of exceptionally scholarly depth. It was a team that was hard to beat over the 24 years in which they were closely associated.

SUMMARY

Although neurochemistry has historical links extending back to alchemy, its modern scientific status with respect to brain metabolism is illustrated by the many contributions of J. H. Quastel. His amazing productivity continued for nearly 60 years. It was Sir Rudolph Peters, however, who related avitaminosis and the "chemical lesion" to clinical disorders with special reference to the vitamin B complex and the nervous system. Dr. Chou Hao Li's great contributions in the neurochemical aspects of the neurohormones of the anterior pituitary closely followed. The radioactive isotopes provided by the invention of the cyclotron by Ernest Lawrence were developed in this same period and have found wide application in neurological research as well as for neurological diagnosis and treatment. Donald Tower's contributions to the neurochemistry of epilepsy and his other studies have bridged the gap between neurochemistry, neurophysiology, and clinical neurology. In addition to Henry Dales's basic studies on neurotransmitters, he bridged the gap between neurochemistry and neuropharmacology. Louis Goodman and his associate Dixon Woodbury represent important aspects of neuropharmacology, with particular respect to the antiepileptic drugs and their mode of action.

The outstanding contributions to the vast field of neurochemistry have been numerous. Those selected to illustrate its main facets have been chosen with difficulty and, in some instances, arbitrarily. With all due apologies to innumerable others, I would refer the interested reader to the articles of Donald Tower, Historian of the American Association for Neurochemistry, and others who have reviewed the historical aspects of neurochemistry and neuropharmacology.

REFERENCES

1. Tower, D.B. Neurochemistry in historical perspective. In: Siegel, G.B., Albers, R.W., Agranoff, B.W., and Katzman, R. (eds): *Basic Neurochemistry.* Boston, Little Brown & Co., 1981.
2. Drabkin, D.L. Thudichum: *Chemist of the Brain.* Philadelphia, WB Saunders, 1958.
3. Garrod, A.E. *Inborn Errors of Metabolism.* 2nd ed. London, Hedder and Stoughton, 1923.
4. Haymaker, W., and Schiller, F. (eds.): *The Founders of Neurology.* 2nd ed. Springfield, IL, Charles C. Thomas, 1970, pp. 285-289, 297-306.
5. Tower, D.B.H. Winterstein. In: Haymaker, W., and Schiller, F. (eds.): *The Founders of Neurology.* 2nd ed. Springfield, IL, Charles C. Thomas, 1970, pp. 307-311.
6. Peters, R.A. The biochemical lesion in vitamin B deficiency. Application of modern biochemical analysis in its diagnosis. *Lancet* 1:1161-1174, 1936.
7. Cannon, W.B. *The Wisdom of the Body.* New York, Norton, 1932.
8. Brown, J.S.L. Otto Loewi. In: Haymaker, W., and Schiller, F. (eds.): *The Founders of Neurology.* 2nd ed. Springfield, IL, Charles C. Thomas, 1970, pp. 293-296.
9. Hodgkin, A.L. *The Conduction of Nerve Impulses.* Liverpool, Liverpool University Press, 1964.
10. Elliott, K.A.C. My colleague. *Q. Can. J. Biochem.*, 43:9:vii-ix, 1965.
11. MacIntosh, F.C., and Sourkes, T.L. Judah Hirsch Quastel. Biographical Memoirs of Fellows of the Royal Society, 36:380-418, 1990.
12. Quastel, J.H., and Wheatley, H.M. Oxidation by the brain. *Biochem. J.*, 26:725-744, 1932.

13. Quastel, J.H. Respiration in the central nervous system. *Physiol. Rev.*, 19:135-183, 1939.
14. Pugh, C.E.M., and Quastel, J.H. Oxidation of amines by animal tissues. *Biochem. J.*, 31:2306-2321,1937.
15. Mann, P.J.G., Tennenbaum, M., and Quastel, J.H. On the mechanism of acetylcholine formation in brain in vitro. *Biochem. J.*, 32:243-261, 1938.
16. Mann, P.J.G., Tennenbaum, M., and Quastel, J.H. Acetylcholine metabolism in the central nervous system. The effects of potassium and other cations on acetylcholine liberation. *Biochem. J.*, 33:822-835, 1939.
17. Jowett, M., and Quastel, J.H. The oxidation of normal saturated fatty acids in the presence of liver slices. *Biochem. J.*, 29:2159-2180, 1935.
18. Mann, P.J.G., and Quastel, J.H. Nicotinamide, cozymase and tissue metabolism. *Biochem. J.*, 35:502-577, 1941.
19. Lahirt, S., and Quastel, J.H. Fluoracetate and ammonia metabolism of the brain. *Biochem. J.*, 89:157-163, 1963.
20. Itoh, T., and Quastel, J.H. Acetoacetate metabolism in infant and adult rat brain *in vitro*. *Biochem. J.*, 116:641-655, 1970.
21. Quastel, J.H., and Wheatley, H.M. Narcosis and oxidations by the brain. *Proc. R. Soc. Lond.*, 112:60,1932.
22. Darlington, W.A., and Quastel, J.H. Absorption of sugars from isolated surviving intestine. *Arch. Biochem.*, 43:194-207, 1953.
23. Quastel, J.H. Molecular transport at cell membranes. *Proc. R. Soc. Lond.*, 163:169-196, 1965.
24. Quastel, J.H., and Wheatley, D.M. Vitamin B and bacterial oxidation. Dependence of acetic acid oxidation on vitamin B. *Biochem. J.*, 35:192-206, 1941.
25. Sung, J.H. J. H. Quastel. *T.I.B.S.* 5:101-102, 1979.
26. Thompson, R.H.S., and Ogston, A.S. Rudolph Albert Peters. *Biographical Memoirs of Fellows of the Royal Society*. London, Royal Society, 1987.
27. Peters, R.A. Pyruvic acid oxidation in brain. I. Vitamin B1 and the pyruvic acid oxidase in pigeon's brain. *Biochem. J.*, 30:2206-2218, 1936.
28. Peters, R.A. *Biochemical Lesions and Lethal Synthesis*. Oxford, Pergamon, 1963.
29. Peters, R.A., Wakelin, R.W., Buffa, P., and Thomas, L. C. The biochemistry of fluoroacetate poisoning. The isolation and some properties of the fluorotricarboxylic acid inhibitor of citrate metabolism. *Proc. R. Soc. Lond.*, 140:497-507, 1953.
30. Peters, R.A., and Walshe, J.M. Studies on the toxicity of copper. I. The toxic action of copper in vivo and in vitro. *Proc. R. Soc. Lond.*, 166:273-284, 1966.
31. Li, C.H., and Oelofsen, W. The chemistry and biology of ACTH and related peptides. In: The Adrenal Cortex. 1967, p. 185.
32. Li, C.H., Yamashiro, D., Tseng, L.-F., and Loh, H.H. Synthesis and analgesic activity of human ß-endorphin. *J. Med. Chem.*, 20:325-328, 1977.
33. Li, C.H., and Evans, H.M., The isolation of pituitary growth hormone. *Science*, 99:183-184, 1944.
34. Sairam, M.R., and Li, C.H. Human pituitary thyrotropin: isolation and characterization of its subunits. *Biochem. Biophys. Res. Commun.*, 51:336-342, 1973.
35. Greenberg, D.M., and Aird, R.B. Blood and spinal fluid magnesium and calcium levels in epilepsy and convulsive states. *Proc. Soc. Exp. Biol. Med.*, 37:618-620, 1938.
36. Sasaki, M., Aird, R.B., Kerber, C., Newton, T.H., and Powell, M. Correlative study of EEG and brain scintiphotography. *Trends Am. Neurol. Assoc.*, 96:299-300, 1971.
37. Davis, N.P. *Lawrence and Oppenheimer*. New York, Simon & Schuster, 1968.
38. Tower, D.B. Neurochemical mechanisms. In: Jasper, H.H., Ward, A., and Pope, A. (eds.). *Basic Mechanisms of the Epilepsies*. Boston, Little, Brown & Co., 1969.
39. Tower, D.B., and Elliott, K.A.C. Activity of acetylcholine system in human epileptogenic focus. *J. Appl. Physiol.*, 4:669-676, 1952.
40. Tower, D.B. Glutamic acid and y-aminobutyric acid in seizures. *Clin. Chim. Acta*, 2:297-402, 1957.
41. Tower, D.B., Wherrett, J.R., and McKann, G.M. Functional implications of metabolic compartmentation in the central nervous system: interrelationships of cellular protein and amino acids, fluid spaces and electrolytes, and oxidative metabolism, as delineated by ammonia. In: Ketty, S.S., and Elkes, J. (eds.). *Regional Neurochemistry*. Oxford, Pergamon, 1961, pp. 65-88.
42. Tower, D.B. Cerebral edema. In: Siegel, G.B., Albers, R.W., Agranoff, B.W., and Katzman, R. (eds.). *Basic Neurochemistry*. Boston, Little, Brown & Co., 1981, pp. 537-554.
43. Tower, D.B. General perspectives and conclusions of the symposium on dynamic properties of glial cells. In: Schoffeniels, E., Franck, G., Hertz, L., and Tower, D.B. (eds.). *Dynamic Properties of Glial Cells*. Oxford, Pergamon, 1978, pp. 443-460.

44. Dale, H.H. The active principles of ergot. BMJ., 2:1610, 1910.
45. Dale, H.H. Chemical transmission of the effects of impulses in the peripheral nervous system: abstract of discussion at the informal meeting of the research group at the dedication of the Lilly Research Laboratories, Indianapolis, Indiana, October 12, 1935.
46. Dale, H.H., Brown, G.L., and Feldberg, W. Chemical transmission of excitation from motor nerve to voluntary muscle. *J. Physiol.*, 87:394-409, 1936.
47. Leake, C. Henry Dale. In: Haymaker, W., and Schiller, F. (eds.). *The Founders of Neurology.* 2nd ed. Springfield, IL, Charles C. Thomas, 1970, pp. 282-285.
48. Goodman, L., and Gilman, A. *The Pharmacological Basis of Therapeutics.* 2nd ed. New York, Macmillan, 1955.
49. Goodman, L.S. Utah Science, Engineering and Medical Archives, Manuscripts Division, Special Collections Department, University of Utah Libraries, University of Utah, Salt Lake City, Utah.
50. Toman, J.E.P., and Goodman, L.S. Conditions modifying convulsions in animals. *Res. Publ. Assoc. Res. Nerv. Ment. Dis.*, 26:141-163, 1946.
51. Swinyard, E. The Goodman era. Award winning pharmacology in global spotlight. University of Utah Rev., November, pp. 101-102, 1968.
52. Aird, R.B. The effect of desoxycorticosterone in epilepsy. *J. Nerv. Ment. Dis.*, 99:501-510, 1944.
53. Gastaut, H., Jasper, H., Bancaud, J., and Waltregny, A. (eds.). *The Physiopathogenesis of the Epilepsies.* Springfield, IL, Charles C. Thomas, 1969.
54. Jasper, H.H., Ward, A.A., and Pope, A. (eds.). *Basic Mechanisms of the Epilepsies.* Boston, Little Brown & Co., 1969.
55. Aird, R.B., and Woodbury, D.M. *The Management of Epilepsy.* Springfield, IL, Charles C. Thomas, 1974.
56. Aird, R.B., Woodbury, D.M. The role of the blood-brain barrier in epilepsy. Presented at the International Congress of EEG and Clinical Neurophysiology, Marseilles, France, September 6, 1973.
57. Aird, R.B., Masland, R.L., and Woodbury, D.M. Hypothesis: the classification of epileptic seizures according to systems of the CNS. Epilepsy Res., 3:77-81, 1989.
58. Aird, R.B., Masland, R.L., and Woodbury, D.M. The Epilepsies: A Critical Review. New York, Raven Press, 1984.
59. Aird, R.B. An Adventure for Adventure's Sake. Privately produced for limited distribution. Bound by University of California Press, San Francisco, 1980.
60. Woodbury, D.M. Physiology of the body fluids and blood-cerebrospinal fluid-brain fluid relations. In: Ruch, T.C., and Patton, H.D. (eds.). *Physiology and Biophysics.* Philadelphia, WB Saunders, 1965, pp. 871-896, 942-950.

CHAPTER 7

Neuroimaging

A number of disciplines closely overlap clinical neurology. Their participation with neurology in the exciting scientific advances that have developed during the flowering period of neurology clearly justifies the inclusion of their contributions in these essays.

Perhaps no other specialty better illustrates the dependence of modern neurology on the technical advances of science than does neuroimaging. Roentgenography made its dramatic entry into the field of medicine in the first decade of the present century. Although Walter Cannon and a few others were experimenting with the technique 2 or 3 years before the turn of the century, the availability of x-ray equipment and its utilization in medical practice came more slowly. I well remember this point because of repeated stories about my marked projectile vomiting in the first year of my life (1903 to 1904), which was before the days of available x-ray. My physician father, an excellent diagnostician, pronounced my condition to be pylorospasm, and sure enough, as expected, the condition slowly cleared after my first year. With spoon feeding, day and night, I survived. Except for the fact that I had no hunger pains and would go all day without eating unless reminded, I became a normal, robust youth. Some 7 to 8 years later, well before World War I, I can recall seeing my father adjusting an early x-ray apparatus as he used the fluoroscopic screen to set broken bones. This would be some 15 years after the original discovery of x-rays.

In the context of reviewing the adaptation of scientific techniques to neurological use, a brief recounting of the story of Roentgen's discovery may be justified. Wilhelm K. Roentgen, a German physicist at the University of Wurzburg, while experimenting with a Crooke's tube (as discussed under Electronics in Chapter 5) in 1895, noted that nearby photographic plates became fogged. He determined that this only occurred when the tube was activated. He dubbed the unknown ray "x-ray" and was able to protect other plates by interposing solid objects. The degree of protection varied with the density of the object, its thickness, and the duration of exposure. In the process of these studies, he obtained the first x-ray image of his own hand. Roentgen very deservedly was the recipient of the first Nobel prize in physics in 1901. It was not until 1905 and 1912, however, that Arthur Schüller published his classic studies on x-rays of the skull (1).

Aside from Cannon's experimental gastrointestinal (GI) studies, the clinical use of contrast media for neuroimaging was first employed by Dandy (ventriculography in 1918 and pneumoencephalography in 1919) and Sicard (lipoidal medium for myelography in 1925) (2-4). It is interesting to note in this connection that isolated reports of air or "gas" had been observed in the cerebral ventricles as early as 1913 (5). This type of observation gave Dandy his inspiration, as discussed in Chapter 8. A tragicomical and possibly apocryphal account of this sort circulated at the Peter Bent Brigham Hospital when I studied there in the late 1920s. Well before Dandy's report, a follow-up x-ray on one of Harvey Cushing's patients revealed gas-filled ventricles. Fearing that Cushing (Professor of Surgery at the Harvard Medical School) might react adversely to their follow-up care, this was not reported. Considering the reaction of many to the "Professor" in his early period at Harvard and also the fact that spontaneous pneumoencephalography can occur in postoperative patients with the loss of cerebrospinal fluid, it might well have been true. However, I never had the courage to ask Dr. Horrax (as discussed in Chapter 8), an associate of Cushing, about this.

I well recall this period of roentgenography as a student under Cushing and Merrill Sossman at the Peter Bent Brigham Hospital in Boston. Also, in the early 1930s, I did pneumoencephalography and myelography with Drs. Van Wagonen and Stafford Warren at the University of Rochester. Later, I became a specialist on pneumoencephalography working with x-rays with Dr. Robert Stone at the University of California, San Francisco (UCSF); this developed from my research work on anesthetic gases as substitutes for air. Seventy percent of air is nitrogen, which was poorly absorbed and greatly prolonged the pain and shock reactions of pneumoencephalography. Good results were obtained with ethylene. The anesthetic gases had no effect on the pain, but ethylene permitted excellent roentgenographic results while shortening the reaction time and hospitalization by an average of 2 days (6). Oxygen was later adopted as a more practical agent because it also foreshortened the pneumoencephalographic reaction period.* Following this experimental work on pneumoencephalography, I did all pneumoencephalograms in the

---

*By way of showing how the multiple and overlapping advances of scientific progress occur, it may be worth recording our demonstration of one form of normal-pressure hydrocephalus as the result of these studies in the late 1940s. With the use of pure gases, detailed studies of their absorption rates followed. Delayed absorption tallied closely with cerebrospinal fluid (CSF) obstructive processes that delayed the flow and reabsorption of CSF. This was documented for both brain tumors and infectious processes. The surgical relief of space-consuming lesions, but more commonly the relief of the inflammation of infectious processes by the new antibiotics, restored a balance between the rates of CSF formation and absorption. Initially, in the acute pressure phase of these conditions, the ventricles were dilated, and the supracortical subarachnoid spaces were reduced or obliterated. Following recovery, the absorption bed and the channels leading to it were adequate to restore a balance between CSF formation and absorption. This was confirmed by normal CSF pressures. In a few instances, studies in the acute phase were obtained, as well as in the late recovery phase (7). The fact that most patients with normal-pressure hydrocephalus obtained a good response to shunting suggests a borderline balance intermittently disrupted. Also, because their background appears to be different from the group reported by Adams and co-workers in 1965, still other mechanisms may be involved (8).

University of California Hospital for a period of over 10 years. As the result of review studies involving a total of some 3,000 procedures, I developed considerable expertise. During this period, I became a close friend of Dr. Stone and reviewed innumerable pneumoencephalograms and other neuroroentgenographic studies with him and his associate, Earl Miller. Although my working relationship with Dr. Stone and his x-ray department had to stop when I was made chair of the new department of neurology at UCSF, teaching relations between us were maintained in a graduate teaching program.

Still others mentioned in these essays besides Dandy were notable for their contributions to neuroroentgenographic imaging. Egas Moniz introduced arteriography, although it did not become practical until better contrast media became available, as discussed in Chapter 13. Graeme Robertson improved the technique of pneumoencephalography to visualize the structures of the posterior fossa better, as discussed in Chapter 14. The radioactive isotopes produced by Ernest Lawrence were used in both neuroimaging, positron emission tomography, and neuroradiation therapy, as discussed in Chapter 6. In addition, Lars Lecksell used several sources of energy for brain imaging, including echoencephalography, and magnetic resonance tomography (MRI), in his efforts to adapt neuroimaging to his therapeutic stereotaxic brain surgery, as discussed in Chapter 8. These many advances, however, for the most part, dealt with the older techniques of neuroroentgenography. They also failed to deal adequately with the problems of radiation therapy, or to explain how the field developed. Nevertheless, because of the very considerable background mentioned, I will limit my additional illustrative, biographical sketches to Lysholm, Sossman, Stone, Newton, and Margulis. This will afford a better sequential picture of how neuroimaging developed and emphasize the importance of the modern techniques of neuroimaging.

ERIK LYSHOLM (1891-1947)

Although Arthur Schüller had been a pioneer in his early studies of the skull and numerous special projections had been reported, considerable lack of uniformity and understanding remained. Lysholm brilliantly addressed and solved this problem.

Lysholm's earlier education was in Uppsala, but he obtained his medical degree in Stockholm. He worked mainly in the Serafimer Hospital throughout his career. Unfortunately, his life was shortened by malignant hypertension, which before and during World War II was treated ineffectively.

His work in radiology did not start until the early 1920s, and his first article on precision radiography of the petrous bone was in 1925. By 1931, he had developed precision techniques for the study of the skull as a whole (9). His technique, which eventually became adopted worldwide, involved a separate skull table from the table supporting the patient's body. Together with a mirror system, which showed the underside of the patient's head, the more precise placement of the head was achieved. The x-ray tube was mounted on a "bucky," which could be rotated around the patient's head and assured that the central beam of the x-rays always impinged on the spherical center of the bucky's motion. The movements of the bucky could be accurately measured in angles, the grid lines always remaining parallel to the beam of the x-rays. This ingenious technique permitted precise planes of study that could be duplicated for follow-up purposes. The engineering aspects of this device were perfected by Georg Schönander and used with great success by Lysholm until his death in 1947.

Lysholm worked closely with Herbert Olivercrona, the Swedish neurological surgeon trained by Cushing. One of his main problems concerned the accuracy of ventriculography, which stemmed from the imprecise studies of partially filled ventricles. This was the next problem in precision radiography that Lysholm solved in 1935 (10-12).

Two other efforts at precision radiography followed. One was by Cornelius Dyke and the neurosurgeon Leo Davidoff in 1937 on the normal pneumoencephalogram, which included the first serious study of cisterns and subarachnoid spaces (13). The second was by Edward Twinning in Manchester, England, on the third ventricle, aqueduct, and fourth ventricle in 1937 (14).

Lysholm's department became a great center of postgraduate study in the 1930s, but this unfortunately was interrupted by World War II and his early death in 1947.

MERRILL CLARY SOSSMAN (1890-1959)

I have selected Dr. Sossman as my second roentgenographer for two reasons. First, although his entry into the field was in that early period when roentgenography was still on trial as a diagnostic entity of sufficient importance to justify its separate departmental status, his career extended on throughout the flowering period of neurology. Indeed, he was one of those prominently involved in its flowering. My second reason involves his modus operandi. Although a great showman, he always was aware that x-rays were a diagnostic aid that had to be integrated with the clinical condition. His process of interpretation involved an exchange with the clinicians, and in this, he was learning as much from them as he was teaching them. He was fortunate in his contacts at Harvard—first with Dr. George W. Holmes at the Massachusetts General Hospital and its outstanding clinical staff and, later, at the Peter Bent Brigham Hospital with such eminent men as Cushing and Horrax in neurosurgery; Christian, Levine, and Burwell in medicine; Quinby in genitourinary surgery; and Cheever, Cutler and Newton in general surgery. He was a keen student, as well as observer, and benefited greatly from the rich experiences of his Harvard setting.

Sossman's great development of expertise in x-ray studies had a most unlikely beginning. He was born in Chillicoth, Ohio, in 1890. After his training at the University of Wisconsin (B.A.) and Johns Hopkins (M.D.), he joined the United States Army in World War I. He was one of those stricken in the great influenza epidemic of 1918 to 1919 and was assigned to roentgenography at the Walter Reed Hospital rather than being sent overseas. In 1921, he obtained further training under Dr. Holmes at the Massachusetts General Hospital, and it was here that his interpersonal exchange technique became fully developed. It also was here that Harvey Cushing, Professor of Surgery at Harvard, recognized his talents and instigated Sossman's discharge from the Army and his appointment as Chief Roentgenographer at the Peter Bent Brigham Hospital in 1922. His rich experience in neuroroentgenography fully developed at the Brigham. Six to 7 years later, as a student, I had contact with him on the surgical service at the Brigham Hospital. By that time, his reputation was well developed. He was a master of repartee. His exchanges with the surgeons were most stimulating and, invariably, gravitated to an interpretation in which the x-ray findings were usually important, although only one facet of the final diagnosis. It was a rich learning experience and especially so from the standpoint of the student.

Sossman's writings were as crisp as his teaching and consultations. Most of his 86 scientific articles involved brief reports of new data rather than lengthy review articles. His articles on the x-ray treatment of pituitary tumors were classics, as were several of his diagnostic reports (15).

Many honors came to Dr. Sossman in his subsequent career. He was president of the principal early roentgen ray societies, chair of the section of radiology of the American Medical Association, and a member of the National Research Council. His close relation to neurosurgery was shown by his election to the presidency of the Harvey Cushing Society (later named the American Association of Neurological Surgery) in 1935. He fulfilled the main lectureships of North America and, in 1957, was awarded the gold medal of the Radiological Society of North America. Following his retirement from the Harvard Medical School in 1956, he was made a consultant in radiology to the Massachusetts General Hospital and was instrumental in establishing there an autonomous department of radiology.

In his late years, he developed a bronchiogenic carcinoma but was cured of this by pneumonectomy. Following his recovery, he successfully undertook a medical lecture tour that circled the globe. His death in February 1959 followed a stroke. Through his original reports and his x-ray treatment of pituitary tumors, Merrill Sossman directly contributed to the flowering stage of neurology. However, even more important was his influence in establishing the new technique of roentgenography as an integral part of modern neurology.

ROBERT S. STONE (1895-1966)

Dr. Stone was mainly known for his pioneering investigative studies on the therapeutic effects of x-rays and neutrons in cancer. However, he was also a superb diagnostician and was internationally known for his work on radiation protection. It was his contributions to radiation therapy and protection that justify his inclusion in this account.

Born in Chatham, Ontario, he received his B.A., M.A., M.B., and M.D. (1928) at the University of Toronto. In World War I, he served with the Royal Canadian Air Force and, directly afterward, was an instructor in anatomy at the Peking American Medical College. Following medical graduation at Toronto, Dr. Stone trained in radiology for 5 years under his uncle Dr. Rollin H. Stevens at the Grace Hospital in Detroit, Michigan. In 1928, he became the first full-time radiologist on the staff of the University of California. He rose from an instructorship to full professor in 10 years and in 1939 became chair of the new Department of Radiology. Except for a period during World War II, he continued as the chair until he retired in 1964. During this period, radiology at UCSF developed from a small, part-time diagnostic service under surgery to a large and modern department.

In 1934, Stone developed a 1,000-kV apparatus for radiation therapy and used it in clinical studies. With Joe Hamilton in 1936, he was the first to use radioactive isotopes, produced by the cyclotron of Ernest Lawrence, for human cancer. In the next 2 years, he worked with Dr. John Lawrence (as discussed in the preceding section about Ernest Lawrence) and Paul Aebersold on the therapeutic effects of fast neutrons (million volts) on human malignancy and reported on this in 1939 to the Radiological Society of North America (16).

Dr. Stone's work on radiation protection started in the cyclotron laboratory of Ernest Lawrence where he found that the laboratory was not using adequate safety measures in its radioactive isotope operation. As Associate Project Director for Health of the Metallurgical (plutonium) Project in World War II (1943 to 1945), Stone was the main force in establishing high standards of radiation protection, which later were adopted by the Manhattan Project (17). Still later, he played important roles on the national and international committees on radiation protection, on the Radiological Safety Advisory Committee to the California State Disaster Council, and the Expert Advisory Panel on Radiation of the World Health Organization.

In his last years, Stone established and directed the 70-million Volt synchrotron for cancer therapy at UCSF. The experimental aspects of his Synchrotron Institute were pursued until his death in 1966. Although the synchrotron proved too cumbersome for routine clinical work, it did result in several significant biological observations (effects of radiation on life span and on some genetic problems) and helped to establish the range of clinically useful radiation energies (radiation dosimetry). Stone produced some 60 scientific contributions in his field. These included a number of articles in the field of clinical diagnosis. However, the bulk of his articles dealt with the subjects of his particular interest—radiation therapy and radiation protection.

Stone received many honors and awards. For his work on radiation protection, he was presented the Gold Medal for Merit, the highest civilian award from the President of the United States. He also was awarded the gold medals of the Radiographic Society of North America, the American Radiation Society, the American Cancer Society, the American College of Radiology, and the Atomic Energy Commission. Stone served as president of the Radiological Society of North America, was an honorary member of the Royal Society of Medicine (London), and fulfilled four honorary lectureships. In 1966, he received an honorary L.L.D. degree from the University of California.

In his private life, Stone was unassuming and shared with his wife the joy of his family, gardening, and music. Mrs. Aird and I enjoyed, along with many others, the gracious hospitality of his home. Stone had a warm personality and was loyally supported by his staff. Again, I experienced this for the 10 plus years that I worked part time in his department. He was a dedicated scientist but, locally, was even better known for his wisdom and abilities as an administrator. He served on the executive committee of the UCSF Medical School Advisory Board and was the first chief of staff of the Moffitt Hospital (in addition to his duties in the Department of Radiology and the Synchrotron Institute).

HANS NEWTON (1925-   )

The career of Hans Newton, a former UCSF medical student, illustrates, in particular, the development of arteriography and, still later, magnetic resonance imaging (MRI). Newton was born in Berlin, Germany, and arrived in the United States in 1938. He obtained his college and medical training at the University of California (Berkeley and San Francisco). An internship at the University of Wisconsin (1953 to 1954) was followed by residency training in radiology at Harvard (Peter Bent Brigham Hospital) from 1955 to 1958. He obtained a Damon Runyon Cancer Research fellowship (1958 to 1959), which provided him with training in the new catheter technique of arteriography at the Karolinska Institute of Stockholm, Sweden, and also for some time at the Kantonspital of Zurich, Switzerland. In 1959, he also spent time as an National Institutes of Health fellow under James W.O. Bull at the National Hospital for Nervous Diseases, Queens Square, London.

When Newton came as the first full-time neuroradiologist at UCSF, he found a difficult situation because one of the senior neurosurgeons had energetically initiated cerebral arteriography several years before and was loath to give it up. Over a period of 2 to 3 years, Newton quietly went ahead with the arteriograms of other services and, in 1960, published two articles dealing with the problems of internal carotid artery occlusion and the failure of carotid artery injections to reveal more proximal defects (18). The greater complications of direct internal carotid artery injections in comparison with those of catheter arteriography were soon highlighted, and the neurosurgeons begrudgingly gave up (19). Quiet persistence won the day and was an excellent object lesson to all because overcoming entrenched interests is often, if not usually, associated with bitter political activity—if not with explosive, disruptive effects. While on a sabbatical leave from UCSF in 1966, additional training was obtained by Newton in Stockholm, Sweden, as a fellow of the Commonwealth Foundation.

The advent of MRI brought another turning point in Newton's career. MRI uses the magnetic alignment of the water molecules of the central nervous system, which when disturbed by radio waves or other magnetic forces, emit energy signals that can be detected by computed tomographic techniques. The radiation effects are minimal, and it is a noninvasive technique, which in many respects is superior to computed axial tomographic (CAT) scans for both the brain and spinal cord. As might be expected of Newton, he quickly mastered the use of MRI and has been in the forefront of its development.

The ability of Newton as a diagnostician, consultant, and innovative research worker became widely known by 1969 when he was promoted to full professor of radiology. His cooperation with neurologists and neurosurgeons in interpreting the neuroradiological complexities of arteriography, CAT scans, and MRI was well recognized as far back as 1969 when he was promoted to the joint professorships of neurology and neurosurgery. The division of neuroradiology slowly grew with the addition of four other full-time staff members, three of whom had been fellows in training. In addition to undergraduate teaching, he supervised the graduate training of over 260 fellows in neuroradiology, including 80 from foreign countries.

His bibliography lists over 200 published articles, mainly dealing with the diagnostic aspects of neuroradiology. He has been the editor of four volumes of *Modern Neuroradiology*, five volumes of *Radiology of the Skull and Brain,* and the author or co-author of 43 chapters in books on various aspects of angiography, neuroophthalmology, computed tomography, and MRI. His articles and invited lectures on MRI have averaged about ten per year over the past 10 years, and he has become a well-recognized expert in this field.

Newton has attained wide recognition in the field of neuroradiology. He was a founding member of the American Society of Neuroradiology in 1961 and was its president from 1973 to 1974. He was made an honorary member of the European Society of Neuroradiology and a fellow of the Société Français du Neuroradiologie, as well as a member of nine other medical societies. Newton was editor of *Radiology* and of the *Journal of Computer Assisted Tomography*, in addition to serving on the editorial boards or as a consulting editor of four other radiological journals.

ALEXANDER R. MARGULIS (1921-   )

In the preparation of these essays, I have considered many individuals in addition to those finally selected. A borderline case for neuroimaging was Dr. Alexander Margulis, who as chair of the Department of Radiology, UCSF, loyally supported the development of Hans Newton and the section of neuroimaging. Dr. Margulis did early research that involved the nervous system and was a pioneer in the development of MRI, which has proved so valuable for the study of the brain and spinal cord. However, it was his value in illustrating some of the administrative difficulties of large radiation and imaging service units that finally tipped the scale for his inclusion.

His career, also, is unusual in that he achieved remarkable success despite early obstacles. Born in Yugoslavia, he attended the University of Belgrade where he began his training in medicine. As World War II polarized the politics under Tito, Margulis escaped in 1946 to America. Completely without resources, he was admitted to the Harvard Medical School and provided with part-time employment. Following basic training at Harvard and an internship at the Henry Ford Hospital in Detroit, he became a resident in radiology at the University of Michigan Hospital, and in 1953 to 1954, he was made a clinical instructor. In 1954, Margulis passed the examinations of the American Board of Radiology.

His career rapidly advanced as an accredited radiologist from instructor at the University of Minnesota to full professor by 1961 at Washington University, St.

Louis. This rapid rise is all the more remarkable in that he served as a captain in the United States Medical Corps from 1957 to 1959. In 1963, Margulis transferred to UCSF to succeed Dr. Robert Stone as chair of the Department of Radiology; he served in this capacity for the next 25 years. Shortly after mandatory retirement because of age, he became an associate chancellor at UCSF, still retaining his professorship.

Margulis did considerable experimental work on the angiography of malignant tumors before and after irradiation, trauma, and chemotherapy, and again after tumor transplantation (20-23). This resulted in the demonstration of specific vascular patterns in different types of tumor (24). His microangiography in experimental cerebral edema was an early basic study of considerable interest (25). His early studies on MRI were mainly directed at the GI system but were basic for the nervous system, as well (26,27).

Margulis authored in 300 articles, the majority of which have dealt with GI studies and the new technique of MRI in neuroimaging. He has been the chief author of three book chapters and two texts. *Diagnostic Radiology*, co-authored with C. A. Gooding, has gone through three editions (28).

The list of his honors now number over 50—too numerous to mention. However, it is not difficult to understand his rapid advancement and the great honors that have been heaped on him when one grasps his brilliance, his efficient industry, and his leadership qualities, which are greatly enhanced by his remarkable diplomacy and accommodating interpersonal relationships. We have all seen the effect of oppression on able and scholarly doctors who have immigrated to the United States to participate in its freedom and opportunities. When this background is combined with brilliance and a charming diplomacy, the end result is a career such as that of Margulis's.

A humorous personal story illustrates some of the qualities of Dr. Margulis, as well as the administrative difficulties of a large department of radiology. As indicated in an earlier section of this chapter, I had a life-threatening GI condition in my first year of life that had been diagnosed as pylorospasm before the days of x-rays but was followed by normal development. In 1925, while in southern France, I suffered from a severe and prolonged GI episode, which I thought was due to "food poisoning" but that might have been related to this earlier incident. Much later, at the age of 65, in answer to the questions of my internist during an annual checkup, I had recalled slight sternal discomfort after working for hours over my desk, taking a snack, and then retiring well after midnight. I had attributed the discomfort to neuromuscular fatigue on a postural basis with growing age, but my internist decided on an upper GI series. Following the custom in the medical school, when such tests are done on chairs of departments, the chair of the department doing the test also conducts it. So it was that the world authority on GI problems was doing my upper GI study.

As Dr. Margulis progressed with the fluoroscopic study, he suddenly became very excited and finally cried, "Bob, when did you have your pain?" My astonished answer was, "What pain? I have had nothing but a mild muscle discomfort after bending over my books for hours." To this, Dr. Margulis replied, "Why, you must have had pain. This is the biggest upside down stomach I have ever seen, and I have seen hundreds." With this, he turned the fluoroscopic screen around so that I could see it, and sure enough, there was my stomach perched above the diaphragm, with the esophagus and intestinal connections through a large hiatal hernia.

Margulis proceeded to take many pictures and finally said, "You must come in at once and have this repaired."

"But Dr. Margulis, I am about to leave on a safari to East Africa."

"Cancel it at once," was Alexander's stern reply. "You have considerable torsion and could be badly caught on one of your trips to far places."

I finally asked him to send his report to my internist and assured him that I would follow Dr. Chamberlain's advice. At that time, Chamberlain was a recent past president of the American Heart Association.

The x-ray films failed to arrive in time for my appointment with Chamberlain, and because of the questionable significance of my symptoms, he agreed that I could take my African safari. However, on my return, an urgent message from Chamberlain requested another appointment. The x-rays had finally arrived, and Chamberlain was stunned by the enormity of my upside-down stomach. This led to consultations with a noted GI expert. Precisely the same sequence of events occurred. The x-rays did not arrive, and he concluded that not much could be amiss with no more symptoms than I had experienced. Again, following his late review of the x-rays, I was excitedly recalled, and this time referred to an outstanding GI surgeon. When the x-rays again failed to arrive in time for my third consultation, the surgeon concluded, "I would not consider doing such a major procedure on a person in good health and with such questionable symptoms." This reaction was perhaps stimulated by the fact that, in the meantime, by propping myself up at night with pillows and reducing my prolonged hours of work, I was symptom free. However, when the great surgeon finally reviewed my x-rays, he too recalled me in consternation.

Six months after the upper GI study, I finally met the four consultants: Dr. Margulis, the internist, the GI consultant, and the GI surgeon. Except for Margulis, they could not make up their minds, and the decision was left up to me. Having no fear of surgery in the hands of the meticulous surgeon, whom I knew personally, I finally agreed to go ahead, fearing that my episode of "food poisoning" in 1925 might actually have been a bout of the type suggested by Dr. Margulis. However, I made the provision that I must have our best anesthetist. He would have to breathe for me for many hours. To make a long story short, the surgeon had to cope with one of the worst case he had ever had—a large stomach firmly adherent to the lungs, which required many hours of careful dissection to free it, to replace it below the diaphragm, and to repair finally my large hiatal hernia. Thanks to my splendid team, surgeon and anesthetist, the next morning I was pushing a cart about loaded with bottles and tubes running to all portions of my anatomy. I was discharged in 9 days.

The main point of this episode concerned the stern reforms that followed in the Department of Radiology. Margulis had planned to use my x-rays for teaching purposes, but his department had lost them! He was outraged! When he was jokingly informed of the late x-ray delivery on three consecutive consultations, his chagrin and fury reached Olympian proportions. Reforms, such as delivering test results on time, often peter out, but I may have had some effect in preserving them by occasionally inquiring of Margulis whether or not his department had found the x-rays. Aside from the reforms instituted by the meticulous and efficient chair of the Department of Radiology, this episode well illustrates the firm convictions of Dr. Margulis, his exemplary diplomatic stance in the conference of specialists, and the high regard of specialists of very different temperaments for him.

SUMMARY

Except for brain scintiphotography (as discussed under Lawrence in Chapter 6) and positron computed tomography (PCT),* the main advances in neuroimaging have been included in this account. In each case, the advances depended on the development of new techniques, which may be summarized as follows: (1) the discovery of x-rays and their potential for medical diagnosis; (2) the use of contrast media; (3) the development of arteriography; and (4) CAT scans, MRI, and PCT.

Only two radiologists were involved in the original discoveries and advances listed. Lysholm made the technique of roentgenography precise, and Stone determined the potential and limits of radiation therapy. Nevertheless, they all contributed notably to the refinement and understanding of clinical neuroimaging. As pointed out in the career of Merrill Sossman, it is the physician trained in neuroimaging, in combination with the neurologist (whether medical, pediatric, or surgical), who remains central to the proper integration of the clinical and neuroimaging data for the benefit of each individual patient. This aspect has been exemplified well by Newton in the case of arteriography and by both Newton and Margulis in the new techniques of CAT for neuroimaging purposes.

REFERENCES

1. Schiller, A. *Röntgen-diagnostik der Erkrankunger des Kopfes Nothnagel Pathologie und Therapie.* Leipzig, Heider, 1912.
2. Dandy, W. Ventriculography following the injection of air into the cerebral ventricles. *Ann. Surg.*, 68:4-11, 1918.
3. Dandy, W. Roentgenography of the brain after the injection of air into the spinal canal. *Arch. Surg.*, 70:344-403, 1919.
4. Sicard, J. A., and Forestier, J. Method radiographique d'exploration de la cavité epidurale par de lipiodol. *Rev. Neurol.*, 37:1267, 1926.
5. Luckett, W.H. Air in the ventricles of the brain, following a fracture of the skull. *Surg. Gynecol. Obstet.*, 17:237-240, 1913.
6. Aird, R.B. Encephalography with anesthetic gases. *Arch. Surg.*, 34:853-867, 1937.

---

*PCT is primarily a research technique that utilizes radioactive biological agents of value in studying metabolic processes. By using agents whose radioactive half-life is brief, their ionizing radiation effects are slight. The technique is of particular value in determining normal cerebral metabolic effects and abnormalities of function in specific cases.

7. Aird, R.B., and Zealear, D. Pneumoencephalographic study of absorptive block mechanisms and of the hydrodynamics of cerebrospinal fluid. *Trends Am. Neurol. Assoc.*, 75:174-177, 1950.

8. Adams, R.D., Fisher, C.M., Hakin, S., et al. Symptomatic occult hydrocephalus with "normal" cerebrospinal-fluid pressure. *N. Engl. J. Med.*, 273:117-126, 1965.

9. Lysholm, E. Apparatus and technique for roentgen examination of the skull. *Acta Radiol.*, (suppl xii), 1931.

10. Lysholm E., Ebunius, E., and Sahlsted, M. *Das ventriculogram*: I. Acta Radiol., (suppl. 24):1-75, 1935.

11. Lysholm, E., Ebunius, E., and Sahlsted, M. *Das ventriculogram*: II. Acta Radiol., (suppl. 25):1-199, 1937.

12. Lysholm, E., Ebunius, E., Lindblom, M., and Sahlstedt, H. Das ventriculogram: III. *Acta Radiol.*, (suppl. 26):1-129, 1937.

13. Dyke, C., and Davidoff, L. The Normal Encephalogram. Philadelphia, Lea & Febiger, 1937.

14. Twinning, E.W. Radiology of the third and fourth ventricles. Part 1. Br. J. *Radiol.*, 12:385-418, 1937.

15. Sossman, M.C. Roentgen therapy of pituitary adenomas. *J.A.M.A.*, 113:1282-1285, 1939.

16. Stone, R.S., Lawrence, J.H., and Aebersold, P.C. Preliminary report on use of fast neutrons in treat ment of malignant disease. *Radiology*, 35:322-327, 1940.

17. Stone, R. Industrial Medicine on the Plutonium Project: Survey and Collected Papers. 1st ed. New York, McGraw-Hill, 1951.

18. Newton, H., and Couch, R.S.C. Possible errors in the arteriographic diagnosis of internal carotid artery occlusion. *Radiology*, 75:766-773, 1960.

19. Humphrey, J.G., and Newton, T.H. Internal carotid artery occlusion in young adults. Brain, 83:565-578, 1960.

20. Margulis, A.R., Carlsson, E., and McAlister, W.H.,, Angiography of malignant tumors in mice. *Acta Radiol.*, 56:179-192, 1961.

21. McAlister, W.H., and Margulis, A.R., Angiography of malignant tumors in mice following irradia tion. *Radiology*, 81:664-675, 1963.

22. McAlister, W.H., and Margulis, A.R., Comparison of effects of chemotherapy and local irradiation on the vascularity of a transplanted mouse lymphosarcoma: a study using angiography and microan giography. Radiology, 82:525-528., 1964.

23. Noonan, C.D., Margulis, A.R., Patt, H.M., et al. Angiographic evaluation of the effect of trauma and irradiation on transplanted lymphosarcoma un mice. *Radiology*, 89:923-929 1967.

24. Milne, E.N.C., Margulis, A.R., Noonan, C.D., et al. Histologic type specific vascular patterns in rat tumors. Cancer, 20:1635-1646, 1967.

25. Perez, C.A., Hodges, F.J.J. III, and Margulis, A.R. Microangiography in experimental cerebral edema in rats. Radiology, 82:529-535, 1964.

26. Margulis, A.R. The lessons of radiobiology for diagnostic radiology, Caldwell lecture. Am. J. *Radiol.*, 117:741-756, 1973.

27. Crooks, L.E., Hoenninger, J., Arakawa, M., Watts, J., McCarten, B., Kaufman, L., Mills, C.M., Davis, P.L., and Margulis, A.R. High resolution magnetic resonance imaging: technical concepts and their implementation. *Radiology*, 150:153-171, 1984.

28. Margulis, A.R., and Gooding, C.A. (eds.). *Diagnostic Radiology*. 3rd ed. San Francisco, UCSF, Radiology Research and Education Foundation, 1989.

Neurological Surgery

There are few specialties in the field of medicine that are as demanding or therapeutically challenging as neurosurgery. I was attracted to this field myself in the 1920s, influenced by my father, John W. Aird, a surgeon, who was one of the founding members of the American College of Surgery and by Harvey Cushing, my professor of surgery at Harvard. One of the attractions to neurosurgery in that early period was the splendid group of men who pioneered the field. Surgeons are said to be men of action, who tend to be decisive and bold. This was doubly so in that small group who entered the field of neurosurgery during and following World War I. I was fortunate to know almost all of that early group. I am still a member of the American Association of Neurological Surgery, which originally was the Harvey Cushing Society, started by my mentor, William P. VanWagonen. In spite of this bias, I believe that my account can be made with perspective because I left neurosurgery over 60 years ago to pursue my interest in neurological research.

Neurosurgery, a remunerative calling, antedated neurology as an independent discipline by some 25 to 30 years. However, because of its reliance on the scientific advances in anesthesia, asepsis, electrocautery, and other technological advances, as well as the improved techniques of neurological diagnosis, it well illustrates the thesis of this account, namely that modern neurological disciplines could not fully mature until the advances of sciences developed.

Brain surgery by Macewen and others, extending back into the 19th century, was known but was rare and based on exceptional circumstances. My father had one such case in 1914, but in general, these usually involved accessible tumors and were rarely reported. Victor Horsley in London was certainly an exception to this generalization, but his surgery was done on highly selected patients.

Cushing, while at Johns Hopkins, approached the problem with the idea of developing the techniques necessary for success on a regular basis. Brain tumors were being diagnosed, but they were considered hopeless conditions. Furthermore, the early neurosurgeons were confronted by terminal patients at a time when anesthesia did not permit prolonged procedures. Cushing's first 15 patients succumbed. By

1930, as the surgical techniques were improved and as earlier diagnosis was achieved, his surgical mortality rate was reduced from 100% to less than 10%. Others, such as Frazier in Philadelphia, soon joined in, but the credit of establishing neurosurgery on a practical basis clearly belongs to Cushing.

HARVEY CUSHING (1869-1939)

Cushing was born and raised in Cleveland, Ohio. He went on to Yale College and then to the Harvard Medical School, from which he graduated in 1895. After an internship at the Massachusetts General Hospital, he worked under William Halsted at the Johns Hopkins Hospital for 4 years. He next went abroad. In Berne, Switzerland, under Theodore Kock and the physiologist Hugo Kronicker, he studied the relationship of intracranial pressure to blood pressure. Also, he helped Sherrington and his group at Liverpool with their studies on the anthropoid motor cortex.

On his return to Hopkins, he undertook the technical improvements necessary for a more successful surgical approach to the central nervous system. In particular, he sought to reduce blood loss. His main focus of work involved patients with pituitary tumors; his famous monograph on this subject, *The Pituitary Body and its Disorders*, was published before he went to Harvard as the Moseley Professor of Surgery (1). The turning point in his career, however, had occurred in 1910 after his operation on Major General Leonard Wood, Chief of Staff of the United States Army. The operation for a meningioma was successful; General Wood returned to his office within 1 month, served throughout World War I, and went on to become the Governor of the Philippines.

At Harvard, Cushing was surgeon-in-chief at the Peter Bent Brigham Hospital, where I first had contact with him. He then was at the peak of his career. Brigham Hospital was a center for many visiting surgical fellows. For example, I was taught to scrub up by Norman Dott of Edinburgh, who later became a neurosurgical celebrity in his own right. Dott's technique involved scrubbing in the dark after applying lamp black to the hands. After the allotted scrub-up time, it was phenomenal how much lamp black still persisted in the crotches of our fingers on the first try.

Cushing's main contributions in his Harvard period were *Tumors of the Nervus Acousticus and Syndromes of the Cerebellar-Pontine Angle, Intracranial Tumors*, and *Meningiomas* (2-4). His studies on the endocrine aspects of the pituitary, however, caused much confusion for years. I well recall watching some of his ventricular injections of pituitary extract and pilocarpine in postoperative patients. He had postulated the probable existence of parasympathetic centers, which could be stimulated by pilocarpine or pituitary extract from the ventricular cerebrospinal fluid (CSF). The implication was that this might be the normal route of pituitary functioning. The responses, however, varied in degree, character, and time. There were no control studies for the reabsorption of the CSF and injected agents through the vascular system. Dr. Mary Montgomery and I showed, in carefully controlled studies, that the stimulation of pilocarpine was a peripheral effect, regardless of the route of administration. It persisted undiminished after section and degeneration of the parasympathetic nerve supply to the salivary glands. We also showed that the salivary response to ventricularly injected pilocarpine was physiologically negligible (5). Our cautious conclusion was that Cushing's hypothesis "must be examined more critically before it can be accepted" (5). From this experience, I quietly concluded that, although a master surgeon and a wonderful teacher, my former professor was not a master experimentalist.

Cushing's name was used for the syndrome produced by adrenal cortical overfunction. This developed as a result of Cushing's thesis that it was due to "pituitary basophilism," i.e., increased secretion from basophilic tumor cells. In spite of this error, the appellation "Cushing's disease" can appropriately be used, inasmuch as he was the one who first delineated this clinical syndrome.

Personally, Cushing was a striking figure—handsome and animated. He was high strung, somewhat of a prima donna, and an obvious perfectionist, who was making every effort to protect his patients and, beyond this, to establish high standards for neurosurgery. Gilbert Horrax *opened and closed* Cushing's neurosurgical operations, leaving the master to handle the cerebral surgery. When Cushing's meticulous approach was thwarted or the vagaries of cerebral surgery took unexpected turns for the worse, his nervous tension vented itself in sharp comments to his associates and, perhaps, rapping the knuckles of a resident if he or she was not holding the retractor as Cushing wanted. Having seen the perfect control of my father under equally trying conditions, I wondered about this. In retrospect, I am sure that it was a matter of temperament. We all tended to forgive Cushing because we realized that he was pushing himself far harder than he was pushing his team. Furthermore, he never stooped to the profanities of his brilliant successor Walter Dandy at Johns Hopkins.

I, along with the other students who elected surgery at Peter Bent Brigham Hospital, greatly admired Cushing. He was most cordial, and his wealth of historical knowledge and depth of subject background made him an impressive teacher. We all worked extra hard on his service, suspecting that our best might show us up as flagrant failures. However, Cushing was fair and usually generous in his handling of students. I personally respected and liked him and was greatly pleased when he later gave me an excellent recommendation.

Cushing and his neurosurgical group dominated the surgical service of Peter Bent Brigham Hospital. The workups and conference discussions on neurosurgical patients were impressive. They were typed and made a permanent part of the patient's record. It was the memory of this practice that led me, at a later date, to initiate the practice of complete discharge summaries on all hospitalized neurologic patients. These typed summaries were used for report purposes as well as for research. Many years ago, this practice slowly spread to other clinical services at the University of California, San Francisco, and finally was made mandatory on all services.

Cushing retired in 1932, the victim of his own ruling. When he first arrived at Harvard, he had promoted the practice of surgical retirement at the age of 65. When his own time came, he regretted this, but the rule was upheld. Perhaps as a result of this and other difficulties at Harvard, Cushing gave his considerable library collection to Yale, being strongly influenced in this by his former pupil John Fulton, who then was professor of physiology and director of the Physiological Institute at Yale. Cushing's final 7 years in New Haven were disturbed by ill health, which included poor circulation in his legs. According to my classmate, John Lawrence, while a resident at Yale, he was used by Cushing for his self-directed care.

Honors, awards, medals, prizes, and lectureships have proliferated over the years roughly in proportion to inflation. Even so, Cushing was one of the most highly honored men in medicine with too many awards, honorary degrees, and memberships in foreign societies to list.

WALTER DANDY (1886-1946)*

My inclusion of Dandy is based on his brilliant contributions—particularly pneumoencephalography, which for years revolutionized the diagnostic aspects of both neurology and neurosurgery. His background can quickly be summarized. Born in Sedalia, Missouri, he later graduated from the University of Missouri; he then spent the rest of his life in Baltimore. In 1910, Dandy graduated from the Johns Hopkins School of Medicine and trained in surgery under Halsted and in neurosurgery with Cushing. His early studies were with Blackfan on the production and absorption of CSF and on the pathogenesis of hydrocephalus.

He introduced ventriculography in 1918 and pneumoencephalography in the following year (6,7). I may be prejudiced on this score, because of the years of further research devoted to this subject (as discussed in Chapter 7), but in my opinion, if Dandy had not accomplished anything else, this achievement alone would have immortalized his name—at least for the next 55 years in which pneumoencephalography revolutionized neurological diagnosis.

However, in addition to this, he developed a posterior approach for section of the trigeminal nerve to relieve tic douloureux (8). Anatomically, this approach was simpler and less complicated than the earlier approach of Frazier and Spiller. In 1928, Dandy reported the differential section of the vestibular portion of the eighth cranial nerve for the relief of Meniere's disease (a procedure suggested 20 years before by Mills) (9).

Dandy's surgical abilities were legendary; his great ingenuity and dexterity accounts for his success with complete resection of acoustic tumors that previously were considered too hazardous. His pioneer work in cerebrovascular surgery was also noteworthy, as exemplified by his successful operation on cerebral aneurysms. Again, he showed that intraventricular tumors could be successfully removed. That he could maintain a relatively low mortality rate while pursuing these daring innovations speaks highly for his surgical skill.

---

*I was tempted to include William P. VanWagonen and Howard C. Naffziger, who both trained with Cushing, in this account. However, to give a broader perspective, I have selected Walter Dandy, Percival Bailey, Donald Matson, Murrary Falconer, and Lars Lecksell. I regret not including such colorful figures as Sir Geoffrey Jefferson, Paul Bucy, Larry Pool, and Irving Cooper, the latter two of whom went with me to Russia in 1965.

Dandy epitomized the brilliant, bold, innovative, and skilled neurosurgeon. Visiting surgeons and students from all parts of the world went to Hopkins to see him operate and to study his methods. In addition, he was a prolific writer.

Aside from his foul language, the only objection I ever had to Dandy was his feud with Cushing; I am not certain where the blame was in this episode. This is a subject that has been hushed up in the medical literature, but I am not certain that it should be forgotten because it throws light on the characters involved. Apparently, Dandy resented Cushing taking certain material, which he considered to be his own, away from Hopkins when the latter went to Harvard—hence the resentments on both sides. Their feud even served to unsettle the rapport and exchange of some of the early meetings that I attended. That such misunderstandings are bound to arise occasionally in human affairs is understandable. That two highly intelligent men could not resolve their difference is more difficult to understand.

PERCIVAL BAILEY (1892-1973)

Another remarkable figure in the early days of neurological surgery was Percival Bailey.* His genius was early recognized by Martha Buck, one of his high school teachers, as I recall, and our debt to her should be acknowledged. With her help, he obtained his B.S. and Ph.D. from the University of Chicago and then his M.D. in 1918 from Northwestern University. Following an internship at the Mercy Hospital, he worked with Cushing in Boston from 1919 to 1928. These were eventful years because it provided him contacts with many of the most outstanding neuroscientists of that time. He worked with the neuropathologist George B. Hassin, the great French neurologist Pierre Marie, the Belgian neurophysiologist Frederic Bremer, the German neurologist Georges Schaltenbrand, and with the French psychiatrists Henri Claude, Gasten Gation de Clerambalt, and Pierre Janet. Remarkably, in all these fields, Bailey excelled and became recognized as a leader. In Boston, he established close friendships with many others, such as Kenneth McKenzie of Toronto, Tracy Putnam of Boston, and Norman Dott of Edinburgh. His main interest, aside from becoming an able neurological surgeon, was the neuropathological study of Cushing's series of brain tumors, from which developed his classic report, *Tumors of the Glioma Group* on a Histogenic Basis with a Correlated Study of Prognosis (12). This was the first attempt to classify the gliomas, and it was an exciting privilege to hear him summarize his study in a talk shortly before he left for Chicago.

In 1928, Bailey went to the University of Chicago and developed a division of neurology and neurosurgery. The vested interests of the Departments of Medicine, Surgery, and Pediatrics, however, created a difficult administrative impasse, as discussed in Chapter 9. This led Bailey to accept a professorship of neurology and neurosurgery at the University of Illinois. During this period, he visited Otfrid Foester of Breslau, Germany, and worked in neurophysiology with J. G. Dusser de

---

*For further reading, see Percival Bailey's own account, Up From Little Egypt (10). Also, Paul Bucy has written a fine obituary on his mentor (11).

Barenne. Later, at the University of Illinois, he worked with Gerhardt von Bonin on the cytoarchitecture of the human cerebral cortex and on the neurophysiology of the primate cerebral cortex with Warren M. McCullock and others (13,14). In 1951, along with Frederic Gibbs, Bailey studied psychomotor epilepsy in a group of patients that exhibited striking psychological and behavioral manifestations; it was this study that rekindled his interest in psychiatry (15).

Visualizing an approach to psychiatric problems through temporal lobe epilepsy, utilizing neurosurgical and stereotaxic techniques, he transferred to the University of Illinois, where he became director of the Illinois State Psychopathic Institute and a professor of psychiatry at the University of Illinois. He persuaded the Governor of Illinois to build the Illinois State Psychiatric Institute, following the lead developed earlier in California, as discussed in Chapter 1. With Schaltenbrand, he developed a massive stereotaxic atlas of the human brain (16). However, again the vested interests of the psychiatrists obstructed progress. Believing that psychoanalysis and its remunerative aspects were the cause of this, he made a study of Sigmund Freud and psychoanalysis. His critical address as the president of the American Psychiatric Association produced a great stir and his later book, *Sigmund the Unserene: A Tragedy in Three Acts*, challenged the scientific basis of psychoanalysis and the old psychiatry (17).

Of all the people that I have known, Percival Bailey was one of the most outspoken and diligently honest, often a hazard to administrative compromise. As Bucy has written, he was a "tolerant man who was rabidly intolerant of cant, hypocrisy and dishonestly" (as discussed in the section on Schaltenbrand, Chapter 15) (18). His successful pursuit of research in neuroanatomy, neurophysiology, neuropathology, neurology, neurosurgery, and psychiatry, in addition to his heavy teaching and administrative workload, as well as other interests as a bibliophile and historian, conveys some impression of his extraordinary scope and abilities. If anyone well illustrates the thesis of these essays, it is Percival Bailey. His employment of the techniques of research and practice clearly depended on the advances of science.

DONALD MATSON (1913-1969)

Donald Matson illustrates the extension of neurosurgery into pediatrics and the establishment of high standards of discipline through his work as secretary and then chair of the American Board of Neurological Surgery.

I first knew Matson as a student of a junior college in Deep Springs, California, that I had attended and of which I was later director.* Deep Springs is a small school on a farm and a ranch near the Nevada border. Students are selected for their all-around abilities, but academic performance (top 2% of College Board examinations results) is necessary because of the problem of transfer to the best universities following their basic training at Deep Springs. In recent years, many have been finalists or semifinalists in the National Merit Awards. The students have unusual

---

*The founding of Deep Springs College was mentioned under Papez in Chapter 4, but its modus operandi, which is pertinent to Dr. Matson, was not explained.

powers and, in effect, feel responsible for the operation of the school. An outstanding academic staff is necessary to "keep ahead of the students." The students work daily on the farm and ranch in jobs of responsibility and develop a keen sense of community welfare. As shown by follow-up studies, the lessons learned at Deep Springs almost invariably are given credit by the school's alumni for their motivation and later direction in life. So it was with Matson, whom I regularly visited on my occasional visits to Boston.

Matson later won scholarships from the Telluride Association and lived in the Telluride House at Cornell University. This pattern and his later medical training at Harvard followed the same mold that I had pursued 10 years earlier. While in medical school, Matson worked with Dr. John Rock and Dr. Thomas Lannan, as a result of which his first two articles were written (19,20). He next took a surgical internship at the Peter Bent Brigham Hospital, followed by a fellowship in neurological surgery (Massachusetts General Hospital, Peter Bent Brigham and Children's Hospitals) in 1943. Army service in World War II (1943 to 1946) interrupted his training. Part of his tour of duty as a neurosurgical consultant in the First Army Group was under Elliot Cutler. As a result of this experience, he wrote his monograph, *The Treatment of Acute Craniocerebral Injuries Due to Missiles* (21). Following the war, he was a neurosurgical fellow under Dr. Gilbert Horrax at the Leahey Clinic, Boston, and then he took a neurosurgical exchange under Barnes Woodhall at Duke University Hospital. He next returned to the Children's Hospital, Boston, and became associated with Franc Ingraham. Matson maintained this connection until Ingraham's retirement in 1964, following which Matson was made chief neurosurgeon of the Children's Hospital. In 1954, Ingraham and Matson published their classic text, *Neurosurgery of Infancy and Childhood* (22). He also served as a neurosurgeon at the Peter Bent Brigham Hospital. His duties were especially heavy at the Children's Hospital when Ingraham developed an essential tremor and depended on Matson to do most of the surgery.

Matson was added to the American Board of Neurological Surgery in the mid-1950s and served as secretary and later as chair. This was a heavy responsibility, which he took very seriously. He became known for his "clarity of thought, fairness and his utter dedication to principle" as Joe Evans has phrased it (23). Matson was equally dedicated to his graduate teaching at Harvard. He wrote many articles in his field. One of his main interests involved CSF shunting procedures through the ureter for hydrocephalus. He followed this with modifications for 20 years (24). He served as co-author with Dr. William German of Dr. Cushing's selected writings. He, also, was a member of the editorial board of the *Journal of Neurological Surgery*.

Matson developed a mysterious disorder in 1967 that was eventually diagnosed as Creutzfeldt-Jakob disease. His increasing disability made it impossible for him to chair the 1969 meeting of the American Association of Neurological Surgeons, of which he had been elected president; he died that year. Had he lived longer, he would have reaped many other honors and awards. As it was, an award for excellence in teaching was named in his honor and is given annually to outstanding teachers by the surgical services of the Brigham and Women's Hospitals in Boston.

In addition, the Donald Matson Lectureship in Neurosurgery at Harvard Medical School was established, which brings distinguished neurosurgeons to the medical school for several days each year.

Franc Ingraham chose exceedingly well in recruiting Matson. Matson leaned over backward to carry Ingraham through his later years; their accomplishments in the development of pediatric neurosurgery were outstanding. Matson was all that Joe Evans has said, but beyond his obvious integrity, advocacy of high standards, and his own neurosurgical abilities, he was an excellent teacher and prodigious worker. In addition, he was a kindly man of great tact and perception. In spite of our long-lasting friendship, I always felt highly honored when he invariably took time off to see me on my visits to Boston.

MURRAY FALCONER (1910-1977)

To show that all neurosurgical talent was not confined to the United States, I considered adding Olivicrona of Sweden and Jefferson and Cairns of Great Britain, but I finally settled on Murray Falconer, of British descent, and Lars Lecksell of Sweden, who illustrate still different aspects of neurological surgery. Like Donald Matson, Falconer was one of the second generation of neurological surgeons directly involved in the flowering period of neurology. He made mainly three contributions: (1) to the development of an excellent teaching service at Dunedin University in New Zealand with consultative clinics at Christchurch, Wellington, and Palmerston North; (2) to the diagnosis and treatment of lesions of the intervertebral discs; and (3) most importantly, to the surgical treatment of temporal lobe epilepsy, working closely with Sir Charles Symonds and the Guys Epilepsy Unit at the Maudsley Hospital. The comprehensive studies of this group were a model of teamwork—neurologists, psychiatrists, and neurorehabilitative workers. Whereas Penfield's group had delineated the potential and limitations of neurosurgery in different cortical regions, Falconer, through the discerning studies of his team on temporal lobe epilepsy and his surgical skill, was able to establish surgery as a successful approach to otherwise intractable victims of this stressful and common form of epilepsy. In this respect, he overlapped with Penfield's group at the Montreal Neurological Institute, as discussed in Chapter 2. As a colonial who was finally accepted into the highest circles of neurology and neurosurgery of Great Britain, Falconer's story is an interesting one.

Falconer was raised in Dunedin, New Zealand, the son of a notable father of Scotch origin, Alexander R. Falconer, who established and ran the Sailor's Rest at Dunedin. After graduation from the Otago Medical School in 1933 and 2 years of hospital training, he obtained a fellowship of the Royal College of Surgeons and, 2 years later, was given a surgical research scholarship to the Mayo Clinic in Minnesota. Back in Dunedin in 1938, Falconer passed the M.Ch. examinations and was awarded a Nuffield Dominion Assistantship in the department of Sir Hugh Cairns at Oxford. After 3 years in this position, he joined the Royal Army Medical Corps and served in World War II. However, in 1943, he returned to Dunedin to develop a neurosurgical department in the Otago Medical School. Over the next 7 years, he established not only an outstanding department, but three strategically located consultative clinics in New Zealand, as previously mentioned. It was also in Otago that he became noted for his surgery on intervertebral discs and subarachnoid hemorrhage. In recognition of his diagnostic and therapeutic work on intervertebral discs, he was appointed Hunterian Professor of the Royal College of Surgeons of England for 6 months in 1947.

In 1950, Falconer was invited to develop a neurosurgical department at the Guy's and Maudsley Hospitals in London. King's College Hospital later joined in this effort. To develop such a service that combined the resources of the teaching hospitals mentioned took great administrative ability. To integrate his new neurosurgical service with other entities in these medical schools, such as Sir Charles Symonds's Epilepsy Unit and the psychiatric service of Sir Dennis Hill at the Maudsley Hospital, required even greater diplomacy. As Sir Charles Symonds aged, Falconer became the undisputed leader of this outstanding research group. Over the years, he amassed a richly documented series of patients with temporal lobe epilepsy, studied carefully before surgery and with excellent follow-up studies. Of his many articles on this subject, I have selected five that illustrate the scope of his interests, which were always fascinating to discuss with him (25-29).

Falconer was meticulous in his surgery and research. He was wise in his integration of neurologic, psychologic, psychiatric, and neuropathologic expertise with neurosurgery in follow-up studies of his patients. His ability to weld a harmonious team involving so many disciplines was perhaps his greatest attribute.

On his trips to the Neurological Institute, University of California, Los Angeles, he invariably visited me in San Francisco because he was interested in my comprehensive approach to the neurological therapy of temporal lobe epilepsy as well as my clinical and electroencephalographic diagnostic efforts in this condition. He was said to be dogmatic, but I never found him so. It was true that he was definitive in his opinions, but this was backed by experience and the comprehensive expertise of his team. He was a very friendly person, and throughout his last 26 years in the highest medical and surgical circles of England, he remained the simple, unassuming colonial. Falconer's main concerns always seemed to me to be the welfare of his patients, the furtherance of his complex research, and the advancement of neurosurgery.

Falconer's neurosurgery was by no means limited to patients with temporal lobe epilepsy; his published articles substantiate this point. Another aspect concerned psychosurgery. He was hailed by the psychiatrists in this respect and was elected a fellow of the Royal College of Psychiatry. He served as a visiting neurosurgeon or neurological consultant to five American universities.

LARS LECKSELL (1907-1986)

Lars Lecksell well deserves inclusion in these essays. Of all the neurosurgeons, he best exemplifies the utilization of new scientific techniques. Lecksell was at his peak during the flowering period of neurology.

Born in Füsberg, Sweden, his early training was in the local schools and in medicine at the Karolinska Institute. His innovative brilliance apparently went unnoticed in his early life and training or, at least, was not mentioned in the reports that I have seen. Starting in 1935, he trained in neurosurgery with Professor Herbert Olivecrona at the Serafimer Laûsarette, Stockholm. He then took advanced training in neurophysiology under Professor Ragnar Granit. In this setting, his brilliance became obvious. His Ph.D. dissertation on the gamma motor system was a basic contribution, which was later pursued by Granit to establish the basis of motor control.

Lecksell became established in neurosurgery at Lund.* By 1958, Lecksell was advanced to the professorship of neurological surgery and, 2 years later, was transferred to head neurosurgery at the Karolinska Institute in Stockholm. Following retirement in 1974, he continued to do research and to monitor stereotaxic surgical procedures for 12 more years.

Lecksell was a perfectionist in developing brain imaging techniques as guides to neurosurgery. This ranged from pneumoencephalography in 1949, echoencephalography in 1955, computed tomography in 1976, to magnetic resonance imaging in 1983 (30,31,32). These advances reflected his belief that essentially all forms of energy could be adapted to the problems of brain imaging in monitoring brain tumor surgery or therapeutic stereotaxic surgery.

His most brilliant innovation in neurosurgery was his "gamma knife." This involved a large array of radioactive cobalt sources arranged so that they could be stereotaxically focused on deep tumors and, thus, bypass much of the stress, hazards, and destructive effects of the traditional approach using the neurosurgical knife (33).

Lecksell was a perfectionist in his writing, as well as in his stereotaxic surgery. He always stressed quality in scientific articles, as opposed to quantity. He was an accomplished linguist (five languages) and was very much the humanist, making himself available to his patients, colleagues, and family. Lecksell had a keen sense of humor. He was a raconteur and, above all, a stimulating teacher and a brilliant innovator.

Lecksell won many international honors. He was decorated by several governments and was elected to honorary membership in many neurological as well as neurosurgical societies. He left a large legacy of new scientific techniques, which had a great impact in advancing the field of neurosurgery.

SUMMARY

The early advances in neurosurgery have been illustrated by the careers of Harvey Cushing, Walter Dandy, and Percival Bailey. They were a brilliant group, who pioneered the surgical approaches to essentially all types of intracranial lesions. Cushing developed the techniques that established neurosurgery as a practical sur-

---

*My junior colleague, Dr. Bertram Feinstein, studied Lecksell's stereotaxic technique at Lund while on a poliomyelitis graduate fellowship with Professor Wohlfart from 1951 to 1952, as discussed in Chapter 15.

gical discipline, and his series of operations on brain and pituitary tumors was most impressive. Dandy developed new approaches to the fifth cranial nerve for tic douloureux, for acoustic neuromas, and cerebrovascular surgery, and he introduced pneumoencephalography and ventriculography. Bailey was extraordinary in his breadth of scope, not only in neurosurgery, but also in his research in essentially all aspects of the basic neurosciences and related clinical fields.

A second generation of neurosurgeons is illustrated by the careers of Donald Matson (pediatric neurosurgery), Murrary Falconer (especially temporal lobe epilepsy and psychosurgery), and Lars Lecksell (stereotaxic surgery, neuroimaging, and his gamma knife).

All exploited the new technical advances of science and materially contributed to the flowering of neurology.

REFERENCES

1. Cushing, H. *The Pituitary Body and Its Disorders. Clinical States Produced by Disorders of the Hypophysis Cerebri, an Amplification of the Harvey Lecture for December.* Philadelphia, JB Lippincott, 1912.
2. Cushing, H. *Tumors of the Nervus Acousticus and the Syndromes of the Cerebellar-Pontine Angle.* Philadelphia, WB Saunders, 1917.
3. Cushing, H. *Intracranial Tumors.* Springfield, IL, Charles C. Thomas, 1932.
4. Cushing, H. *Meningiomas.* Springfield, IL, Charles C. Thomas, 1938.
5. Aird, R.B., and Montgomery, M.D. Studies upon the site of stimulation of salivation by intraventricularly injected pilocarpine in dogs. *J. Pharmacol.* Exp. Ther., 56:290-306, 1936.
6. Dandy, W. Ventriculography following the injection of air into the cerebral ventricle. *Ann. Surg.,* 68:5-11, 1918.
7. Dandy, W. Roentgenography of the brain after injection of air into the spinal canal. *Ann. Surg.,* 70:397-403, 1919.
8. Dandy, W. Section of sensory root of trigeminal nerve at the pons. *Bull. Johns Hopkins Hospital,* 36:105-106, 1925.
9. Dandy, W. Meniere's disease: its diagnosis and method of treatment. *Arch. Surg.,* 16:1127-1152, 1928.
10. Bailey, P. *Up From Little Egypt.* Chicago, Buckskin Press, 1969.
11. Bucy, P. Percival Bailey. Trans. *Am. Neurol. Assoc.,* 99:276–278, 1974.
12. Bailey, P., and Cushing, H. *A Classification of the Tumors of the Glioma Group on a Histogenic Basis with a Correlated Study of Prognosis.* Philadelphia, JB Lippincott, 1926.
13. Von Bonin, G., and Bailey, P. *The Isocortex of Man.* Urbana, IL, University of Illinois Press, 1951.
14. Bailey, P., von Bonin, G., Garol, H.W., and McCullock, W.S. Functional organization of temporal lobe of monkey (*Macaca mulatta*) and chimpanzee (*Pansatyrus*). *J. Neurophysiol.,* 6:121-128, 1943.
15. Bailey, P., and Gibbs, F. The surgical treatment of psychomotor epilepsy. *J.A.M.A.,* 145:365-370, 1952.
16. Schaltenbrand, G., and Bailey, P. *Introduction to Stereotaxis with an Atlas of the Human Brain.* New York, Grune & Stratton, 1959.
17. Bailey, P. *Sigmund the Unserene: A Tragedy in Three Acts.* Springfield, IL, Charles C. Thomas, 1965.
18. Bucy, P. *Percival Bailey* (1892-1973). New York, *Springer,* 1975, pp. 357-361.
19. Rock, J., Barttlett, M.K., and Matson, D.D. The incidence of anovulary menstruation in patients of low fertility. *Am. J. Obstet. Gynecol.,* 37:3-12, 1939.
20. Matson, D.D. Lung abscess. *N. Engl. J. Med.,* 222:15-21, 1940.
21. Matson, D. *The Treatment of Acute Craniocerebral Injuries due to Missiles.* Springfield, IL, Charles C. Thomas, 1948.
22. Ingraham, F., and Matson, D. *Neurosurgery of Infancy and Childhood.* Springfield, IL, Charles C. Thomas, 1954.
23. Evans, J. Donald Darrow Matson. *Trans. Am. Neurol. Assoc.,* 95:339-340, 1970.

24. Matson, D.D. Hydrocephalus. In: Gellis, S.S., and Kagan, B.M. (eds.). *Current Pediatric Therapy.* Philadelphia, WB Saunders, 1968.
25. Falconer, M.A., et al. Treatment of temporal lobe epilepsy by temporal lobectomy. Survey of findings and results. *Lancet*, 1:827-835, 1955.
26. Falconer, M.A. The pathological substrate of temporal lobe epilepsy. *Guy's Hospital Report.* London, Guy's Hospital 119:40-60, 1970.
27. Falconer, M.A. Genetic and related aetiological factors in temporal lobe epilepsy. A review. *Epilepsia*, 12:13-31, 1971.
28. Falconer, M.A. Reversibility by temporal lobe resection of the behavioral abnormalities of temporal lobe epilepsy. *N. Engl. J. Med.*, 289:451-455, 1973.
29. Falconer, M.A. Electrophysiological correlates of pathology and surgical results in temporal lobe epilepsy. *Brain*, 96:129-156, 1975.
30. Lecksell, L. Stereotaxic apparatus for intracranial surgery. *Acta Chir. Scand.*, 99:229-233, 1949.
31. Lecksell, L. Echo-encephalography: detection of intracranial complications following head injury. *Acta Chir. Scand.*, 110:301-315, 1956.
32. Lecksell, L., Herner, T., Lecksell, D., Person, G., and Lindquist, C. Visualization of stereotaxic radiolesions by nuclear magnetic resonance. *J. Neurol. Neurosurg. Psychiatry*, 9:797-803, 1983.
33. Lecksell, L., Stereotaxic radiosurgery, *J. Neurol. Neurosurg. Psychiatry*, 9:797-805, 1983.

CHAPTER 9

Pediatric Neurology

Having participated in a minor way in Dr. Stephen Ashwal's major editorial under-taking, *The Founders of Child Neurology*, I can approach this subject with some degree of confidence (1). The pleasure of Ashwal's book derives from the delightful characters portrayed in it. In this connection, when a granddaughter once voiced inter-est in going into pediatric neurology, I enthusiastically encouraged her. I assured her that, as her studies progressed, her world of friends and acquaintances would narrow in one sense, but in another sense, the quality of contacts that are important in life would greatly expand. More explicitly, I added that, if she did finally go into pediatric neurology, she would enter a world of charming, superior people who are dedicated to understanding and helping those children who will determine the future as well as to caring for the great majority of less fortunate ones.

Although pediatric neurology has much in common with the broad field of neurol-ogy, its developmental aspects definitely set it apart. Inherited defects, infancy, growth, and childhood involve special problems of genetics, metabolism, hormonal, neurological, and behavioral development.

I became very conscious of this problem as a consultant neurologist before the days when pediatric neurology became established in academic medicine. I worked for nearly 20 years on two successive University of California, San Francisco (UCSF), chiefs of pediatrics to give recognition to the special problems involved, which an adult neurologist could not adequately cover. However, they assured me that my expertise in epilepsy, electroencephalography, and so forth was fine and was all that was needed. In a limited sense, they were correct, inasmuch as they already had staff members interested in pediatric psychology, mental retardation, cerebral palsy, and others. These were "old-time" pediatricians, however, who meant well but were not fully trained in the modern neurological sciences.

It took me a long time to realize the probable interconnection of the following two facts: (1) about one third of pediatrics involves neurology and (2) pediatrics is not a highly remunerative specialty. Perhaps the assignment of this important subspecial-ty to a new staff specialty trained in both neurology and pediatrics was similar to what I previously had observed in the separation of neurology from the former neuropsychiatry of medicine at UCSF. Unvoiced, practical considerations initially eluded my academic and research thinking. Finally, the pediatricians relented and agreed to joint appointments for superior staff trained in both fields. This occurred after the American Boards of Neurology and Pediatrics established guidelines for pediatric neurology. At that time, pediatricians were overwhelmingly generalists, as formerly was true of medicine in general, and as is still the case in the field of family medicine.

A few outstanding pediatricians developed special interests in aspects of pediatric neurology and served important roles in the establishment of it as a separate discipline. Of those that I have selected to illustrate the different phases of pediatric neurology, Frank Ford best illustrates some of difficulties of this transition period.

FRANK FORD (1892-1970)

The careers of some physicians defy categorization in accordance with the usual cubbyholes of classification—such was that of Ford. As an academic person at Johns Hopkins, he was never head of a department, never had a bed service, and never had residency training. That a brilliant man would serve his entire career in such a subservient position in which he did not even have patient admitting privileges is explained by his unusual personality, his background, the early rigid academic pattern at Hopkins, and the circumstances of the time. In spite of this, Ford was a teacher, had special pupils, and became recognized as one of the outstanding pediatric neurologists of his time. Ford had an aversion to administrative detail; he derived satisfaction from his early commitment to undergraduate and graduate teaching on the Hopkins medical service and his primary interest in case study. He entered neurology well ahead of its scientific flowering phase when it was generally accepted that neurologists had to combine neurology with some other means of support. By the time the Great Depression and World War II had passed and the great expansion of neurology had developed with the aid of generous grants from the National Institutes of Health for research and training, Ford was approaching retirement.

As in most departments of medicine in the early decades of the 20th century, there was great resistance to the splitting off of neurology (let alone pediatric neurology). This attitude was particularly strong at Hopkins, as had been the case at UCSF, as discussed in Chapter 1, and continued past Ford's time, causing Ford's successor, David Clark, to leave Hopkins in 1965. The pediatrics department also had obstructed Clark's development of pediatric neurology. It was not until 1969 that Guy McKhann finally obtained a separate department of neurology.

Born in 1892, Ford was mainly educated in Baltimore and graduated from Hopkins in medicine in 1920. He was a resident in psychiatry under Adolph Meyer at Hopkins, where he obtained a good grounding in neuroanatomy and neuropathology. He next served as a resident in neurology under Foster Kennedy at the Bellevue Hospital in New York, but in 1923, he returned to Hopkins as a neurological house officer in the Department of Medicine. He was made head of a division of neurology (still under medicine) in 1932 and maintained this position until his retirement in 1958.

Ford was an excellent consultant who worked closely with Frank Walsh in his neuroophthalmological conferences and with Walter Dany in neurosurgery at Hopkins. Nevertheless, he was somewhat of a "lone wolf," a role that was accentuated by his eccentricities. Aside from his neurological interests, one of the principal features of Ford was his close attachment to Baltimore and the medical school of Johns Hopkins University. He was averse to travel and never attended medical meetings. Ford was a chain smoker, informal in his dress and manner, had a slight limp, spoke quietly, and was the antithesis of the former German academic showman. In his 3rd year of teaching, he presented the basic aspects of neurology in a clear and effective manner. Students showing interest were encouraged and helped; others were tolerated, and few demands were made of them. Graduate students were accepted if he liked them, but it was not a regular program of Hopkins with financial support.

His reputation rested mainly on his remarkable diagnostic skill that depended largely on the details of the patient's history and his keen observation. His neurological examinations were brief and usually made to settle questions that were unresolved by the history or his observations.

The other and perhaps the main basis for his great reputation depended on his monumental book, *Diseases of the Nervous System in Infancy, Childhood and Adolescence* (2). This was the result of his early interest in developmental neurology and his systematic record keeping over many years. One of the early neurological texts to be based on etiological classification, his book systematically presented a definition, etiology, pathology, clinical picture, diagnosis, prognosis, and treatment for each condition. First published in 1937, it went through six revisions over the next 33 years, grew to an encyclopedic 1,500-page length, and was translated into three languages. Even his text, however, illustrates another Ford anomaly—he never had training in pediatrics.

Although the career of Ford illustrates how his brilliance overcame many of the limitations of his time and setting, his impact in pediatric neurology rests largely on his text, a few graduate students, and his brilliance as a consultant. He was a glorious, but reclusive paradox, and his career illustrates some of the early problems of both neurology and pediatric neurology.

Another early pediatric neurologist, Douglas Buchanan, who in many respects was the opposite of Ford, is included in this account, because he understood the impact of science on modern neurology and probably trained more pediatric neurologists than any other teacher in the United States.

DOUGLAS BUCHANAN (1901-1983)

Buchanan's background in neurology and neurophysiology was unusual. He was born in Glasgow where he received his early training and medical education (M.A., 1922; B.Sc., 1922; M.R. and Ch.B., 1925). Following a Barbour Fellowship in physiology of the nervous system at the University of Glasgow for 2 years (1923 to 1925), he went to Trinity College, Cambridge, and spent the next 5 years as a lecturer in neurophysiology and research investigator for the Medical Research Council. He then turned to clinical work and spent 1929 through 1931 as a resident physician at the National Hospital, Queen Square, London, where he developed his enthusiasm and skill for case demonstrations. During this period, his devotion to Kinier Wilson as a teacher was notable, and this considerably influenced his later career. Through arrangements made by Percival Bailey in Chicago and Paul Bucy, who was studying neurology at the National Hospital at that time, Buchanan was invited to the University of Chicago as a pediatric neurologist. Starting in 1931, Buchanan rose to the highest academic levels over the next 35 years and, following retirement at the mandatory age of 65, continued to teach for another 15 years.

Buchanan's scientific publications were limited. He was not a ready scribe, which probably explains his earlier transfer from physiological research to clinical work. Only two physiological articles were written in his earlier period. With Bailey and Bucy, he produced an excellent monograph on *Intracranial Tumors of Infancy and Childhood* (3). His later clinical publications were chiefly case reports. However, he wrote nine chapters and reviews on epilepsy, the motor unit, and demyelinating diseases, which were well received.

As a teacher, Buchanan was superb. For decades, he held graduate teaching sessions in the amphitheater of the Children's Memorial Hospital, Chicago, where he would take histories, examine, and discuss the problems of selected children. Most of the patients were from the outpatient clinic of the hospital, but hospitalized patients were included when the residents requested it. As he dictated his examination and discussed the problem, a house officer summarized the case report in the medical record. Buchanan always made a diagnosis—although with follow-up visits, this might be modified.

Another teaching session, primarily for undergraduate medical students at the University of Chicago, was popularly attended by graduate students and visitors as well. Whereas in the clinic he mainly saw new patients, the patients for undergraduate teaching were carefully preselected. In both cases, his remarkable memory and his skill at eliciting histories and performing the neurological examinations were enthusiastically hailed by many generations of students at the University of Chicago. His ability to summarize the findings, to discuss differential diagnostic aspects, and to arrive at a final diagnosis was exceptional. Buchanan was fascinating to his audience, and his amphitheaters were always filled.

Buchanan was a member of several societies in England, as well as in the United States, and the latter included the American Neurological Association and American Pediatric Society. He served on the National Institutes of Health Study Sections for years. The University of San Carlos (Guatemala) awarded him an honorary Doctor of Medicine. In 1970, the University of Chicago School of Medicine awarded him its Gold Key.

Buchanan was also noted for his inspiration to undergraduate students. For a decade, he was selected to administer the Oath of Hippocrates to graduating classes.

As Nicholas J. Lenn has written of Buchanan, "his clinical skill and knowledge, his scholarly devotion to history, and the great warmth of his personality, combined to form the essence of this inspiring physician-teacher" (4).

PHILIP ROGERS DODGE (1913-   )

Dodge's career, like that of Sidney Carter in New York, dovetailed nicely with the widespread recognition of pediatric neurology in the United States. Both men were excellent examples of the new discipline, but I have selected Dodge because of his greater commitment to basic mechanisms underlying disease processes, which contributed to the flowering of neurology.

Dodge was born in Beverly, Massachusetts, and raised in northeastern Massachusetts. He obtained his undergraduate education at the University of New Hampshire and Yale and his medical education at the University of Rochester. After internship at the Strong Memorial Hospital, Rochester, he trained in neurology and neuropathology under Denny-Brown at the Harvard Neurological Unit of the Boston City Hospital. He then continued his training in Raymond Adam's set-up at the Massachusetts General Hospital (MGH). This was particularly important to Dodge's career, because it was to this service that he returned after Army service from 1950 to 1956. Adams had perceptively recognized Dodge's warm rapport with children and their parents and his abilities and potential in pediatric neurology. Dodge proceeded to create the pediatric neurology service at the MGH, which eventually won international recognition. His trainees later headed similar services throughout the United States and abroad. His dedication to his service, his expert handling of difficult patients, and his excellent teaching abilities were hailed by his graduate students. When he transferred to Washington University in 1967, a large number of the MGH house officers followed him.

Dodge's post at St. Louis was professor and chair of the Mallinckrodt Department of Pediatrics at the Washington University School of Medicine. He also was medical director of the St. Louis Children's Hospital. In these positions, Dodge's leadership expanded into several other facets of pediatrics as well as pediatric neurology. He served on several of the leading national scientific advisory committees, councils, and commissions in the field of pediatrics. He was active in national and international societies of both pediatrics and neurology. In addition, he was on the editorial boards of the *Journal of Pediatrics, Pediatric Research Neurology*, and *Developmental Medicine and Child Neurology*. He received many awards, including the prestigious Hower Award of the Child Neurology Society in 1978.

Dodge later relinquished his duties as chair of the department of neurology to devote his time to research and teaching in pediatric neurology. To this end, he continued as head of the Division of Child Neurology at Washington University. His studies on the neurological complications of fluid and electrolyte abnormalities, water intoxication, the battered child, acute encephalitis, bacterial meningitis, myasthenia gravis, and subdural effusions were basic contributions to pediatric neurology (5-11). In addition, his reviews and chapters of books often contained original observations.

Heads of teaching services usually possess outstanding qualities of leadership and teaching abilities, as well as organizational and administrative abilities. When research potential is added to this, a truly distinctive end result develops, as was the case with Dodge.

NEIL SIMPSON GORDON (1918-   )

Aside from Bronson Crowthers, whom I knew as a medical student at Harvard Medical School, the pediatric neurologist I have known best was Neil Gordon. Our warm friendship has persisted for over 40 years.

Gordon came to UCSF as a visiting assistant professor of neurology in early 1952. It was a difficult period for the UCSF neurology department because of the lack of qualified academic neurologists. As chair of the department, I had managed to develop a good 3-year undergraduate curriculum in neurology, but our postgraduate program was limited in spite of the good potential with three teaching hospitals. The National Institutes of Health was just starting, but its promise for the future still lay several years ahead. My strategy to overcome this difficulty was to import one or two well-trained men from England, where the National Health Service had created a glut of able young neurologists. Macdonald Critchley had already recommended Donald Macrae, and we also had Sigvald Refsum from Norway (later professor at Oslo and president of the World Federation of Neurology, as discussed in Chapter 12), who was spending 1 year with us in neurology at UCSF. Unfortunately, budgetary limitations made it impossible for us to recruit Gordon, but considering his later outstanding career in England, it was just as well that he returned to London. Certainly, it was a great gain for pediatric neurology in Great Britain.

He was raised in Bath, England, where his father, Ronald Grey Gordon, was a consultant in neurology, pediatrics, and psychotherapy. Gordon's father was one of the founding members of the Association of British Neurologists. His older brother, Ian, was also a physician, who became a distinguished radiologist and wrote a book on the subject. In connection with his earlier life in Bath, I well recall his eerie stories of the haunted house in one of the Bath Crescents where he was raised.

Gordon's higher education was in Edinburgh, where he graduated in 1940. Following two postgraduate posts in Edinburgh, he was swept into the British army in World War II. He was a squadron medical officer of a mobile field hospital, which followed the advances of the Allied army from North Africa to Italy and, finally, France. In spite of this, he managed to complete a thesis, which won him his M.D. in 1943. Following the war in 1946, he passed the membership examinations of the Edinburgh College of Physicians, and on moving to London in 1947, he also passed the examinations of the London, Royal College of Physicians. Both colleges elected him to their fellowship during the 1960s. Gordon went through the training program in neurology at the National Hospital, Queen Square, and it was immediately after this that he came to California.

On his return to London, he worked in the clinic at Moorfield's Eye Hospital from 1952 to 1958, and from 1955 to 1958, he was the senior registrar at St. Mary's Hospital in London. In 1958, he obtained an appointment as a neurologist in Preston, 35 miles northwest of Manchester, and a joint appointment as pediatric neurologist to the Royal Children's Hospital of Manchester. This made Gordon the first English pediatric neurologist outside of London, and he served in this post for 25 years until retirement from the National Health Service in 1983. Through his father, he had an early interest in pediatric neurology; this was further stimulated by Charles McNeil in Edinburgh and Thomas Stapleton in London. In addition to developing the pediatric neurology service in Manchester, he established three pediatric neurology centers in the Manchester area. Following this, he relinquished his adult neurology connection in Preston. J. P. M. Tizard has described Gordon's setup as "what must be regarded as the best staffed and organized hospital and community based child neurology service of any health region in the country" (12).

Gordon has published a number of articles (three with myself), but I believe his main contributions have been made in the form of annotations, published in *Developmental Medicine and Child Neurology*. His annotations have covered a wide range of clinical problems in pediatric neurology and have had the effect of summarizing the forefront of clinical opinion on them. In 1976, his text *Pediatric Neurology for the Clinician* was published, and a revised second edition came out in 1991 (13).

An interesting sidelight was Gordon's role in establishing pediatric neurology societies in both England and Europe. He participated in the pediatric neurology meetings of Ronald MacKeith in Oxford and elsewhere. These were an outgrowth of support contributed by the Spastic Society. Foreign pediatric neurologists were invited to the Oxford meetings, from which the European Federation of Child Neurology developed. Gordon was elected honorary secretary for 4 years and then president for 2 years. This society meets in different countries every 2 years. When the British Association of Pediatric Neurology was organized in 1974; Gordon was elected the first chair of this group and then was president for 6 years. A few representative pediatric neurologists are invited to the British meetings from other European pediatric neurology groups.

Perhaps even more significant was Gordon's influence in the Neurological Committee of the Royal College of Physicians for the establishment of pediatric neurology as an independent specialty. This was accomplished conjointly with the support of Sir Peter Tizard in the Pediatric Committee of the Royal Society and Ian McKinlay's negotiations with the British Department of Health.

Gordon's other honors include two traveling fellowships. On his retirement in 1988, 60 colleagues from 33 centers in Great Britain attended a symposium in his honor at the Royal Manchester Children's Hospital to celebrate his 70th birthday and his career in pediatric neurology. In 1985, he was presented the James Spence Medal by the British Pediatric Association.

In spite of the tragic deaths of his wife and daughter, Gordon has carried on in his quiet and yet very effective way. His dedication and abilities are known far beyond his group in pediatric neurology. Years ago, Dr. MacDonald Critchley informed me that Gordon undoubtedly was the foremost pediatric neurologist in Great Britain.

JEAN AICARDI (1926-   )

I have been unfortunate in missing Jean Aicardi in my many visits to France. He was a medical student in Paris in 1949, when I attended the International Neurological Congress that met at the medical school of the University of Paris in September of that year. After graduation in 1951, Aicardi served as an intern under Raymond Garcin at the Hôpital de la Salpêtrière and became interested in child neurology under Stephane Thieffry at the Hopital des Enfants Malades in Paris. His thesis on convulsive disorders in the first year of life had kindled his interest in Henri Gastaut and Joseph Roger, but he did not contact these Marseilles neurologists until 1960, long after my sabbatical period with Gastaut in 1957. In 1955 to 1956, Aicardi worked with Charles Janeway, William Lennox, and Caesare Lombroso in the seizure unit of the Children's Hospital Medical Center of Harvard Medical School, but again I missed him there. Nevertheless, through our common interest in epilepsy, I have been well aware of Aicardi for many years and have often quoted his studies. His great abilities and productivity have made him one of the most outstanding pediatric neurologists of the world. Because he contributed so much in the flowering period of neurology, he must be included in my account.

Aicardi was born in Rambouillet, France in 1926. Following his early training, he became the pediatrician in the department of infantile surgery at the Hôpital des Enfants Malades, and from 1964 to 1969, he worked as the assistant to Thieffry in the Department of Child Neurology of the Hopital Saint Vincent de Paul. As a member of the Institut National de la Santé et la Recherche Médicale, he developed a research group in child neurology and established a new unit at the Hôpital des Enfants Malades in 1979.

Aicardi is the epitome of the modern pediatric neurologist, who works closely with his team of neurosurgeons, neurodevelopmentalists, electroencephalographic workers, pathologists, and biologists. The team has been most productive and published over 250 articles. His interests have ranged widely from encephalitis, Rett syndrome, the Aicardi syndrome (a cerebral malformation), several other malformations (such as the Walker-Warburg and Joubert syndromes), and the progressive encephalopathies (14-18). However, over 50% of his studies have been in the area of his original interest—epilepsy in infancy and childhood. Following his thesis on epilepsy in the first year of life, he worked with Thieffry to show the important difference between cryptogenic and symptomatic forms of infantile spasm (19). His group intensively studied the effects of adrenocorticotropin and the corticosteroids on infantile spasms following the original favorable report of Gibbs and co-workers. His studies have ranged into all aspects of childhood epilepsy, such as myoclonic seizures, status epilepticus, febrile convulsions, and partial seizures (20-23). In 1986, he published *Epilepsy in Children*, which summarized his 25 years of work in this field (24). Notable in many of Aicardi's studies has been the collaboration of his loyal colleague, Jean Chevrie.

Aicardi participated with the Oxford group in the development of the European Study Group in Child Neurology in 1970. As explained in the previous essay on Gordon, this developed into the European Federation of Child Neurology, which soon had branches in most European countries; Aicardi became president in 1990. He also is a member of the Council of the International Child Neurology Association. Aicardi's other honors have included the Cornelia de Lange Medallion of the Dutch Society of Child Neurology in 1985 and the Hower Award of the American Child Neurology Society in 1986. Like Gastaut, Aicardi has a Gallic intensity of interest (passioné) and drive, which have now catapulted him into the forefront of his field. In the field of pediatric neurology, he personifies those aspects of modern neurology that have produced its flowering—the integration of neurological science with clinical neurology.

J. GORDON MILLICHAP (1928-   )

Few neurologists have equaled J. Gordon Millichap's productivity or have had his extensive background and training. My main point in including him in this series of essays is to document the close interrelationship between clinical neurology and the neurological sciences. Millichap's background in neuropharmacology, neurochemistry, and neurophysiology were particularly strong, and he closely integrated these with his clinical work.

Millichap's early schooling was at Rugby. His basic medical training was in England from 1942 to 1953; he obtained seven degrees, not including his F.R.C.P. (London) in 1971. He was a product of St. Bartholemew's Hospital and Medical College, University of London, where he obtained his M.S. and B.S. (honors) in 1946. In this same period, he passed the examinations of the M.R.C.S. (England) and L.R.C.P. (London). Other diplomas were obtained in 1947 (M.R.C.P., London, in internal medicine) and in 1948 (D.C.H., England, in Child Health). Following his military duty (1948 to 1950), he obtained his M.D. degree in 1950.

Having developed an interest in childhood epilepsy, he came to America in 1953 and spent 1 year as a fellow in pediatric neurology at the Harvard Medical School with Dr. William G. Lennox at the seizure unit of the Children's Hospital, as discussed in Chapter 2. This was followed by 1 year of studying the neuropharmacology of anticonvulsants at the University of Utah with Dr. Louis Goodman, as discussed in Chapter 6. In the following year, he was a pediatric neurologist at the National Institute of Neurological Disease and Blindness at Bethesda, Maryland, and he also served as an assistant clinical professor of neurology at George Washington University in Washington, D.C. Two more years followed (1956 to 1958) at the Albert Einstein College of Medicine, New York, where he was an associate professor of pediatrics and pharmacology. He finally completed his training in 1960 as a fellow and assistant resident in neurology and neuropathology at the Massachusetts General Hospital with Raymond Adams, Phillip Dodge, and Edward Richardson. Thus, except for his 2 years in the military and 2 years at the

Einstein College of Medicine, Millichap was engaged in medical training for 14 years from 1942 to 1960. During this period, he wrote 39 papers, 29 of which dealt with his primary interest in epilepsy.

In 1960, Millichap served as the pediatric neurologist of the Mayo Clinic in Rochester, Minnesota, and was made associate professor of pediatric neurology at the University of Minnesota Graduate School of Medicine in 1962 to 1963. In 1963, he transferred to Northwestern University in Chicago, where he became a professor in the departments of neurology and pediatrics. He became the pediatric neurologist of the Children's Memorial Hospital, and from 1963 to 1970, Millichap was the head of the Division of Neurology at Northwestern and attending neurologist at the Northwestern Memorial Hospital.

After his retirement at Northwestern, Millichap started the pediatric neurology service at the Southern Illinois School of Medicine in Springfield. He served as a visiting professor, the chief of pediatric neurology, director of the Children's Epileptic Clinic, and co-director of the Muscular Dystrophy Clinic. In addition, he served as the pediatric neurologist on the staff of St. John's Hospital in Springfield.

Following his development of pediatric neurology in Springfield, Millichap returned to his posts at Northwestern University and the Children's Memorial Hospital in Chicago, where as professor emeritus of neurology and pediatrics, he edits Pediatric Neurology Briefs, a monthly review and commentary of the current literature on pediatric neurology.

Millichap's thorough and broad preparation is reflected in his passing the examinations of four American specialty boards (pediatrics, neurology, pediatric neurology, and electroencephalography). He also passed six state medical licensing boards. Reflecting again his diverse interests, he is a member of 18 medical societies.

Millichap's 156 articles indicate his primary interests. Ninety-three articles and 11 book chapters deal with the various aspects of epilepsy, such as antiepileptic drugs (46 articles) and febrile convulsions (16 articles). Particularly notable are his 29 articles and 3 book chapters on the underlying pathophysiology of epilepsy. Two examples of the latter are "Systemic Electrolyte and Neuroendocrine Mechanisms in Epilepsy" and "Metabolic and Endocrine Factors in Epilepsy" (25,26). Although he wrote very broadly in the field of pediatric neurology, his other main interests have been in the hyperactive child and minimal brain damage (23 articles and 7 book chapters) and dyslexia (11 articles and 2 book chapters) (27). Some of his work and interests in epilepsy are summarized in Modern Treatment Symposium, in which he wrote five chapters. In addition, Millichap was author and editor of eight books; the last one was Progress in Pediatric Neurology, published in 1991 (28).

Some neurologists rise to notable success with limited backgrounds, as in the case of William G. Lennox. Others spend many years in preparation, such as Denny-Brown. The latter, perhaps, are searching for their proper niche and opportunity but also tend to be perfectionists. Among the pediatric neurologists, it has been my impression that Millichap belonged in this latter group—a group notable for its close synthesis of clinical studies with the basic disciplines.

SUMMARY

Frank Ford illustrates the difficult transitional period of pediatric neurology from pediatrics. Douglas Buchanan and Philip Dodge in America and Neil Gordon in Great Britain were the brilliant leaders who led in the early development of pediatric neurology. Many others were involved in this exciting flowering period, through the decades from about 1940 to 1970, as is well-illustrated in the final section of Ashwal's *The Founders of Child Neurology* (1).

Two additional pediatric neurologists, Jean Aicardi of Paris and J. Gordon Millichap of Chicago, have been included because they brilliantly exemplify the close interaction of pediatric neurology with modern science. The future of pediatric neurology will hinge on this connection as neurogenetics develops and as the normal and abnormal neurological aspects of physiology, chemistry, and immunology of infancy and youth are clarified.

REFERENCES

1. Ashwal, S. *The Founders of Child Neurology*. San Francisco, Norman Publishing, 1990.
2. Ford, F. *Diseases of the Nervous System in Infancy, Childhood and Adolescence*. Springfield, IL, Charles C. Thomas, 1939, pp. 718-725.
3. Bailey, P., Buchanan, D.N., and Bucy, P.C. *Intracranial Tumors of Infancy* and Childhood. Chicago, University of Chicago Press, 1939.
4. Lenn, N.J. Douglas Buchanan. In: Ashwal, S. (ed.). *The Founders of Child Neurology*. San Francisco,Norman Publishing, 1990, pp. 666-671.
5. Crawford, J.D., and Dodge, P.R. Complications of fluid therapy in patients with neurologic diseases: with special emphasis on water intoxication and hypertonic dehydration. *Pediatr. Clin. North Am.*, 6:257-279, 1959.
6. Dodge, P.R., Crawford, J.D., and Probst, J.H. Studies in experimental water intoxication. *Arch. Neurol.*, 3:513-529, 1960.
7. Dodge, P.R. *Medical Implications of Physical Abuse of Children: Protecting the Battered Child*. vol. 21. Children's Division, Englewood, Colorado, The American Humane Society Publications, 1962.
8. Lyon, G., Dodge, P.R., and Adams, R.D. The acute encephalopathies of obscure origin in infants and children. *Brain*, 84:680-708, 1961.
9. Swartz, M.N., and Dodge, P.R. Bacterial meningitis: a review of selected aspects. *N. Engl. J. Med.*, 272:725-731; 842-848; 898-902; 954-960; 1003-1010, 1965.
10. Millichap, J.G., and Dodge, P.R. Diagnosis and treatment of myasthenia in infancy, childhood and adolescence: a study of 51 patients. *Neurology*, 10:1007-1014, 1960.
11. Rabe, E.F., Flynn, R.E., and Dodge, P.R. A study of subdural effusions in an infant with particular reference to factors influencing prognosis and the efficiency of various forms of therapy. *Neurology*, 18:559-570, 1962.
12. Tizard, J.P.M. James Spence Medalist: Neil Simpson Gordon. *Arch. Dis. Child.*, 60:603-604, 1985.
13. Gordon, N.S. *Pediatric Neurology for the Clinician, Clinics in Developmental Medicine*. nos. 59/60. London, Spastics International Medical Publications, Heinemann, 1976.
14. Aicardi, J., et al. Acute measles encephalitis in children with immuno-depression. *Pediatrics*, 59:232-239, 1977.
15. Hagberg, B., et al. A progressive syndrome of autism, dementia, and loss of purposeful hand use in girls: Rett's syndrome: report of 35 cases. *Ann. Neurol.*, 14:471-478, 1983.
16. Aicardi, J., Chevrie, J.J., Rousalie, F. Le syndrome spasmes en flexion, agénésie calleuse, anomalies choriorétiniennes. *Arch. Fr. Pediatr.*, 26:1103-1120, 1969.
17. Bordarier, C., Aicardi, J., and Goutieres, F. Congenital hydrocephalus and eye abnormalities with severe developmental defects: Warburg's syndrome. *Ann. Neurol.*, 16:60-65, 1984.
18. Aicardi, J., and Goutieres, F. A progressive familial encephalopathy in infancy with calcifications of the basal ganglia and chronic cerebrospinal fluid lymphocytosis. *Ann. Neurol.*, 15:49-54, 1984.

19. Thieffry, S., et al. Les spasmes in flexion du nourrisson. 36 observations. Etude critique. *Semin. Hip. Paris,* 34:1167-1178, 1959.
20. Aicardi, J., and Chevrie, J.J. Myoclonic epilepsies of childhood. *Neuropediatrie,* 3:177-190, 1971.
21. Aicardi, J., and Chevrie, J.J. Convulsive status epilepticus in infants and children. A study of 239 cases. *Epilepsia,* 11:187-197, 1970.
22. Aicardi, J., and Chevrie, J.J. Febrile convulsions. Sequelae and mental retardation. In: Brazier, M.A.B., and Coceani, E. (eds.). *Infantile Febrile Convulsions.* New York, Raven Press, 1976, pp. 247-257.
23. Aicardi, J., and Chevrie, J.J. Atypical partial benign epilepsy of childhood. *Dev. Med. Child Neurol.,* 24:281-292, 1982.
24. Aicardi, J. *Epilepsy in Children.* New York, Raven Press, 1986.
25. Millichap, J.G. Systemic electrolyte and neuroendocrine mechanisms in epilepsy. In: *Basic Mechanisms of the Epilepsies.* Boston, Little Brown, 1969, pp. 709-736.
26. Millichap, J.G. Metabolic and endocrine factors in epilepsy. In: *Handbook of Clinical Neurology.* vols. 9 and 10. Amsterdam, North-Holland Publishing, 1974.
27. Millichap, J.G. Minimal brain dysfunction. In: *Learning Disabilities and Related Disorders.* Chicago, Year Book Medical Publishers, 1977.
28. Millichap, J.G. *Progress in Pediatric Neurology.* Chicago and London, Pediatric Neurology Briefs and Publishers, 1991.

Neurological Rehabilitation

Perhaps no other field approximates the high goals of patient care than those proclaimed by neurological rehabilitation. The chronic nature of the disabilities commonly dealt with by this discipline and the psychological factors involved in their care demand a high level of patient support and physician empathy, if the rehabilitation efforts are to be successful. I used to say that any doctor "worth his or her salt" would study patients thoroughly and handle their problems in a comprehensive fashion. No doubt this was influenced by the ideals and practice of my dedicated father. I refer to this earlier period to emphasize the point that, although the flowering of rehabilitation has largely developed since World War II, the concept of rehabilitation and its basic values are by no means new. My father was an exceptional diagnostician and maintained great rapport with his patients. His reputation grew both community wide and in the medical profession, which latter led to his election as the president of his state medical association. He also was a surgeon, and the reputation of his surgical skill drew patients from distant areas. His hospital served the needs of the community, a community, however, that contributed nothing to its support. In spite of this, before the days of modern inflation, he kept the patients as long as necessary, and his idea of "necessary" included rehabilitation when required and adequate arrangements for follow-up care with family and community. This was supported by his surgical fees, which now would be considered ridiculously low. I could quote many examples, some with severe injuries that required repeated operations and unpaid hospital stays for months, but an abbreviated account of one example will serve to illustrate the point I want to make.

A young man was brought to my father's hospital following a dynamite explosion, in which both his hands were blown off, both eyes were blinded, and his face and body were horribly mutilated. He was near death for days, but with heroic medical care, he finally slowly recovered. Mental depression and despair followed. My father soon discovered his pride of family and underlying sense of Western self-sufficiency, and he appealed to these values. One of the young man's grandfathers was a first cousin of Lincoln's wife, Nancy Hanks, and the other on his mother's side was a nephew of General Stacy, who fought at Bunker Hill in the American Revolution. Finally he read to him the poem of Edward Vance Cooke "How did you die? " (1).

> Did you tackle that trouble that came your way
> With a resolute heart and cheerful?
> Or hide your face from the light of day
> With a craven soul and fearful?
> Oh, a trouble's a ton, or a trouble's an ounce,
> Or a trouble is what you make it.
> And it isn't the fact that you're hurt that counts,
> But only how did you take it?
>
> You are beaten to earth? Well, well, what's that!
> Come up with a smiling face.
> It's nothing against you to fall down flat,
> But to lie there—that's disgrace.
> The harder you're thrown, why the higher you bounce;
> Be proud of your blackened eye!
> It isn't the fact that you're licked that counts;
> It's how did you fight—and why?
>
> And though you be done to the death, what then?
> If you battled the best you could;
> If you played your part in the world of men,
> Why the Critic will call it good.
> Death comes with a crawl, or comes with a pounce
> And whether he's slow or spry,
> It isn't the fact that your dead that counts,
> But only how did you die?

This may seem harsh to modern ears but not to the rugged self-sufficiency of the West two and three generations back, and young Hanks responded to it. With help, he learned to dress and to take care of himself. He kept a copy of the poem with him as a treasured reminder of his heritage and personal fortitude.

By hiring a small boy to lead him, he made a living by door-to-door selling and paid his hospital bills. A friendly teacher taught him, and he went to Stanford University for 2.5 years. He took courses in history, languages, literature, public speaking, and lectures from the then-President, David Star Jordan.

When he wrote his story, which is unique in its poetic prose form, he had developed seven lectures, memorized "50,000 words of classical literature," and lectured in high schools, colleges, and universities all over the country. He became independent, married a nurse who had befriended him in his darkest hours (my father inspired his staff as well as his patients), owned two houses, and traveled over 10,000 miles per year (2).

Mr. Hanks gave a copy of his book to my father, who he always credited for saving both his life and spirit. The poem was the spark, but my father had laid the groundwork of hope and support before that. Mr. Hanks was in the hospital for a long period, and the medical bills he paid were for actual hospital costs, not professional fees.

The medical and lay literature are full of inspiring accounts of this sort, but as Dr. Howard Rusk has pointed out, relatively few were rehabilitated before World War II. Although millions were disabled, rehabilitation was "catch as catch can" (3). The secret of rehabilitation is hope and motivation. The many aspects of motivation have been brilliantly analyzed by Drs. Esbönsson and Olle Höök (4).

Modern rehabilitation, however, involves an entirely different operational approach than the rehabilitation techniques of my father, or even of my own of 30 to 50 years ago. It is concerned with the teamwork of many medical disciplines as well as paramedical groups. Depending on the nature of the disability, neurological surgeons, orthopedic surgeons, cardiologists, rheumatologists, urologists, and others may be involved as well as neurologists. In addition, psychological studies may be required, or the help of brace or prosthetic experts, special nursing care, physiotherapists, speech therapists, occupational therapists, social service workers, and so forth. The director of rehabilitation services is responsible for an evaluation of each patient's problems, the organization of an appropriate rehabilitation program, and the coordination of effort to achieve it. Since much depends on the patient's motivation, a continuity of rapport and support is essential, which only superior teamwork, headed by a wise director, can attain.

Even one-half century ago, rehabilitation had greatly advanced, and I was fortunate in having three rehabilitation units. The one at the University Hospital (University of California, San Francisco [UCSF]) was closely affiliated with orthopedic surgery, as was common of old. A second one, affiliated with neurology, dealt with the wartime disabilities of veterans at the local Veterans Administration Hospital under the control of the Combined Dean's Committee (University of California and Stanford, when the latter was in San Francisco), of which I was the first chairman. We organized a third center to deal with the chronic and geriatric problems at the Laguna Honda Hospital, a city institution that handled San Francisco's indigent patients. In addition, resources were available for several other types of rehabilitation—our multiple sclerosis, epilepsy, and pain clinics utilized a private rehabilitation agency with excellent industrial outlets. Still other resources involved state rehabilitation agencies, rehabilitation in the public school system, and volunteer groups interested in special problems.

I mention this background to illustrate the fact that the scope of rehabilitation a generation ago was relatively broad. Even then, patient referral was a problem of the first magnitude, which often fell short of a comprehensive evaluation, optimal programing, and social service expertise in mobilizing available community resources and supportive follow-up care.

Following World War II, the problems and field expanded several fold. Dr. Richard Masland, while serving as the president of the World Federation of Neurology, quoting the data of Dr. J. F. Kurtzke, stated, "Every year, in the U.S.A. alone, over 30,000 people are killed on the highways. Approximately 200,000 receive a head injury of sufficient severity to require hospitalization and 370,000 have at least transient post-concussive syndromes. Injury is the major cause of death up to the age of 40 years. An almost equal number of the elderly suffer from strokes. These figures can be duplicated throughout the world. The toll of disability that derives from these accidents and illnesses is incalculable"(5).

Reflecting the great growth of rehabilitative needs is the increase of workers in the field. The American Speech-Language-Hearing Association increased in membership from 1,623 in 1950 to 35,000 in 1980 and by January 1990, to 60,000 (6). This, of course, was only one aspect of the overall problem in one major country.

Judging from the comments of my friend, Dr. Sedgwick Mead, the problems in rehabilitation medicine have grown more or less in proportion to the expansion of the field. Mead is a graduate of Harvard Medical School (1938) and then did postgraduate work at Washington University in St. Louis, where he advanced to the associate professorship. In 1954, he became the medical director of the Kaiser Foundation Rehabilitative Center at Vallejo, California. Using the Kabat techniques, he developed a large rehabilitative center for the Kaiser Medical insurance system. Still later, he was chief of neurology at the Kaiser-Permanente Medical Center in Vallejo, and after retirement, he became the medical director of the Easter Seal Rehabilitative Center in Oakland, California.

From this very considerable background in rehabilitation and in spite of the previous discussion of the high goals of rehabilitation, Mead has commented on a number of problems, as follows.

1. "In California, beginning roughly in the 1980s, rehabilitation has been mandated by law to those individuals who have received a final judgment under the Worker's Compensation Act as being permanently partially disabled. This has greatly increased the cost to insurers and is ridden with abuses. Most of the work is carried out in store-front type of facilities, some of which are limited to hand clinics. Results are spotty because clients are encouraged by labor attorneys to maximize symptoms and minimize recovery."

2. "Some aspects of compensation law are completely nonsensical, such as the assumption that heart attacks in firemen and policemen are automatically compensatable because of the stress of those jobs."

3. "The government programs are burdened with bureaucratic waste of time, money, and personnel."

4. "...(For Profit Centers) are often single diagnosis limited, such as head injury, having treatment areas combined with dormitory facilities. They depend on insurance coverage and injury awards for financing, and dismiss their clients when their money runs out."

5. "Sheltered workshops are debatably rehabilitative, since they finance protected, highly restricted, terminal employment. They are highly useful sociologically, especially for the mentally retarded."

After nearly one-half century following the flowering of neurology and neurorehabilitation, these are disturbing comments by a superior participant (Mead S., personal communication, 1992). His conclusions place much of the difficulty on the widely dispersed facets involved in rehabilitation. Mead states, "Rehabilitation medicine is a horizontal specialty unlike neurology or ophthalmology. It crosses many areas. Its practitioners must be conversant with many fields, including neurology, psychiatry, orthopedics, pediatrics, urology, and dermatology." He also places the blame on "...the lack in this country (USA) of a comprehensive health care system."

Another friend, Professor Dr. Med., Olle Höök, who also has spent his entire career in neurology and rehabilitative medicine and was the professor and chair of the Institute of Rehabilitation in the University of Göteborg, Sweden (see later section), has had an entirely different experience (Höök O., personal communication, 1992). Although Mead admits that there are some good rehabilitative centers and Höök agrees that there are many problems in rehabilitation, their reactions to their specialty vary considerably. No doubt the situation is much better in small countries of less affluence and greater ethnic homogeneity, where the pattern of rehabilitation is influenced by academic institutes, such as in Sweden. Even there, Professor Höök tells me that a perennial problem in rehabilitation concerns its necessary coordination of many elements—what Mead has referred to as its "horizontal" character. Also, they both agree as to the difficult integrating role of the medical director of rehabilitation.

So diverse are the elements of medical rehabilitation, it is difficult to present them in a unified fashion. However, by limiting the account to neurological rehabilitation during the exciting period of its flowering, which coincided with that of neurology, its principal aspects can be illustrated.

The early phase of rehabilitation in America was usually covered by physical medicine, as a rule closely affiliated with orthopedic surgery. Physiotherapy was its mainstay, although diathermy and other forms of treatment were added as they were introduced and became popular. It was in this stage of development that Dr. Howard Rusk initiated his rehabilitative efforts after World War II.

HOWARD RUSK (1901-   )

The story of Howard Rusk is an extraordinary one and is selected to illustrate an important aspect of rehabilitation—the need of this discipline for broad public understanding and adequate support. Rusk has given recognition to Dr. George Deaver for first showing that paraplegic patients could be trained to walk and, especially, for his ability in training physicians in rehabilitation. It is not overstating the case, however, that the several developments in rehabilitation that occurred after World War II would not have been possible without the career-long impetus given to this field by Rusk.

Born in Missouri and with 2 years of medicine in the University of Missouri, he completed medical school at the University of Pennsylvania. He interned in St. Louis and developed a thriving practice there with a teaching connection with the Washington University School of Medicine. He joined the Medical Corps of the United States Air Force in World War II. Having developed an interest in rehabilitation in his earlier career and now confronted by the tremendous number of disabilities of the war, he conceived the idea of an Air Force Rehabilitation Center. With the backing of General Henry H. Arnold and the expertise of Dr. George Deaver in New York City, he succeeded in developing such a center at Pauling, New York. Lowell Thomas, Jr. and Sr., Eleanor Roosevelt, and several others aided in this. This became the model for 12 other Air Force Rehabilitation Centers in the country, and eventually, 250 such centers were developed (3).

At the end of the war, he decided to stay in rehabilitation instead of going back to private practice in St. Louis. A department of physical medicine and rehabilitation was established in the reorganized Medical School of New York University with the help of Dr. Sheahan and Alan Gregg of the Rockefeller Foundation. A rehabilitative setup at Bellevue Hospital followed that demonstrated the needs of civilian rehabilitation. Four other centers were developed in New York City hospitals and others were planned.

To fill the needs of private rehabilitation, in addition to the city-supported centers, Rusk developed a rehabilitative center with the support of the Milbank Memorial Fund, the United Mine Workers Union, Bernard Baruch, and many others. In addition to training doctors in rehabilitation in the United States, the Institute trained over 1,000 doctors from 85 other countries. This led to Rusk's international role in developing centers in such countries as Poland, Rumania, and Thailand.

A permanent rehabilitation center was established in New York City in 1951, and Rusk was instrumental in gaining recognition of the American Medical Association for rehabilitation as a medical specialty.

The institute provided a comprehensive approach to rehabilitation, which included occupational therapy and industrial rehabilitation needs. To meet the employment needs of rehabilitative patients, "Abilities, Inc." was started, which eventually hired hundreds of people. Surveys proved that the rehabilitated patient had a higher production rate, lower absentee rate, and nine times less turnover than did other groups. He was enabled with the help of "Wild Bill" Donovan, Mrs. Albert Lasker, and many others to organize in 1955 a nonprofit rehabilitation agency, the purpose of which was to launch rehabilitative programs all over the world, supported by the World Rehabilitation Fund.

His final Rehabilitation Institute (eight stories high) was opened in New York City in 1968, and this included a broad spectrum of research in the fields of rehabilitation. I had the pleasure of hearing his talk to the Medical Advisory Board of the National Multiple Sclerosis Society on December 6, 1970 and had lunch with him and Houston Merritt following this. His engaging personality, encyclopedic knowledge of rehabilitation, and obvious dedication to his cause were most impressive.

In addition to his personal qualities, which attracted patients and gave them a great sense of support, Rusk was a clever entrepreneur in advancing his cause. He developed many contacts, whose wealth and influence greatly advanced his rehabilitation efforts. Whereas a number of fragmented and limited efforts at rehabilitation had existed before (poorly supported by even the medical profession), following his efforts, the need of comprehensive rehabilitation became widely recognized, and both the number of such centers and their support increased a 1,000-fold.

Another early development that closely overlapped with the career of Rusk, but which gave an entirely different impetus to rehabilitation, was the research of my brilliant colleague, Dr. Verne Inman. Because Inman was a spur to the field of prosthesis and the study of human locomotion in the early flowering period of neurology, his story is pertinent and of considerable interest.

VERNE INMAN (1905-1980)

Inman was a product of the San Francisco Bay area. Born and raised in San Jose, he obtained A.B. and M.A. degrees at the University of California (Berkeley) and M.D. and Ph.D. (Anatomy) degrees at the UCSF. From 1936 to 1939, his internship and residency training was at the University of California Hospital, San Francisco, following which he obtained an orthopedic fellowship at the San Francisco Hospital. He was certified in Orthopedic Surgery in 1943 and, by 1948, had advanced to the associate clinical professorship of Orthopedic Surgery.

Stimulated by the problems of amputees in World War II, he recruited physiologists and engineers to study human locomotion and to design more functional prosthetic devices. Although this effort was initiated as early as 1943, it was not until 1957 that the Biomechanics Laboratory was finally established. In the meantime, with the cooperation of professor H. D. Eberhart of the School of Engineering (University of California, Berkeley), basic studies on the nature of human locomotion were undertaken and resulted in ten reports. In addition, there were six studies on the problems of prosthesis, the locomotion of amputees, and so forth (7). This had a great impact in stimulating further research in this field, which eventually obtained the support of the National Institutes of Health (NIH), when this latter became available. Inman became known as Dr. Biomechanics by NIH committees and others in the fields of orthotics and orthopedic surgery.

Pain, as a complication of amputations and the use of prosthetic devices, as well as in other orthopedic conditions, greatly interested Inman. This, in part, had been stimulated by his earlier studies on sensation, one of which had been his thesis for a Master's degree. This was further stimulated by the studies of J. H. Kellgren in England (8). With J. B. de C. M. Saunders, he made a study of referred pain from "skeletal structures" (9), and with our recruitment of Dr. Francis Schiller, a pain clinic was started at UCSF in the early 1950s. Patients were studied by psychiatrists and physiologists, as well as neurologists and orthopedic surgeons. It was the first pain clinic in the country and established a pattern for the study of pain problems. With Inman, Professor H. J. Ralston of Anatomy, Ben Libet of Physiology, and H. F. Albronda of Psychiatry, we organized three symposiums on pain with the participation of neurologists from the East and Europe (10-10b). This resulted in four articles by Inman and others.

Another active area of study was muscle physiology, which in part, was related to locomotion problems. Dr. Bertram Feinstein, who had received training at Oxford and who also had a connection with anatomy, was recruited for this purpose (as discussed under Gunnar Wohlfart in Chapter 15). He and Ralston worked closely with

Inman. More than a dozen articles developed from this effort. This was quite aside from the routine electromyography (EMG) and nerve conduction studies on patients in our electroencephalography and EMG laboratory.

A later interest of Dr. Inman concerned foot and ankle problems, and he published 22 articles in this special field. Still other reports involved studies on the shoulder, intervertebral discs, spasticity, and other orthopedic conditions.

I should add that Inman was a superb teacher and excellent clinician. Although not primarily an administrator, he was very good in organizing comprehensive research programs. He served as director of the Biomechanics Laboratory for 16 years and was Chair of the Department of Orthopedic Surgery for 13 years. He also was very successful in obtaining research grants—some 15 grants for the study of locomotion and 9 for studies on prosthesis. Primarily, he was noted for his clinical research, and in his field of locomotion and prosthesis, he became nationally and internationally known. He belonged to 11 orthopedic societies and was a founding member of the Orthopedic Research Society and American Orthopedic Foot Society. He served on several prestigious committees and councils in his field. Whereas Howard Rusk was the entrepreneur, who led the explosive development of rehabilitation following World War II, Inman was an early stimulus to its research and succeeded in placing locomotion and prosthesis on a more scientific basis.

LUDWIG GUTTMANN (1899-1980)

The career of Ludwig Guttmann is especially significant in showing the importance of combining scientific research with patient support in the development of rehabilitation of spinal cord injuries. Starting as the son of orthodox Jewish parents in Poland, he studied medicine in Breslau, Germany, and worked up to being the first assistant to Otfried Foerster in research and neurosurgery. Having withstood the early persecutions of Hitler's Gestapo, he migrated to England with his family in 1939. He became the Head of the Spinal Injury Unit at Stoke Mandeville in 1942 and, over the next 20 years developed techniques, which transformed this hopeless condition to successful rehabilitation. He ended up as a knighted Englishman, highly revered for his distinguished accomplishments. The story is filled with surprising aspects, and Whitteridge, in his obituary, has gone so far as to indicate that Guttmann's "mission" can be compared to that of Isaiah of Biblical fame (11).

Consider the following highlights of Guttmann's career that aided him in the preparation for his mission, some of which were of an unusual and propitious character.

1. While waiting to be inducted into the German Army at the age of 17 (World War I), he worked as an orderly in the local accident hospital. He was greatly impressed by the treatment of a severe back injury with its then-hopeless prognosis. His work as an orderly influenced him to a medical career and served him well in later life with respect to the direct care of patients. A severe throat infection, picked up from a patient and requiring tubal drainage, saved him from military induction in both 1917 and 1918.

2. Intent on applying for postgraduate specialty training in pediatrics, he switched at the last moment to neurology, when he discovered that there were many applications for the one open post in pediatrics. It was this that brought him to the service of Foerster.

3. Foerster encouraged his students to use exercises as a form of therapy in neurological disorders. The influence of Foerster in the study of paraplegia, pain pathways, and the symptomatology of spinal cord injuries was both basic and clinically important (12).

4. Although under the observation of the German Gestapo in the 1930s and restricted by them, he and his immediate family were never subjected to physical harm. His position with Foerster, early renunciation of Jewish orthodoxy, reputation, and probably, patient influence, protected him until he migrated to England in 1939. In the meantime, however, his parents, sister, and brother-in-law had been liquidated by the Nazis.

5. Although recognized as one of the foremost neurosurgeons of Europe and sought in consultation in other countries than Germany, he later was not permitted to do surgery by the British and was shunted off into neurological research at Oxford. Guttmann's research, while at Oxford (1939 to 1943) included studies on nerve regeneration and the beneficial effect of galvanic stimulation of paralyzed muscles in staying their atrophy (13,14).

6. Guttmann published reviews for the Medical Research Council on rehabilitation after injuries of the nervous system and the surgical aspects of injuries of the spinal cord and cauda equina (15). These were read by George Riddoch, Consultant Neurologist to the Emergency Medical Service in World War II. Riddoch and Head had written a classic paper on spinal injuries during World War I (1917). Riddoch offered Guttmann the directorship of a new spinal unit at Stoke Mandeville, established for the casualties of the invasion of Europe in World War II. The impetus for this came from one of my former professors at Harvard, Dr. Donald Munroe. His experience on the rehabilitation of paraplegic patients at the Boston City Hospital indicated that bed sores could be avoided by turning the patient every 2 hours. This ray of hope, combined with Guttmann's background of research and clinical experience, were the inspiration of Riddoch's providential decision.

7. Guttmann's meticulous training of orderlies to turn patients every 2 hours and his strict aseptic catheterization of bladders greatly improved the prognosis of spinal cord injuries. These efforts were markedly aided by the recent availability of penicillin and later streptomycin.

8. Guttmann was formidable in his insistence on reforms with respect to older procedures, which experience proved were inadequate. These included the transportation of paraplegic patients on plaster beds as practiced by orthopedic surgeons, the suprapubic cystostomy of urologists, and the immediate operation on patients with spinal cord injuries with mechanical fixation of the vertebrae by spinal plates, as practiced by ambitious orthopedic surgeons.

9. Much research was done, but Guttmann ruled out invasive procedures, except where there was much to learn, when the procedure was explained to the

patients, and after obtaining their consent. The viscera-cutaneous reflex, triggered by distention and contraction of the bladder, produced vasodilatation of the head and neck, vasoconstriction of the lower extremities, slowing of the heart rate, and a sharp rise of blood pressure. This appeared in patients whose lesions were above T-6 but, minimally, with lesions at T-6 or below.

10. Guttmann was very supportive to his patients and paid close attention to their psychological problems and the morale of his wards. The depression of patients was improved when they realized that other patients, worse than themselves, were responding to Guttmann's meticulous treatment. Their devotion to him was expressed by calling him "Papa."

Morale and rehabilitation were greatly stimulated by wheelchair sports and industrial rehabilitation, both of which Guttmann stimulated. The former led to Olympic Games for the paralyzed patient and the latter, to the establishment of industrial rehabilitation centers in various parts of the country by the Ministry of Labor in Great Britain.

Recognized for his great contributions, Guttmann received the O.B.E. in 1950, the C.B.E. in 1960, and was knighted in 1966. Rehabilitation centers were named for him in three countries, and he was elected to membership in the Royal Society in 1976. He was given honorary degrees by three universities, made an honorary member of many societies, and received state awards from eight countries. His main contributions were summarized in 1976 (16). He founded the journal Paraplegia and served as its editor from 1962 to 1980. His influence in developing high standards of rehabilitation for spinal cord injuries resulted in incalculable benefits.

WILLIAM BRYAN JANNETT (1926-   )

Jannett's main research interest has been in the care of head injuries, and because of his original contributions and outstanding expertise in this field, he has been selected to illustrate this aspect of rehabilitation.

His extensive background admirably fitted him for his research on head injuries. His original training was at the University of Liverpool (M.B., 1949, and M.D., 1960). He became a Fellow of the Royal College of Surgeons in 1952. Following several postgraduate posts, which included registrar posts at Oxford with Sir Hugh Cairns, and at Cardiff, his academic career in neurosurgery started in 1957 at the University of Manchester. In 1958 to 1959, as a Rockefeller Fellow, he worked at the Neurological Institute and in Neurosurgery at the University of California, Los Angeles. In 1961, he was Hunterian Professor in the Royal College of Surgeons of England, and 2 years later, he transferred to Glasgow, where he was a consultant neurosurgeon in the West of Scotland Regional Neurosurgical Unit. He was appointed to the first chair of neurosurgery in 1968.

His interests in head injuries and posttraumatic epilepsy were kindled at Oxford, and he completed a monograph on the latter subject while at Manchester (17). However, it was at the University of Glasgow that he was able to exploit several favorable opportunities. With Sloan Robertson, the Institute of Neurological

Sciences was developed (18). With Murray Harper, he utilized a cerebral blood flow method of predicting and avoiding permanent hemiplegia in patients following temporary carotid artery clamping. This and other blood flow studies led the Medical Research Council to establish a "Group for Study of the Cerebral Circulation" under the co-directorship of these two (19). With Gordon McDowell, he demonstrated that halothane anesthesia produced a rise of intracranial pressure that was dangerous for patients with brain tumors (20). With Ian Ledingham and co-workers, he showed that hyperbaric operating conditions failed to produce a benefit either in the surgery of intracranial cerebrovascular lesions or experimental brain injuries.

It was his follow-up studies on head injuries, however, that have been of particular value for rehabilitation. With a group of statisticians headed by Wilfred Card, Jannett developed a method of predicting the outcome of severe head injuries (21). Because this required large numbers of patients, collaborative studies were established with two Dutch and two American centers. The results were found to have significant prognostic value and have been adopted internationally. This also led to studies of coma and persistent vegetative states (22). With Reinder Braakmann of Rotterdam, he also did a study of posttraumatic epilepsy in patients with depressed skull fractures (23).

In addition, he has written widely on medical ethics and how to establish priorities for the use of limited beds, equipment, and highly trained personnel (24). In particular, he has assessed the cost to the patient, family, and society of neurological disabilities and the value of rehabilitation (25).

The Institute of Neurological Sciences has become an important center of research and postgraduate training. Jannett's reputation as an outstanding teacher and investigator have spread worldwide, and he has established an excellent academic department of neurosurgery that has successfully integrated programs of clinical and laboratory research. He is known for his crisp, clear writing and his "An Introduction to Neurosurgery" illustrates this very well (26).

In summary, Jannett is not just another neurosurgical technician. His career well documents his creative abilities and, at the same time, his outstanding talents as a teacher, administrator, and research worker. His kind handling of patients and interest in medical ethics might well have qualified him for inclusion in Chapter 14 on the Art of Medicine in Neurology.

A good counterpart to Jannett's studies on head injury is Dr. Derick Wade's research on stroke, a field in which he has developed an enviable reputation. Both conditions are common brain disorders requiring prolonged rehabilitation. However, stroke usually involves an older age group, which often constitutes a limiting factor to their rehabilitation.

DERICK TREHAME WADE (1948-   )

Dr. Wade well illustrates the prolonged and variable training of modern medical academicians. Following 4-year stints at Pembroke College, Cambridge (M.A., M.B., and B.Chir., 1973) and the St. Thomas Hospital and Medical School, London

(M.R.C.P., 1976), he served in over a dozen posts that gave him postgraduate training in neurology, neurosurgery, psychiatry, general medicine, and general practice. This extended from 1973 to 1985, when he obtained his M.D. degree from Oxford. His M.D. thesis concerned an assessment of domiciliary care for acute stroke (27).

His appointments at Oxford are as lecturer in clinical neurology and consultant in neurological disabilities. He has considerable clinical responsibilities at both the Rivermead Rehabilitation Center, Radcliffe Infirmary Unit, Oxford, and the in- and outpatient units of the Richie Russell House, Churchill Hospital Unit.

In addition to a dozen chapters in books that deal with all aspects of stroke, their medical care, and rehabilitation, he has authored or co-authored six books on the subject. He has published nearly 50 original articles on stroke involving research and more than a dozen review articles, again covering a wide spectrum of interests on stroke and its treatment. He has been particularly interested in the rehabilitation of poststroke patients and methods of evaluating the various forms of disability caused by stroke (28). He also wrote several articles on visuospatial neglect (29).

Beyond his heavy clinical, teaching, research, and service duties, he is an associate editor of *Clinical Rehabilitation* and referee for five other neurological journals. He serves in important capacities to six organizations and was a founding member of two of them. His commitment to the problems of stroke, in both its clinical and research aspects, are impressive, as are his interests in rehabilitation. Considering his extensive background and dedication to the problems of stroke and rehabilitation, it would be difficult to find a better representative of this important field.

OLLE HÖÖK (1918-   )

One could go on almost endlessly with those who have illustrated the many aspects of neurorehabilitation, but I will end with Olle Höök, who so successfully exemplifies many of its expanded facets in the flowering period of neurology.

Höök's background is unusual in several respects. One grandfather was a member of the Swedish Parliament, and he married Kerstin Lundevall, the daughter of a member of the Swedish Supreme Court, who became a professor of psychiatry in her own right. Raised in Uppsala, he has spent his active career in Stockholm and Göteborg.

Primarily, Höök was a neurologist, trained in the Karolinska Institute, where he rose to be assistant professor of neurology at the Serafirmerlasarettet (1957 to 1963). Bit by bit, his interests in neurorehabilitation increased, and he was made head of the department of neurological rehabilitation at the Karolinska Hospital, Stockholm, in 1963. It was at this time he came to work with me and completed an interesting neurophysiological study (30).

Höök's rehabilitative interests were greatly intensified when, in 1966, he was promoted to be professor and chair of the Institute of Rehabilitative Medicine at the University of Göteborg, Sweden. This was the first rehabilitative institute in Sweden, and he headed it for 17 years until retirement in 1983. His partial bibliography (to 1981) includes 15 articles on tetraplegia and spinal cord injuries and 12 on technical aids for rehabilitation. His other reports have included studies on head injuries, speech problems, stroke, and patient motivation with a total of some 250 articles, reviews, and addresses pertaining to the subject of rehabilitation. A few of his more notable articles in English involved "Motivation—some concepts" (4), "Organization of medical resources for rehabilitation in neurological disease" (31), "Rehabilitation" in the Handbook of Clinical Neurology (32), "Economics and epidemiology of workplace injuries" (33), and "Head injury: Integrated rehabilitation approach: Optimal adaptation to disability" (34). He founded the Scandinavian Journal of Rehabilitative Medicine in 1968 and served as its Chief Editor for over a quarter of a century,

Since 1974, his activities have expanded on an international scale, when he became a member of the Executive Committee of the International Rehabilitation Association and also a member of the Executive Committee, Research Group of Neurology Rehabilitation of the World Federation of Neurology. He also has served as a member of the Advisory Board of the United States National Aphasia Association since 1987. Several international assignments have followed, and he has been an invited lecturer in several European and other countries.

One of his main side activities has been the Royal Scandinavian Air Force, in which he was a consultant in neurology from 1953 to 1970. Since 1966, he has also served as a member of the Medical Science Council of the Swedish Civil Board of Aviation.

Many other national appointments have been fulfilled, including the Swedish Insurance Court, the National Board of Health, and the Medical Board of the Armed Forces. He has headed all of the Swedish organizations in his field and, in addition, was Chairman of the Swedish Neurological Society.

Following retirement, the Hööks have returned to their ancestral home in Uppsala, and Dr. Höök works out of his office of the Scandinavian rehabilitation journal in the Department of Rehabilitative Medicine, Uppsala University. Steeped in the background of all phases of neurorehabilitation, he is a modern version of Howard Rusk in his promotion of all aspects of rehabilitation, and this has been greatly implemented by his editorship of the Scandinavian Journal of Rehabilitative Medicine. Beyond all this, he has trained a whole generation of leaders in rehabilitation and has edited or co-authored 20 books on the subject. His approach, supported by solid experience, has been comprehensive, ranging from physiotherapy, basic physiological studies of muscle activity, injuries of the head and spinal cord, stroke, speech disabilities, and occupational rehabilitation to organizational, economic, and social studies, studies of patient morale, and their psychological reactions. His impact on Scandinavian and international rehabilitation has been enormous, and he is optimistic that the political and bureaucratic problems of this vast discipline can slowly be ironed out. This has included neurologic and public recognition of the rights and economic desirability of rehabilitation for the disabled. Recently, in the United States, this culminated in the "Americans with Disabilities" Act. How effective this governmental act proves remains to be seen, but there is no doubt about the strong tide of understanding initiated by Dr. Rusk and sustained by Höök and many others since World War II.

SUMMARY

Neurological rehabilitation is a hodgepodge of many medical and paramedical groups, which must be skillfully integrated, if the disabled patients are to be motivated and enabled to achieve their optimal recovery. The ideals of the discipline are superb, and practical results have been good, when not bogged down by bureaucratic interests, politics, and the poor cooperation of multiple specialties, as so often is required in serious disabilities. Using the experience of Sedgwick Mead, some of these problems were considered.

Neurorehabilitation constitutes the most important and difficult phase of rehabilitation and has developed in the flowering period of neurology as scientific advances have made this possible. Although the discipline defies simplistic description, some of its principal facets have been illustrated by the careers of a few of its leaders, who have made outstanding contributions in their efforts to develop and improve the field.

As shown by the skillful entrepreneur, Howard Rusk, rehabilitation also requires the understanding and concerted support of society. Earlier fragmented medical efforts had failed. By taking advantage of the conditions during and following World War II, Rusk was eminently successful. Guttmann accomplished much the same thing in Great Britain with his rehabilitation of previously hopeless spinal cord injuries. At the same time, Inman was advancing the scientific aspects of the field by his studies on prostheses, locomotion, skeletal pain, and others.

More recently, notable advances have been made by Jannett on head injuries and by Wade on stroke problems. Olle Höök, the head of the first rehabilitation institute in Sweden has continued these efforts. His comprehensive approach has been successful in advancing both the scientific and social aspects of rehabilitation. These advances, his training program, and the Scandinavian Journal of Rehabilitative Medicine have achieved recognition on an international scale.

REFERENCES

1. Cooke, E.V. How did you die. In: Markham, E. (ed.) *The Best Loved Poems of the American People*. Garden City, NY, Garden City Books, 1936, p. 118.
2. Hanks, N.C. *Up from the Hills*. Chicago, Hammond Press, 1921.
3. Rusk, H. *A World to Care For*. New York, Random House and The Reader's Digest Association, 1977.
4. Esbjörnsson, E., and Höök, O. Motivation—some concepts. Scand. J. Rehabil. Med., 10: (suppl 6):114-126, 1978.
5. Kurtzke, J.F. *Mortality and morbidity data on epilepsy*. In: Alter, M., and Hauser, W.A. (eds.). The Epidemiology of Epilepsy: A Workshop. Bethesda, MD, Department of Health, Education, and Welfare, 1972. Publication no. 73-340.
6. Sarno, M.T., ed. *Acquired Aphasia*. 2nd ed. San Diego, Academic Press, 1991.
7. Eberhart, H.D., Elftman, H., and Inman, V.T. *The Locomotor Mechanism of the Amputee*. In: Klopsteg, P.E., Wilson, P.D., et al. (eds), Human Limbs and their Substitutes. New York, McGrawHill, 1954, pp. 472-480. revised 1968.
8. Kellgren, J.H. On the distribution of pain arising from deep somatic structures with charts of segmental pain areas. *Clin. Sci.*, 4:35-46, 1936.
9. Inman, V., and Saunders, J.B. de C.M. Referred pain from skeletal structures. *J. Nerv. Ment. Dis.*, 99:660-667, 1944.

10. Aird, R.B., et al. Symposiums on pain: I. Basic concepts. *Calif. Med.*, 86:289, 1957.

10a. Aird, R.B., et al. Symposiums on pain: II. Pain in clinical medicine. *Calif. Med.*, 86:357, 1957.

10b. Aird, R.B., et al. Symposiums on pain: III. Headache problems. *Calif. Med.*, 87:12, 1957.

11. Whitteridge, D. Ludwig Guttmann. London, The Royal Society, 1970.

12. Bumke, O., and Foerster, O. Handbuch der Neurologie. Berlin, *Springer-Verlag*, 1936, vol. 5, pp. 1-403, vol. 8, pp. 316-414.

13. Guttmann, L. Study on sweat disturbances in peripheral nerve lesions. *J. Neurol. Psychiatry*, 3:197-210, 1940.

14. Guttmann, E., and Guttmann, L. The effect of galvanic exercise and reinervated muscles in the rabbit. *J. Neurol. Neurosurg. Psychiatry.* 71:7-17, 1944.

15. Guttmann, L. Rehabilitation after injuries to the central nervous system. *Proc. R. Soc. Med.*,35:305, 1942.

16. Guttmann, L. Spinal Cord Injuries: Comprehensive Management and Research. 2nd ed. Oxford, Blackwell, 1976.

17. Jannett, W.B. Late epilepsy after blunt head injuries: a clinical study based on 282 cases of traumatic epilepsy. Assoc. R. Coll. *Surg. Engl.*, 29:370-384, 1961.

18. Miller, J.D., and Jennett, B. *Surg. Neurol.*, 10:213-215, 1978.

19. Jannett, W.B., Harper, A M., and Gillespie, F.C. Measurement of regional cerebral blood flow during carotid ligation. *Lancet,* 2:1162-1163, 1968.

20. Jannett, W.B., Barker, J., Fitch, W., and McDowall, D.G. Effect of anesthesia on intracranial pressure in patients with space-occupying lesions. *Lancet*, 1:61-64, 1969.

21. Jennett, B., Teasdale, G., Braakman, R., Minderhoud, J., Heiden, J., and Kurze, T. Prognosis of patients with severe head injury. *Neurosurgery*, 4:283-289, 1979.

22. Jannett, B., and Plum, F. Persistent vegetative state after brain damage. A syndrome in search of a name. *Lancet*, 1:734-737, 1972.

23. Jannett, B., Miller, J.D., and Braakmann, R. Epilepsy after non-missilic depressed skull fracture. *J. Neurosurg.*, 41:208-214, 1974.

24. Jannett, B. High technology medicine and quality of life. J. Technol. Assess. *Health Care*, 3:51-60, 1987.

25. Jannett, B. *High Technology Medicine, Benefits and Burdens.* 2nd ed. Oxford, Oxford University Press, 1986.

26. Jennett, W.B. *An Introduction to Neurosurgery.* 4th ed. London, W. Heinemann Medical Books, 1983.

27. Wade, D.T. *An Assessment of Domiciliary Care for Acute Stroke.* M.D. thesis, Cambridge University, 1985.

28. Collen, F.M., Wade, D.T. Robb, G.F., and Bradshaw, C.M. The Rivermead Mobility Index: a further development of the Rivermead Motor Assessment. Int. Disabil. Studies, 13:50-54, 1991.

29. Halligan, P.W., Burn, J.P., Marshall, K., and Wade, D.T. Visuospatial neglect: qualitative differences and laterality of cerebral lesion. *J. Neurol. Neurosurg. Psychiatry*, 55:1060-1068, 1992.

30. Höök, O., Rubinstein, M., and Aird, R.B. Relation of blood pH and CO2 to central stimulatory effects of saline on dogs. *Am. J. Physiol.*, 205:723-726, 1963.

31. Höök, O., Organization of medical resources for rehabilitation in neurological disease. Scand. J. Rehabil. Med., 4:137-139, 1972.

32. Höök, O. *Rehabilitation: Part II. Injuries of the brain and skull.* In: Vinken, P.J., and Bryun, C.W. Handbook of Clinical Neurology. vol. 35. Amsterdam, Elsner Press, 1976, pp. 683-697.

33. Höök, O. *Economics and epidemiology of workplace injuries.* In: Ferrara, F., and Nordin, M. (eds.). Proceedings of the First International Conference on Injuries in the Workplace. New York, NY, World Rehab. FI,1984.

34. Höök, O. Head injury: integrated rehabilitation approach: optimal adaptation to disability. In: *Advances in Neurological Rehabilitation and Restorative Neurology.* O. Höök and M.R. Dimitrijerk (eds.) Uppsala, Sweden, Almqvist & Wicksell Tyckeri 1988.

Infectious Processes
of the Nervous System

The antibiotic therapy of bacterial infectious disorders of the nervous system reached its peak in the flowering period of neurology, which justifies its inclusion in this account. However, revolutionary changes in our understanding of certain delayed infectious diseases (for example, scrapie, kuru, and Creutzfeldt-Jakob disease) have occurred more recently. Because of the latency of these diseases, plus their relationship to genetic and novel replication processes, they have been placed in this "continuing" phase of neurological research. By providing background data, the necessary antecedents of this on-going aspect of the neuroinfectious processes can be covered.

BACKGROUND

The story of the sulfa drugs and antibiotics is so well known that it may seem redundant to review it. However, few seem to remember that there was a gap of 12 years between the original observation of Alexander Fleming on the bacteriocidal effect of penicillin in 1928 and its purification to a practical form in clinical trials at Oxford by Howard Florey and Ernst Chain in 1940 to 1941. They all shared in the Nobel prize of 1947; Fleming and Florey were knighted.

Again, how many remember the discoverer of the sulfa drugs? Gerhard Demagh, a German bacteriologist, reported the chemotherapeutic effect of prontosil, a sulfanilamide agent, on streptococci in 1935. He was awarded the Nobel prize in 1939 but was not permitted to accept it by the Nazi regime. Hitler was on the move, and World War II was so imminent that it disrupted the International Congress of Neurology in Copenhagen in September of that year.

The real story in retrospect, however, was the effect of these bacteriocidal agents on the world's population. The old mortality figures were greatest in pneumonia— 20% to 25% of patients diagnosed with pneumonia died. The sulfa drugs reduced this to 5%, and later, penicillin reduced this figure to under 1%. Similar spectacular results were obtained in other infectious disorders, including those of the nervous system, as a result of which the population explosion took off. Although the bacteriocidal agents were introduced only one-half century ago, along with improved public health measures, they have already transformed our world. From a population of approximately 2.2 billions in 1945, we are now contending with more than double that number. Famine now threatens the peoples of Africa and Asia. Wasteful and careless economic exploitation is despoiling the world's resources of fertile topsoil, forests, and animal wildlife. The ecological balance of the earth is now threatened by human pollution of its streams, seas, and skies. Major adjustments must be made within the next few decades. If science can develop an effective method of avoiding conception, as well as greatly accelerating food production, an ecological balance to ensure a habitable world may still be possible (1-1b).

This is a poor introduction to the heroes of medical science, who have achieved miracles of disease control. There was no way that they could foresee the astonishing magnitude of population growth and its secondary effects, famine and ecological disaster. While few want to forgo the gains of science, which now underlie almost every facet of our modern civilization, many, ignorant of the appalling conditions of life two centuries ago, have developed a false nostalgia, which finds expression among religious conservatives and antiintellectual groups. Social and religious mores change slowly, as they are passed from parent to child. The effects of science, on the other hand, have progressed more rapidly and, in the case of the population growth, are approaching crisis proportions. Necessary adjustments may well have secondary effects on all aspects of our social, economic, and political lives. Because the advances of science have not been curbed for long in the past century, it seems likely that the only possible solution will be more science.

Like Fleming, those who have pursued and extended the life-saving measures in the case of the nervous system have been superb individuals. Their praiseworthy efforts have been in the finest tradition of medical science and should not now be condemned because of the secondary effects of their great successes, which have become apparent only within the last decade or so. As indicated, the solution, if there is a solution, will be in terms of more science and education.

Infectious processes, such as parasites, fungi, and viruses, have not responded to the bacteriocidal agents, and more recently, viroids and prions have been discovered. Among those I have known who have worked in this field, Hans Zinsser, Karl Meyer, Wendel Stanley, Ernest Jawetz, Carleton Gajdusek, and Stanley Prusiner have been outstanding and will serve to illustrate different phases of the field of the infectious disorders. Innumerable others might have been selected because this has been a field of intense activity over the past half century. As in other specialty fields, the control of infectious processes has had dramatic effects in the case of the nervous system, and this can be demonstrated by the few men that I have selected.

HANS ZINSSER (1878-1940)

The story of Zinsser has been included in this section to illustrate the application of early microbiological research to human disease. He was a well-trained physician who, in the early decades of the 20th century, turned to bacteriology and, because of his success in bridging the gap between bacteriology and clinical medicine, became a noted public figure and professor of bacteriology at Columbia, Stanford, and Harvard. He was a transitional figure in one sense but clearly overlapped into the period of the flowering of neurology.

His college and medical training were at Columbia, where he served a 2-year internship at Roosevelt Hospital from 1903 to 1905. However, his interests in bacteriology had already developed, and he served as a bacteriologist at Roosevelt Hospital and as an assistant bacteriologist at the College of Physicians and Surgeons at Columbia.

From 1905 to 1908, he started private medical practice but still maintained his bacteriological connections at Roosevelt Hospital and Columbia. During this period, he also published with Dr. Philip Hiss the first edition of their *A Textbook of Bacteriology* in 1910 (2). When offered an instructorship of bacteriology at Columbia in 1908, he gave up his private practice. In 1913, he accepted an appointment at Stanford University as associate professor of bacteriology, a great jump academically. As President David Star Jordan of Stanford described him at that time, he was "a live wire" and "probably would go further than the others considered for the position" (3). His career well bears this out.

Before World War I, his studies were chiefly on immunology, anaphylaxis, and antibodies. He published two books, *Infection and Resistance* in 1914 and *A Laboratory Course in Serum Study* in 1916. His interest in typhus was kindled when, in 1915, he served as a member of the American Red Cross Sanitary Commission to Serbia and again, in 1917 to 1919, as an officer in the Medical Corps of the United States Army. Still later (1923), as a representative of the League of Red Cross Societies, he encountered epidemic typhus in Russia. His war record was distinguished, and he rose to the rank of colonel in 1918. During this period, he served with the American expeditionary Force in France and, after the war, was awarded the Distinguished Service Medal.

Dr. Zinsser was at his peak at Harvard and this was when I, as a student, had the good fortune of knowing him. He has been described as "exceptionally energetic and alert," and this was the impression he gave us students. If physical activity enhances good health, Zinsser must have been "in the pink." Energetic walking seemed to be a stimulus to his energetic lecturing or, more likely, a secondary offshoot from his "geared-up" state. Certainly, he had no cervical arthritis as he turned his head from side to side to face the audience while striding back and forth in the pit of the auditorium. Several of us jokingly estimated the distance he traversed in his lectures. The methods of estimation varied considerably, as did their results (from 1 to 3 miles), but I have always believed that the lower figure was probably the more accurate.

Immunological research was one of Zinsser's main interests. However, his research was by no means limited to immunology. He was widely known for his research on typhus, a rickettsial infection that involves severe and diffuse damage to the cerebrovascular system and brain. He became interested in this as a result of the epidemics previously mentioned and returned to the study of typhus in 1930. He and his collaborators developed techniques for the culture of the rickettsia and vaccines to control it. Different forms of typhus and its mode of transmission complicated the study. Much of the early basic work on typhus was done by Zinsser and his group. One of Zinsser's best known books was *Rats, Lice and History.*

In addition, his studies on herpes encephalitis and syphilis were notable, as was his concept of the pathogenesis of sensitizing, toxic agents that were elaborated in bacterial and other infectious foci. In this category, he believed that the widespread effects of streptococci caused rheumatic fever.

Of his 185 articles, 75 dealt with immunology and over 45 involved other scientific subjects. Nearly 30 were on educational and other nonmedical subjects. Most of his books concerned the problems of immunity, and three were texts of bacteriology (two with Hiss and one with Bayne-Jones).

Zinsser was involved in innumerable activities. He was on many committees and boards, including the editorial boards of five scientific and medical journals. He was a member of 36 scientific societies, of which he was president of 3. He received honorary degrees from five universities and four honorary decorations or awards. Considering the inflation of honorary awards since his day, this list might have been tripled in more recent years.

His personal life is revealed in his book "As I Remember Him," and the best biographical sketches were written by J. Howard Mueller and S. Burt Wolbach (4-6). His poetry should be mentioned in this connection. Under the anonymous title "R.S.," he published poems from time to time; these were collected in the volume *Spring, Summer and Autumn* (7). Although not a connoisseur of poetry, I have heard his poetry highly praised, most recently by a lay neighbor. His writings on education were also notable, which conveyed his conviction that education in science should rank high along with instruction in the humanities.

Few people have equaled Hans Zinsser in his great abilities, his remarkable memory, his fascinating teaching, his research, and the wide diversity of his interests. His brilliance and appealing personality were widely recognized, and this was especially true among his colleagues and students.

KARL F. MEYER (1884-1974)

Except for his honorary degree, Karl Meyer was not even a doctor of medicine, let alone a neurologist. Nevertheless, he represents an aspect of infectious diseases that was of importance to neurology and medicine in general and that should be included in this series of essays. Although not heralded in neurological circles, he was one of the greatest men that I have had the pleasure of knowing. Experts have ranked him along with Theobold Smith as one of the top "microbe hunters" (8).

Because my research facilities at the University of California, San Francisco (UCSF), were immediately adjacent to the Hooper Foundation building, of which he was the director, I came to know Dr. Meyer quite well over a period of some 40 years. Although we both were very busy in our respective orbits of activity, research and university committee assignments provided occasional contacts, in addition to endless greetings and brief exchanges in the halls. I have always been grateful to Karl Meyer for his help in many ways.

My summary of Meyer's contributions to infectious processes of neurological interest will necessarily be highly selective. His curriculum vitae, which covers his training, posts, activities, and honors, involves seven pages that merely list all the items. Perhaps his accomplishments, as summarized in the Lasker Award by the American Public Health Association in 1951, will convey the gist necessary for the purpose of this essay.

Brilliant scientist, dynamic teacher, inspired humanitarian, his influence now extends over two generations of students of medicine, biology and the allied health sciences. His research and leadership have benefitted all classes of people for four generations (9).

Paul de Kruif, the author of *The Microbe Hunters* has described Meyer as a "champion among microbe hunters " (8).

Students for 30 years at Berkeley and UCSF would be unanimous in their description of Meyer's unique teaching and dynamics. His lectures were carefully prepared and presented with great gusto. He hypnotized the students with his vast knowledge, laced with intriguing side comments, and all aimed at providing them with a solid background of the goals of microbiology, its techniques, problems, and accomplishments. According to report, his lectures extended for a minimum of 2 hours and, often, were much longer. His explosive delivery caused all students to sit three or four seats from the front row; as an expert on bacterial transmission, Meyer never resented this.

He was a rebel to old world authoritarian ways, too brusque for the ultrapolite scientific exchange of Philadelphia, but as he mellowed, he found a receptive and challenging career in California. Simon Flexner had warned him while he was still at the University of Pennsylvania, "If you go to California, you will disappear in the Pacific Ocean, because the intelligentsia of the U.S. lives within a hundred miles from New York" (9). This expressed the provincial opinion of Eastern people in the early 19th century, and only was outmatched by the early Bostonians, who thought the West started shortly beyond the Hudson River. However, Flexner had a point in the sense of the scientific and public recognition of the time. The West was not fully recognized until the period of World War II, when Lawrence and his cyclotron made history in helping to develop the atom bomb. In much the same way, the East had suffered a lack of recognition in Europe in the first decade or so of the 20th century, judging by the Nobel prize awards. This may have been another factor that determined the limited recognition of Walter Cannon in the East and, later, of Herbert Evans and Karl Meyer in the West. On the other hand, from the standpoint of opportunities to do good research and accomplish something in his chosen field, Flexnor could not have been more incorrect. Because this was what Meyer was interested in, he went against Flexnor's advice and found his bright niche in the far West.

The bare facts of Meyer's background are as follows. He was born in Basel, Switzerland, and trained in the classic *Swiss gymnasium* of the 19th century. He later attended the Universities of Basel, Zurich, Munich, and Bern. His rebellious and yet creative spirit was shown at Bern in his exchange with Professor Paul Langerhans, who discovered the islets of Langerhans. Meyer had requested a few feet of laboratory space for his microtome, paraffin oven, and so forth, but Langerhans refused to accommodate him. Shortly thereafter, he watched Langerhans do an autopsy on a child with a tumor of the jaw. Meyer suspected a teratoma, and when Langerhans's attention was diverted, Meyer "snitched" a bit of the tumor. His beautifully stained section, which confirmed Langerhans's diagnosis, so impressed Langerhans that he changed his position and gave Meyer the space he needed. Later, he recommended Meyer to Professor William Kolle, a former assistant to Robert Koch and then the head of the Institute for Infectious Diseases in Bern. It was there that Meyer did his doctoral thesis, granted in veterinary medicine by the University of Zurich in 1909.

Professor Kolle advised Meyer to pursue an academic career and found him a position as a pathologist in a new institution in South Africa. In addition to his routine work, Meyer accomplished much research in the evenings. However, he soon ran into the autocratic rule of Arnold Theiler, the Director of the Institute, and he returned to Basel in 1910 when his 2-year contract ended. Through a friendly Swiss ambassador to Austria, Meyer soon obtained an assistant professorship of pathology and bacteriology in the School of Medicine at the University of Pennsylvania.

Meyer's period in Philadelphia was a stormy one. As he expressed it himself, "...I was darned critical; I had too sharp a tongue and I never cloaked anything in a lot of praises when I knew perfectly that the work which was done was a five-cent kind of hash piece. That they didn't like." (10). However, Meyer found some friends, such as Frederick Novy, the brilliant microbiologist of the University of Michigan, and Theobold Smith, professor of comparative pathology at Harvard, who greatly impressed Meyer. Dr. Richard Pearce of the University of Pennsylvania advised Meyer to go to California where Pearce had heard of an opening in a new Institute for Medical Research, the Hooper Foundation at UCSF.

His brilliant lectures as Professor of Bacteriology in California soon attracted 286 students, but with laboratory space for only 65 students, shifts in the laboratory had to be arranged to manage this impasse. According to Professor Horstmann, Professor of Epidemiology and Pediatrics at the Yale School of Medicine, who had been a student under Meyer, "The lectures started on Fridays at 1 p.m. and ended anytime between 4 and 6 p.m. But he was always interesting to listen to—and gave scholarly yet colorful lectures. Their main impact for me was due to his tremendous knowledge of pathology and pathogenesis. It was this that stimulated my interest in infectious diseases, and directed my course from then on. I owe Dr. Meyer a great deal" (9). On occasion, his lectures ended with a burst of applause from the students.

In 1914, Dr. George Whipple, the new Director of the Hooper Foundation in San Francisco and later Nobel Laureate in medicine, invited Meyer to join his staff as associate professor of tropical medicine in charge of the section on infectious diseases and immunology. Because this provided him with more time and better facilities for research, Meyer accepted. However, he still continued his teaching three or four times per week in Berkeley, where he retained his title of professor of experimental pathology until his retirement 40 years later.

As professor of tropical medicine and, later, professor of bacteriology, Meyer organized the Department of Bacteriology at the Medical School, UCSF, and launched into his brilliant research career on typhoid, brucellosis, botulism, plague, ornithosis, and Western equine encephalitis. When Whipple departed in 1921 to organize the new medical school at the University of Rochester, Meyer was made acting director of the Hooper Foundation and, in 1924, became its director. His activities in public health soon involved the whole state and beyond. It was to this aspect of his career that the words of Paul de Kruif applied. One episode related to encephalitis will serve to illustrate his activities beyond the laboratory and give some flavor of the critical thinking of a decisive scientist.

In the summer of 1930, many horses in the San Joaquin Valley were reported to be dying of botulism. Meyer, suspicious of this diagnosis (because botulism does not occur in the summer), investigated and found that the horses had encephalitis. At the same time, human cases of so-called "poliomyelitis" were being reported, whose symptoms were suggestive of encephalitis. When inoculated suspensions in horses and rabbits failed to produce infections, Meyer decided that he must try inoculations from fresh specimens, rather than from the brains of animals long dead. However, by late October, the horse epidemic was waning. When Meyer got wind of a horse that was ill with the typical findings, he took action. Unfortunately, the farmer was opposed to selling his horse and had warned "I won't sell the horse, and if you do anything to this horse, I shoot you." Meyer, armed with a 20-dollar bill, managed to talk with the farmer's wife while the farmer was engaged by his associates. His account of the episode went as follows (10).

Meyer, "Look here, this horse is going to die anyhow; and when it's dead you haven't anything. It just goes to the rendering plant and you get a couple of dollars. On the other hand, you see, you could contribute to the knowledge of what this is and perhaps to its prevention."

Housewife, "Well my husband is just irate about this."

Meyer, "Yes, I can readily understand, but look here, suppose I trust you, and I give you $20 and the next morning you will find in the back yard the horse without a head?"

Housewife, "How are you going to do that?"

Meyer, "Look here, about nine o'clock at night when it is dark, I'll be over here behind some bushes...(where) I can see the window of your house. When your husband is sound asleep, you lift up the shade."

Meyer's account followed: "...sure enough about twenty minutes past nine the shade went up. Within about two minutes I was over the fence and in another two minutes the strychnine was under the skin of the horse and in another two or three minutes, the horse went down, and in another five minutes the head was off."

A careful dissection of the brain followed under flashlight in an abandoned chicken coop at some distance, and Meyer was on his way home by midnight.

Suspensions of the brain material were prepared in his laboratory starting about 6:30 a.m. He then went to Berkeley and, by 10 a.m., had made two inoculations into horses, mice, guinea pigs, and monkeys (10). "This gave us the virus."

This was the Western equine encephalitis virus, which later was shown to be the virus that caused the human encephalitis. When an epidemic of human encephalitis hit St. Louis in 1933, Meyer went there, and the same techniques he had developed in California were employed for the St. Louis virus. Later, a similar technique was employed for the virus of human Japanese B encephalitis in monkeys and mice.

Meyer had suspected transmission by mosquito. The intricate ecological cycle and proof of this for both the Western equine encephalitis and the St. Louis encephalitis were entrusted to Dr. William McDowell Hammon, an entomologist, and Dr. William C. Reeves, whom he brought to the Hooper Foundation for this purpose because he had become deeply involved and committed by that time to his studies on psittacosis and sylvatic plague. Hammon and Reeves were eminently successful, and each at a later date served as Dean of the School of Public Health of the University of California, Berkeley.

Because of his background, few scientists have been better prepared than Karl F. Meyer to unravel the complicated interrelationships between humans, domestic animals, wildlife, and the entomological aspects of the environment. This background, combined with his great drive and critical thinking, explain the brilliant results he achieved, several aspects of which were important to neurology. It was Meyers's employment of the new techniques of microbiology and his development of still newer techniques that made possible the very considerable advances he accomplished. Meyer was later involved in extensive studies on the therapeutic effects of the new antibiotics and prophylactic immunization of plague, psittacosis, and brucellosis (11-13). Following his official retirement in 1954, he carried on with his research for another 20 years, his last article appearing in 1975.

There is little to add to what has already been said about this remarkable man. His early brusqueness had certainly mellowed by the time I knew him in the 1930s. It is true that he brooked no nonsense, was demanding of his graduate students, and was feared by the incompetent. He was respected and admired for his vast knowledge, abilities, and accomplishments. To me, he was a good friend, who went out of his way to help me.

Microbiology with "KF" was always intense and interesting and, at times, could be exciting and stressful. On reviewing the notes and comments in his old file at UCSF, which were made by many distinguished doctors and scientists who formerly worked with him, it is obvious that their experiences with him were the most rewarding and often the crucial, determining influences of their careers.

WENDELL MEREDITH STANLEY (1904-1971)

Dr. Stanley has been included in this account, not only because of his basic studies on viruses, for which he won the Nobel prize in 1946, but also to illustrate the importance of technological advances in achieving scientific progress. Stanley was quick to exploit the latest techniques, and because of his background of training in biochemistry and biophysics, he was able to do this very successfully. However, like all the other physicians and medical scientists selected for these essays, Stanley was far more than a technician. His creative research abilities were matched by his skills of interpersonal relations, which made him a proficient ambassador for science on television.

Born in Indiana, he took his early training there and obtained his B.S. degree from Earlham College in 1926. He transferred to the University of Illinois at Urbana and received his M.S. and Ph.D. degrees after 3 more years. At Urbana, he worked closely with Professor Roger Adams, and from 1927 to 1933, they published 12 articles dealing mainly with the stereochemistry of bacteria.

His career had started at the University of Illinois as a research associate and instructor, where he spent an additional year. He then obtained a fellowship from the National Research Council for 1 year in Munich, Germany, and for the next 17 years, he served in various capacities with the Rockefeller Institute. He started as an assistant with the institute in New York City and then in the institute at Princeton, where he worked up to be a member by 1940.

His celebrated studies on tobacco mosaic virus started at Princeton; he reported obtaining the crystalline form of the virus in 1935 (14). He demonstrated that it had the properties of a molecule rather than a living organism. Forty-three articles were published on this subject between 1934 and 1946 (when he won the the Nobel prize) (15). Another major subject of research was the influenza virus, on which he published 12 articles in the 1940s. He purified the virus and produced an effective vaccine against it (16).

In 1948, he accepted a professorship of biochemistry and directorship of a new virus laboratory at the University of California, Berkeley. Hundreds of students and postgraduate fellows received their training in the virology laboratory, and Stanley became noted for the guidance and inspiration he gave while still allowing great freedom in the research of the graduate students on bacterial, plant, and animal viruses. He was chairman of the Department of Biochemistry until 1953. A separate Department of Virology was established for him in 1958, which he chaired until 1964 when it was expanded to establish the Department of Molecular Biology.

Stanley's research interests in Berkeley concerned the crystallization and characterization of the poliomyelitis virus and the determination of the complete 158-amino acid sequence of the tobacco mosaic virus protein (17,18). In addition, he wrote 19 articles on the relationship of viruses to cancer and, for this, won two prizes from the American Cancer Society. In 1970, he was made President of the 10th International Cancer Congress.

Stanley became somewhat of a celebrity on television. This had started while he was still at Princeton but was greatly extended in Berkeley. His video efforts culminated in a series of lectures and demonstrations on "Viruses and the Nature of Life" for educational television. These had an important impact on the understanding of the lay public for science, its objectives, and methods.

When his administrative role was reduced with the establishment of the Department of Molecular Biology in 1964, Stanley more vigorously assumed the role of a scientific statesman. He was a consultant to the National Institutes of Health (NIH) and appeared in Congressional hearings, which were effective in raising the standards of research and increasing the support for fundamental research.

Although I had met Stanley during the 1950s and had followed his career at Berkeley, it was not until the mid-1960s that I saw him in consultation as a patient for his neurological complications of diabetes. He was an excellent patient and bore his illness with great fortitude. I had the impression that, fundamentally, he was an optimist and carried on in his many efforts for science in spite of his difficulties.

His personal life was serene, thanks to Marian Jay Stanley, who had collaborated with him as a graduate student while at Urbana. His son, Wendell, Jr., followed him in biochemistry and molecular biology and became a professor on the Irvine campus of the University of California. His oldest daughter married a former student of mine, Dr. Robert Albo, who worked up to be a clinical professor of surgery in the East Bay as well as a very able and popular "magician" on the side.

The honors won by Dr. Stanley were numerous and prestigious. These included prizes, medals, lectureships, honorary memberships in many societies, and six honorary degrees.

Stanley achieved great success in three overlapping fields: his basic research on viruses, which included the virus of poliomyelitis; as an administrator of departments and the renowned Virus Laboratory with its research and teaching; and finally, as a distinguished scientific statesman, influencing both public education and governmental agencies.

The other notable thing about Stanley was his adaptation of all new scientific techniques to further his research. These included stereochemistry, crystallizing techniques, ultracentrifugation, electron microscopy, electrophoresis, and the chemical identification of amino acid sequences at the molecular level. He emphasized the importance of these for science in a book, and they were frequently mentioned in the titles of his articles (19). He exemplifies in full measure the thesis of these essays.

ERNEST JAWETZ (1916-   )

Jawetz was born in Vienna, but migrated with his family to America in the 1930s. His advanced training included a M.S. at the University of New Hampshire in 1940, a Ph.D. in microbiology at UCSF, and an M.D. from Stanford University School of Medicine in 1946. He served in the United States Army from 1943 to 1946 and was a senior assistant surgeon in the Public Health Service from 1946 to 1948.

He picked up prizes throughout his career, ranging from the Alpha Omega Alpha and Wolfson prizes at Stanford, the LeRoy Briggs Award for teaching excellence, and the Distinguished Faculty Teaching Award at UCSF to the American Representative of the 50th Anniversary of the Discovery of Penicillin at St. Mary's Hospital, London, in 1978, and the Flory Memorial Lectureship of the University of Adelaide, Australia, in 1981.

He participated in the meetings of seven scientific societies, was on the editorial boards of four journals dealing with infectious diseases and immunology, and was a consultant and member of five national boards or councils in his field.

His academic career was entirely in the School of Medicine, UCSF, where he rose from the assistant professorship of microbiology and lecturer in the Departments of Medicine and Pediatrics in 1945 to the professorship in 1953 and chair of the Department of Microbiology from 1962 to 1978, when he retired.

His bibliography contains 320 publications. Jawetz fortunately worked with Karl Meyer in the early 1940s and published ten articles with him on the problems of plague. By the late 1940s, and from then on, he had collaborators in ever-increasing numbers. His studies were of wide scope, involving essentially all the new antibiotics on different forms of bacterial infection. He was particularly interested in the synergism and antagonism of combined antibiotic therapy, which had important implications for all infections, including those of the nervous system (20-23). He was the Almroth Wright Lecturer on this subject in London in 1952 (24). Numerous articles were published on herpes simplex, a virus causing keratoconjunctivitis, the trachoma virus, and adenovirus 8 (25,26). He analyzed the infectious problems of the local blood bank and wrote several papers on the effect of adrenocorticotropin on infectious processes (27).

I have included this short sketch on Jawetz as an example of the many scores of bacteriologists, virologists, and immunologists that taught and did research in the flowering period of neurology. Jawetz was primarily a clinical microbiologist who worked closely with the clinicians dealing with infectious disorders. However, following his early work with Meyer, he continued to do some experimental research. He well illustrates the principal facets of research on the infectious diseases in the past few decades.

The story of microorganisms as the cause of disease has been a fascinating one, from the time of Pasteur and Robert Koch through the advancing research periods of bacteriology and virology. The story has been continued by Gajdusek and Prusiner as a result of their studies on the elusive causes of delayed infectious processes. It has been known for many years that such conditions existed, but the etiological factors involved and nature of the latent process remained unknown. This aspect of the infectious disorders has placed them in the continuing research category of the neurosciences.

D. CARLETON GAJDUSEK (1923-   )

The opening wedge of discovery came from an unsuspected source. D. Carleton Gajdusek, while on a trip in the South Pacific, heard of a strange disorder uniquely affecting a small, Stone Age people of the remote Eastern Highlands of New Guinea. This area had been placed under the administrative control of Australia following World War II and was opened up to missionaries, miners, and others only in 1957. The first report of kuru was made by Dr. Vincent Zigas, the medical officer stationed in the Eastern Highlands. He described kuru as "a form of encephalitis" among the Fore people. Gajdusek was in the area to conduct studies of child growth, development, and disease patterns in primitive cultures, but he joined the study of kuru under the enthusiastic influence of Dr. Zigas (28).

A viral origin was not corroborated by the usual techniques at the Hall Institute of Medical Research in Melbourne, Australia. The lack of fever, pleocytosis, and elevated protein in the cerebrospinal fluid of affected patients, plus the lack of perivascular cuffing or other evidence of an inflammatory reaction in their brains, also seemed to rule out an infectious process. Cannibalism had early been suspected as a probable source of infectious transmission, but the delayed onset and the process involved remained a puzzle.

Following the suggestion of Dr. William Hadlow of the Rocky Mountain Laboratory in 1959 that kuru had a similar pathology and had many features in common with scrapie (an infectious and chronic disease of sheep and goats), Gajdusek pursued this possibility (29). It was this background, which led to his central nervous system inoculation of primates and long-term observations, that finally, in 1966, demonstrated the latent infectious nature of kuru (30). This was the first human disease shown to be due to a "slow virus" infection with unusual features similar to the scrapie disease of sheep and goats.

Dr. Igor Klatzo had drawn Gajdusek's attention to the similarity of the neuropathology of kuru to that of Creutzfeldt-Jakob disease, and the latent transmission of this disease, similar to kuru and scrapie, was established in 1968 (30) (Jackson, E., personal communication, 1992). Creutzfeldt-Jakob disease is a rare, worldwide disorder of potential danger to surgeons, as in the case of my friend, Dr. Donald Matson, as discussed in Chapter 8. These studies have led to many others, including those of Dr. Stanley Prusiner, which now indicate that a protein is capable of both replication and infectiousness and, in addition, has genetic properties (see next section) (32-34). Dr. Gajdusek received the Nobel prize in 1976 (31).

The background of Dr. Gajdusek is almost as amazing as the story of his medical achievements (30). Born in Yonkers, New York, his father was a Slovak farm boy, who migrated to America and became a butcher in Yonkers. His mother was a first-generation American of Hungarian extraction with scholarly interests and attainments. A maternal aunt was an entomologist who stimulated Carleton's early training. By the age of 10, he aspired to an education in mathematics, physics, and chemistry in preparation for a career in medical science.

Carleton attended the University of Rochester from 1940 to 1943, where he graduated with a B.S. degree summa cum laude in biophysics. In 3 more years, he graduated from the Harvard Medical School, where he worked under Dr. John Edsall in protein physical chemistry and Dr. James Gamble of the Children's Hospital in his laboratory of electrolyte balance. Here, also, he turned to pediatrics and later did postgraduate work in this field.

In 1948 to 1949, he was a senior fellow in physical chemistry at the California Institute of Technology under Dr. Linus Pauling and others and made life-long friendships with this outstanding group. He returned to pediatrics at the Children's Hospital, Boston, and qualified in the American Board of Pediatrics in 1951. He also was a research fellow in pediatrics and infectious diseases under Dr. John Enders of Harvard during this period and up to 1952, when he was inducted into the Army and did viral and rickettsial disease studies under Dr. Joseph Smadel of the Walter Read Army Institute of Research. According to my friend, Elizabeth Jackson, it was Dr. Enders who early recognized Gajdusek's ability and arranged his military service under Dr. Joseph Smadel in the Walter Reed Army Medical Graduate Service. Because she worked under Dr. Smadel both in the Walter Reed setting and later when he transferred to the NIH as assistant director, she knew Gajdusek and had the opportunity of following his career (Jackson, E., personal communication, 1992).

Gajdusek's military assignment at Walter Reed involved virological research, and following this, he studied virus diseases in the Near East (Pasteur Institute of Teheran and also in Afghanistan and Turkey) and in the Hall Institute of Medical Research in Melbourne, Australia (1955 to 1957). In the meantime, Dr. Smadel had transferred to the National Institute of Neurological Disease and Blindness (NIND&B), and in 1958 with the blessing and protection of Dr. Richard Masland, director of the NIND&B, Gajdusek was given a new position for the study of child growth and development and disease patterns in primitive cultures. No doubt Dr. Smadel's support and Masland's interests in Gajdusek's appealing pediatric objective had much to do with this. Now, with a base that supplied excellent support, he initiated his studies on primitive youth, which centered mainly in the islands of the South Pacific and especially in New Guinea. This led to his contact with Dr. Zigas and to picking up the kuru project, as previously explained. With the support of both Drs. Smadel and Masland, he developed still another entity at the NIH. This involved the Laboratory of Slow, Latent and Temperate Virus Infection. According to Jackson, Gajdusek used her (Smadel's) laboratory at nights on his return from the South Pacific to get his project started. She felt that he was very fortunate to recruit Dr. Joseph Gibbs, who had also worked at Walter Reed, to run the new laboratory. It was this series of extraordinary and fortunate circumstances that led to his kuru inoculations on primates and long-term observations.

Several other aspects of Gajdusek's career deserve mention. His linguistic abilities almost exceeded his scientific skills. He can speak five European languages in addition to Neo-Melanesian and has a limited knowledge of several languages of Papua New Guinea and other Melanesian and Micronesian islands. Because of my own limitations in this respect, I have always been amazed at the abilities of those in central and eastern Europe to speak several languages. His exposure in early life to the polyglot of languages in his home and Yonkers probably aided this, but a genetic facility may also have fostered it. Certainly, this ability greatly helped in his work and later lectures and travels.

Gajdusek developed a "family" of 54 adopted children (30). This was an extraordinary sideline, which must have taken a great deal of time, energy, and financial support. Probably, his attraction to youth, training in pediatrics, and foreign study of human development contributed to this remarkable venture. A worthy, additional project for Dr. Gajdusek would be to record how he managed so many children, the training and education they received, and the results in terms of the children's careers in later life.

Gajdusek's scientific productivity was enormous. Including his publications, lectures, and other activities, some 1,100 articles have been published. His articles grew from an average of 18 publications per year from 1961 to 1976 to about 47 per year over the next 16 years. The secret of this probably involved Dr. C. J. Gibbs, Jr. as previously explained. Starting in 1964, Gibbs appeared as a co-author and, no doubt, assumed much of the load of research supervision and the operation of the laboratory. This, plus review articles and book chapters could explain the later great productivity of Gajdusek's unit. Multiple authorship was the rule and increased from an average of 2 to 3 in the early days of the laboratory to 6 or 7 later, the peak being 18 authors on one article in 1984. Usually, Gajdusek was listed last, but Gibbs also was the anchor man in many.

The number of lectures undertaken by Gajdusek is astounding (30). In the 7 years before he won the Nobel prize, he averaged seven lectures per year. In the 9 years after the Nobel prize, this jumped to an average of over 25, and from 1986 through 1991, the average was 47 per year.

I thought I was doing a considerable amount of work when I averaged 15 to 16 trips per year for lectures, meetings, and so forth, but this pales in comparison with the effort of Dr. Gajdusek. This can only be explained in terms of a well-organized team that functioned with limited supervision and a series of articles and lectures, which readily could be rescrambled in various forms. Such are the pressures exerted on Nobel laureates. We were favored by nine visits from him in the Bay Area, and when he came as the Hitchcock Professor at the University of California in Berkeley, he gave three lectures.

The honors received by Dr. Gajdusek are too numerous to list. He is a member of 31 societies (most of them honorary) and is on 22 boards and councils, again mostly honorary. These include the editorial boards of seven journals and three honorary professorships. In addition to his lecture invitations (over 1,000), he has received some 16 awards and prizes and honorary degrees from almost as many universities. His honors have come from essentially all parts of the world—their great numbers probably reflecting the novelty of his contributions on kuru and Creutzfeldt-Jakob disease.

STANLEY B. PRUSINER (1942-   )

Although the great majority of neurologists and neuroscientists selected to illustrate the various aspects of the flowering of neurology were active in the 1925 to 1975 period (and especially in the 1935 to 1965 decades), it must be understood that neurology is a rapidly advancing field and in no way is confined to a particular period. It is still flowering in such fields as neurogenetics, the delayed infectious processes, neurochemistry, and behavioral neurology. The delayed onset of several genetic, degenerative, and infectious conditions has long been known. Gajdusek opened the door in the case of kuru and Creutzfeldt-Jakob disease, and now, Prusiner is rapidly expanding it with respect to the underlying processes that are involved. This is a complex problem overlapping into several disciplines, including genetics, cell biology, and experimental neurology. Although trained in neurology, Prusiner is also a professor of biochemistry and has had to master biophysics, virology, microbiology, immunology, and neurogenetics as well. The story of Prusiner is particularly pertinent to the thesis of these essays and, especially, so to illustrate the continuing research aspects of neurology and the neurosciences.

Born and raised in the Midwest, Prusiner graduated from the University of

Pennsylvania cum laude and with such additional honors as Phi Beta Kappa and Alpha Epsilon Delta (premedical honor society). He then went through the University of Pennsylvania School of Medicine (1964 to 1968), graduating with the AOA and the Roy G. Williams Basic Science Research Award. Military service followed as a Research Associate, Lt. Commander, in the Public Health Service, NIH, National Heart and Lung Institute, Laboratory of Biochemistry, Section on Enzymes. With medical licensure in California, he obtained training in our Department of Neurology (UCSF) and was certified by the American Board of Psychiatry and Neurology in 1979.

Prusiner's research career started as a medical student, and by the time he graduated, he was a co-author of eight articles. This trend continued while he was in the Public Health Service. By 1968, his research involved metabolic and neurochemical work. Between 1970 and 1972, an additional seven or eight articles were published. His first on the scrapie agent was published in 1977, and further studies resulted in his development of the concept of prions by 1982 (32).

The background for Prusiner's concentration on the scrapie disease of sheep and goats is of considerable interest. Following the report of Klatzo, Gajdusek, and Zigas on the pathology of kuru, Dr. William Hadlow of the Rocky Mountain Laboratory had noted its close similarity to the pathology of scrapie and suggested kuru transmission to primates (29). As recorded in the previous section, Gajdusek accomplished this in 1966 and in 1968 showed that Creutzfeldt-Jakob disease was a similar delayed infectious disorder (30). The nature of the scrapie agent and its latent infectious process remained unknown. Gajdusek thought it was due to a "slow virus," but intense research failed to confirm this. It was to these problems that Prusiner devoted his research.

Because of the unprecedented aspects of Prusiner's studies and their complexities, a brief summary of the advances achieved by his research group is listed with a few key references.

1. The successful transmission of scrapie to hamsters provided a better animal model and greatly accelerated the rate of studies by reducing the latency period of infection (33).
2. The scrapie agent was shown to be a protein. Procedures that caused degradation of nucleic acid and genetic particles had no effect on its infectiousness. It was not a virus or viroid, as previously thought. It was inactivated by agents that alter proteins. To distinguish these features, Prusiner coined the term "prion" for the new agent (32,34).
3. The purification of the prion finally approximated 100%. With Dr. Leroy Hood, the amino acid sequence of the prion protein (PrP) was determined, and pieces of DNA were synthesized (34).
4. With Dr. Charles Weissmann, the synthetic DNA pieces were used to isolate a prion protein gene, which was coded by the genes of cells. This was in contrast to viruses, which are encoded by the genes that they carry. This study led to the unexpected discovery of the normal, cellular prion proteins found wide-

spread in the body but with the highest levels in brain tissue. Two forms of prion protein were established, PrP^{c} and PrP^{Sc} (35). Mass spectrometry and protein sequencing studies have shown that the cellular and scrapie prions are indistinguishable. Prusiner has theorized that modifications of the scrapie prion protein structure occur through altered folding, and this may account for its infectivity (36).

5. Further studies suggested that the scrapie protein is a component of the infectious prion protein.

   a. Scrapie protein infectivity was not blocked by degradation of nucleic acids or genetic material (37).

   b. A genetic linkage between the prion protein gene and incubation times of infection were established (38).

   c. PrPSc was found only in animals with scrapie and in humans with kuru, Creutzfeldt-Jakob disease, and Gerstmann-Sträussler syndrome (39).

   d. Antibodies to PrpPSc blocked its infectivity (40).

   e. Prpc was found to accumulate within cells and degraded relatively quickly. PrPSc accumulated within lysosomes and degraded slowly (41).

6. Scrapie prion proteins were found to aggregate into amyloid rods and plaques. This has stimulated much research because such plaques are found in Alzheimer disease (42).

7. Localization of PrP gene was made to the short arm of human chromosome 20 (43). Using genetic engineering techniques, Prusiner has conclusively identified the specific gene that produces mutant forms of the prion protein, which can be inherited and causes familial Creutzfeldt-Jakob disease among Libyan Jews and other people worldwide. The genetic transformation that produced the pathogenic prion was found to involve a single amino acid of the mutated prion protein.

Prusiner's research has stimulated great interest, and doubt has slowly changed to acceptance as the studies of his UCSF research group have been confirmed by other workers. Several other developments have added support, including the failure to identify a slow virus in kuru or Creutzfeldt-Jakob diseases. Nevertheless, he had a rough time during the early period of his scrapie studies. He, Hadlow, and their coworkers reported the brain tissue of Creutzfeldt-Jakob disease caused a scrapie-like encephalopathy in goats (44). Further studies showed that Prusiner's prions lacked nucleic acid, which the prevailing wisdom accepted as the exclusive carriers of genetic transmission. Viruses and gene particles were thought to be necessary for mutation, which proteins could not do. Accordingly, Prusiner's theory of prion pathogenicity was challenged as "unscientific." Prusiner remained undaunted, having shown that scrapie-infected brain material remained infectious after treatment to destroy the nucleic acids, which are the hereditary material of viruses (44). Scrapie-infected brain material lost its infectivity, however, when treated with reagents that destroyed proteins (36).

I was amazed on reviewing Prusiner's bibliography at the number of scientific fields and techniques he had to master in his research. An early technique was electron microscopy, with which I was acquainted through an old Deep Springs College friend, Dr. Robley Williams, who had gained an international reputation as an expert in its use. Sure enough, Prusiner found him and used it. To this, he added all the pertinent techniques of biochemistry, ultracentrifugation, chromatography, mass spectroscopy, electrophoresis, and sedimentation analysis. Then there were the techniques of microbiology and immunology, such as immunological antibodies, immunoaffinity purification, and cell culture. Genetic research techniques were another necessary approach, involving molecular genetics and gene cloning, genetic engineering, and transgenetic studies.

What sort of man could master such complex approaches and possess the drive to achieve significant results? Brilliance, youthful energy, flexibility, drive, interpersonal skills in developing a strong research team and contacts, and in addition, vision, motivation, determination, and fund-raising skills are some of the obvious characteristics that come to mind.

Prusiner, although still relatively young, has already won some 15 awards, including the Cotzias Award and election to the National Academy of Science. He is a member of 20 medical and neuroscientific societies and has served on some 20 boards and committees as an advisor or ad hoc referee. He also is an ad hoc referee in biochemistry for 15 journals, plus being on the editorial board of 6 others. Many invited lectures have been given and review articles published, and one can only guess what future honors on an international scale will come his way.

In spite of all this, Prusiner has remained his simple and unaffected self. His rapport with his colleagues has been excellent. I am happy to report that we share one strong characteristic, although it may be regarded by some as of dubious importance. We both have a considerable antipathy to the American press for its biased sensationalism.* Prusiner's brilliance and drive have been outstanding, and he has successfully mobilized an amazing number of scientific techniques in the pursuit of his research. In this respect and for his great accomplishments, he personifies those characteristics, which have accomplished the flowering of neurology.

Whereas Gajdusek's research opened the door on the delayed infectious onset of kuru and Creutzfeldt-Jakob diseases, Prusiner has opened a whole new world on the underlying mechanisms involved. The pathogenicity of his prion protein, and its relation to genetic factors, replication, and infectiousness constitute a revolution in our older concepts. Wendell Stanley carried the study of viruses to the molecular level, but Prusiner's prion approach involves nonvirus proteins at a submolecular level, which have many of the properties of viruses.

SUMMARY

The culmination of humanity's struggles with infectious diseases, which historical-

---

*I will never forget the difficulties I had on one occasion eluding reporters when I was taking care of the Governor of Arizona.

ly extended back to Pasteur, Jenner, and into still earlier centuries, finally developed during the flowering period of neurology with the introduction of the modern antibiotics. Sanitation, quarantine, and enhanced body immunity have played important secondary roles in human defenses. So great has been the success of these measures, the world's population has more than doubled in the past half century and now threatens the ecological balance of the planet.

The advances of bacteriology, virology, and immunology are illustrated by the careers of Zinsser, Meyer, Stanley, and Jawetz, who dealt with typhus, typhoid, botulism, brucellosis, Western equine encephalitis, plague, psittacosis, poliomyelitis, influenza, the rickettsial disorders, trachoma, and many other infectious processes.

Because modern science has now extended these advances to a new level of particular importance to the central nervous system, the research of Gajdusek and Prusiner has been added. The infectivity of prions explain several degenerative diseases of humans and animals, their delayed onset, novel method of replication, and relation to genetic factors. We hope this will open the door to a better understanding of other degenerative diseases, such as Alzheimer disease, parkinsonism, and amyotrophic lateral sclerosis. The story of the prion studies has been added because they well illustrate the ongoing research of neurology and the importance of science in achieving these advances.

REFERENCES

1. Koshland, D.E., Jr. Preserving biodiversity. *Science*, 253:737, 1991.
1a. Mann, C. Extinction: are ecologists crying wolf? *Science*, 253:736-738, 1991.
1b. Soule, M.E., Erwin, T.L., Morowitz, H.J., Jablonski, D., Ehrlick, P.R., and Wilson, E.A. Conservation: Tactics for Constant Crisis, *Science,* 253:744-762, 1991.
2. Hiss, P.H., and Zinsser, H. *A Textbook of Bacteriology*. 1st ed. New York, D. Appleton & Co., 1910.
3. Jordan, D.S. Quoted by S.B. Wolbach in Biographical Memoir of Hans Zinsser. Washington, D.C., *National Academy of Science*, 1947, p. 327.
4. Zinsser, H. As *I Remember Him*. Boston, Little Brown & Co., 1940.
5. Muller, J.H. Hans Zinsser. *J. Bacteriol.*, 40:747-753, 1940.
6. Wolbach, S.B. Hans Zinsser. *Proc. Natl. Acad. Sci.* U.S.A., 23:321-360, 1947.
7. Zinsser, H. *Spring, Summer and Autumn*. New York, Alfred A. Knopf, 1947.
8. de Kruif, P. Champion among microbe hunters. *Reader's Digest,* 56 (338):35-40, 1950.
9. Sabin, A.B. Karl Friedrich Meyer, biographical memoirs. Proc. *Natl. Acad. Sci.* U.S.A., 52:268-332,1980.
10. Meyer, K.F. *Medical Research and Public Health, Oral History*. Berkeley, Bancroft Library, University of California, 1976.
11. Meyer, K.F. The rise and fall of botulism. *Calif. Med.*, 118:63-64, 1973.
12. Meyer, K.F. Effectiveness of live or killed plague vaccines in man. Bull. World Health Organ., 42:653-666, 1970.
13. Meyer, K.F. and Eddie, B. Feather mites and ornithosis. *Science*, 132:300, 1960.
14. Stanley, W.M. Isolation of a crystalline protein possessing the properties of tobacco-mosaic virus. *Science*, 81:644-645, 1935.
15. Stanley, W.M. *The isolation and properties of crystalline tobacco mosaic virus*. Les Prix Nobel, Kungl. Boktryckeriet. Stockholm, P.A. Norstedt and Soner, 1949.
16. Stanley, W.M. The preparation and properties of influenza virus vaccines concentrated and purified by differential centrifuge. *J. Exp. Med.*, 81:193-218, 1945.
17. Schwerdt, C.E., Williams, R.C., and Stanley, W.M. Morphology of type II poliomyelitis virus (MEF) as determined by electromicroscopy. *Proc. Soc. Exp. Med.*, 86:310-312, 1954.
18. Tsugita, A., Gish, D.T., Young, J., Fraenkel-Conrat, H., Knight, C.A., and Sranley, W.M. The complete amino acid sequence of the protein of tobacco mosaic virus. *Proc. Natl. Acad. Sci.* U.S.A, 46:1463-1469, 1960.

19. Stanley, W.M., and Lauffer, A. *Chemical and Physical Procedures Virus and Rickettsial Infections of Man.* 2nd ed. Philadelphia, JB Lippincott, 1952.
20. Jawetz, E., Gunnison, J.B., and Speh, R.S. Antibiotic synergism and antagonism. *N. Engl. J Med.*,245:966-968, 1951.
21. Jawetz, E. Antibiotic synergism and antagonism. A review of experimental of experimental evidence *Arch. Intern. Med.*, 90:301-309, 1952.
22. Jawetz, E., Kimura, S., Nicholas, A., Thygeson, P., and Hanna, L. A new type of APC virus from epidemic keratoconjunctivitis. *Science*, 122:1190-1101, 1955.
23. Hoshiwara, I., Cutler, H.B., Hanna, L., Cignetti, P., Coleman, V.R., and Jawetz, E. Doxycycline treatment of chronic trachoma. *JAMA.*, 224:220-223, 1973.
24. Jawetz, E., and Merrill, E.R. The effect of cortisone upon the therapeutic efficacy of antibiotics. *Science*, 118:549-550, 1953.
25. Gajdusek, D.C., and Zigas, V. Degenerative disease of the central nervous system in New Guinea. The endemic occurrence of "kuru" in the native population. *N. Engl. J. Med.*, 257:974-978, 1957.
26. Hadlow, W.J. Scrapie and kuru. *Lancet*, 2:289-290, 1959.
27. Gajdusek, D.C., Gibbs, C.J., and Alpers, M. Experimental transmission of a kuru-like syndrome to chimpanzees. *Nature*, 209:794-796, 1966.
28. Klatzo, I., Gajdusek, D.C., and Zigas, V. Pathology of kuru disease. *J. Neuropathol. Exp. Neurol.*, 18:335-336, 1959.
29. Gibbs, C.J. Jr., Gajdusek, D.C., Asher, D.M., Alpers, M.P., Beck, E., Daniel, P.M., and Mathews, W.B. Creutzfeldt-Jakob disease (subacute spongiform encephalopathy). Transmission to the chimpanzee. *Science*, 16:388-389, 1968.
30. Gajdusek, D.C. *Unconventional Viruses and the Origin and Disappearance of Kuru.* Stockholm, P.A. Norstedt & Soner, 1977.
31. Gajdusek, D.E. *Curriculum Vitae, Lectures and Awards, Journals, Bibliography.* Bethesda, MD, National Institutes of Health, 1992.
32. Prusiner, S.B. Novel proteinaceous infectious particles cause scrapie. *Science*, 216:136-144, 1982.
33. Prusiner, S.B., Goth, D.F., Cochran, S.P., Masiarz, F.R., McKinley, M.P., and Martinez, H.M. Molecular properties, partial purification and assay by incubation period measurements of the hamster scrapie agent. *Biochemistry*, 19:4883-4891, 1980.
34. Prusiner, S.B., Goth, D.F., Bolton, D.C., Kent, S.B., and Hood, L.E. Purification and structural studies of a major scrapie prion protein. *Cell*, 38:127-134, 1984.
35. Oesch, B., Westaway, D., Walchli, M., McKinley, M.P., Kent, S.B.H., Aebersold, R., Barry, R.A., Tempst, P., Teplow, D.B., Hood, L.E., Prusiner, S.B., and Weissmann, C. A cellular gene encodes scrapie PrP 27-30 protein. *Cell*, 40:735-774, 1985.
36. Basler, K., Oesch, B., Scott, M., Westaway, D., Walchli, M., Groth, D.F., McKinley, M.P., Prusiner, S.B., and Weissmann, C. Scrapie and cellular PrP isoforms are encoded by the same chromosomal gene. *Cell*, 46:417-428, 1986
37. Bellinger-Kawahara, C., Cleaver, J.E., Diener, T.O., Prusiner, S.B. Purified scrapie prions resist inactivation by UV. *Virology*, 61:159-166, 1987.
38. Westaway, D., Goodman, P.A., Mirenda, C.A., McKinley, M.P., Carlson, G.A., and Prusiner, S.B. Distinct prion proteins in short and long scrapie incubation period mice. Cell, 51: 651-662, 1987.
39. Prusiner, S.B. Prions and neurodegenerative diseases. *N. Engl. J. Med.*, 317:1571-1581, 1987.
40. Gabizon, R., McKinley, M.P., Goth, D.F., and Prusiner, S.B. Immunoaffinity purification and neutralization of scrapie prion infectivity. *Proc. Natl. Acad. Sci. U.S.A.*, 85:6617-6621, 1988.
41. Borchelt, D.R., Scott, M., Taraboulos, A., Stahl, N., and Prusiner, S.B. Scrapie and cellular prion proteins differ in their kinetics and topology in cultured cells. *J. Cell Biol.*, 110:743-775, 1990.
42. DeArmond, S.J., McKinley, M.P., Barry, R.A., Braunfeld, M.B., McColloch, J.R., and Prusiner, S.B. Identification of prion amyloid filaments in scrapie-infected brain. *Cell.*, 41:221-235, 1985
43. Sparkes, R.S., Simon, M., Cohn, V.H., Foumier, R.E.K., Lem, J., Klisak, I., Heinzmann, C., Blatt, C., Lucero, M., Mohandas, T., DeArmond, S.J., Westaway, D., Prusiner, S.B., and Weiner Assignment of the human and mouse prion protein genes to homologous chromosomes. *Proc. Natl. Acad. Sci. U.S.A.*, 83:7358-7362, 1986.
44. Hadlow, W.J., Prusiner, S.B., Kennedy, R.C., Race, R.E. Brain tissue from persons dying of Creutzfeldt-Jakob disease causes scrapie-like encephalopathy in goats. *Ann. Neurol.*, 8:628-631, 1980.

Neurogenetics

The field of genetics has rapidly expanded since molecular chemists have unraveled the mystery of the double helix structure of DNA (1). However, many other developments had preceded and set the stage for this advance. These early developments can be summarized under two broad headings as follows: (1) the medical study of inherited traits and medical disorders, which involved the study of familial disorders and was greatly facilitated by full and precise family history taking, as well as by the availability of family records in stable populations extending over several generations, such as in Scandinavia, and (2) pioneering biochemical studies, such as Garrod's "inborn errors of metabolism" and Morgan's later investigations on gender chromosomes, sex linkage, and mutations.

Neurogenetics constitutes only one phase of the broad field of genetics, and yet, because of the vital role of the nervous system, it is by all odds the most important.

To convey the idea that research marches on in the case of neurogenetics is relatively simple, but its precise implementation in terms of the many advances that have been made, and their application to neurobiological disorders is by no means as easy. It is a complex subject of great magnitude. Well over 500 genetic conditions that involve the nervous system were listed in Pratt's 1967 edition of *The Genetics of Neurological Disorders* (2). Again, considerable progress has been made in deciphering the complex molecular changes (for example, enzymatic changes, protein synthesis, and the mutations of recessively inherited disorders) of a handful of these conditions. Technical advances in chromosomal mapping and genetic engineering have opened promising leads to the control and even therapy of a number of neurogenetic conditions.

Exciting as these advances have been, they still do not adequately address the common problems of neurological practice. Afflicted patients and their families are concerned about the hereditary aspects of their conditions—will they occur again and can they be prevented? This is genetic counseling, and the answers depend on the countless family studies of the more mundane, clinical aspects of neurology. Thus, in sketching the background of neurogenetics, it is necessary to present this very practical aspect of hereditary disorders. At the same time, the essential step-by-step, scientific progress that underlies the molecular basis of genetics must be presented if the promising advances of the latter are to be understood. Some aspects, such as genetic insulin production and neonatal diagnostic techniques, are already established, and the promise of therapeutic possibilities greatly adds to the alluring prospects of genetics. Nevertheless, wise genetic counseling and prevention will still constitute an important and essential phase of the field. The importance of this aspect of genetics has been recognized for centuries. The cultivation of plant life and animal breeding extends back into prehistoric times, as does the recognition of familial physical and mental traits in humans. Even the endless efforts of Communist ideology could not wipe out the inequalities of the latter.

The devastating inheritance of many medical conditions, in particular, has emphasized the importance of human genetics and the main categories of those that involve the nervous system may be listed as follows:

1. Congenital malformations (cerebral, skull, and vertebral)
2. Dementias (e.g., Huntington's chorea, Pick's, Creutzfeldt-Jakob)
3. Various disorders of cranial and peripheral nerves (e.g., peroneal muscular atrophy, syringomyelia, Morvan's syndrome)
4. Lipidoses (e.g., amaurotic family idiocy, Niemann-Pick disease, Refsum's sydrome)
5. Leukodystrophies, including several demyelinating conditions
6. The spinal muscular atrophies (myotonia congenita, progressive spinal muscular atrophy, motor neuron disease)
7. Hereditary muscle diseases (dystrophies, myotonia syndromes, familial periodic paralysis, glycogen storage diseases)
8. Disorders of metabolism (e.g., porphyrias, phenylketonuria, maple syrup urine disease)
9. Other conditions, such as Von Recklinghausen's disease, absence epilepsy, and Lafora-body type of epilepsy

The underlying, basic biochemical advances that have been made are sequentially listed below (those neurogenetically important are indicated by asterisks):

BASIC ADVANCES IN GENETICS
1865 — Mendel: laws of heredity (not recognized until 1900)
1906 — Garrod: inborn errors of metabolism (alcaptonuria)
1919 — Morgan: sex chromosomes and linkage mutations
1934 — Folling: phenylketonuria*
1944 — Avery, et al.: DNA carries genetic information
1952 — Cori and Cori: glycogen storage disease, an enzyme defect*
1953 — Watson and Crick: molecular structure of DNA (Nobel prize)
1958 — Beadle and Tatum: one gene, one polypeptide (Nobel prize)
1961 — Nirenberg: genetic code (triplet nucleotide codons)
1963 — Gajdusek and Gibbs: kuru, scrapie, and Creutzfeldt-Jakob disease infections, primate transfer (Nobel prize for Gajdusek)*

1965 — Brady: sphingolipidoses, enzyme defect and replacement therapy

1967 — Seegmiller: enzyme defect in Lesch-Nyhan syndrome

1970 — Neufeld: mucopolysaccharidoses, enzyme defects

1970 — Nathans and Smith: endonucleases cut DNA into fragments

1972 — Berg: recombinant hybrid DNA from DNA of two viruses

1973 — Boyer and Cohen: inserted human gene into bacterial plasmid, start of genetic engineering*

1974 — Brown, et al.,: molecular defect in hypercholesterolemia

1975 — Bishop and Varmus: oncogenes (Nobel prize)*

1977 — Gilbert and Sanger: techniques of sequential analysis of recombinant DNA

1977 — Rutter, et al.: Isolate gene for insulin, bacterial transplant

1979 — Genentech, Inc.: human growth hormone synthesis*

1979 — Kan and Chang: prenatal study, beta-thalassemia mutation*

1980 — Botstein, D., et al.: genetic linkage map in humans*

1981 — Transgenic mice and flies: study of mutations*

1982 — Palmitter: rat growth hormone introduced into mouse zygotes and produced giant mice

1983 — McClintoch: shifting genes (Nobel prize)

1983 — Gusella: DNA polymorphism of Huntington's disease (mutant gene on chromosome 4)*

1984 — Prusiner: prions replicating infectious protein subunits that cause scrapie, Kuru, Creutzfeldt-Jakob, and Gerstmann-Sträussler disorders*

1984 — Friedman: possibility of enzyme therapy for Lesch-Nyhan disease

1990 — Human Genome Project: mapping chromosomes*

1992 — Schellenberg, et al.: Familial Alzheimer disease (chromosome 14)*

Aside from Mendel, the scientific aspects of genetics date back to Sir Archibald Garrod.

SIR ARCHIBALD GARROD (1858-1936)

Archibald Garrod, a transitional figure, was a Victorian Englishman of the upper crust—well educated, impeccable in his dress and manners, and imposing in appearance with his broad brow, dark eyes, bushy eyebrows, and walrus mustache. He was a kindly physician of the old school. However, he went well beyond this characterization, and it is likely that his family background had much to do with this. His father, Sir Alfred Garrod, and his brother were scientifically inclined physicians. The three of them constituted a rare phenomenon—three members of one family elected to the Royal Society. The father was the first to relate a medical disorder to its chemical cause—uric acid to gout (1848). Archibald Garrod, although primarily a physician, sustained his interests in biological chemistry throughout his life, and his studies on the "inborn errors of metabolism" went far to stimulate the biochemical aspects of genetics and medicine in the early decades of the 20th century. His approach was the spectrographic analysis of the urine in unusual medical disorders.

His training was dictated by family tradition—Marlborough College and The House at Oxford, where he took first-class honors in natural science. He did his medical studies at St. Bartholomew's Hospital, London, qualified (M.R.C.S.), and graduated from Oxford (M.B.) in 1889. Two years later, he obtained his doctorate from Oxford. Various medical posts followed, including lecturer in chemical pathology at "St. Barts," but he had to wait some 19 years before there was a vacancy on the medical staff of the hospital and medical college. During this period, he obtained pediatric training, serving on the staffs of the Alexandrian and Great Ormond Street hospitals. This prepared him for a joint appointment as head of a new outpatient clinic for children at St. Barts in 1904. He was made a full physician to St. Barts in 1912. His interests in pediatrics were climaxed in 1913 by publication of *Diseases of Children* by various authors. He co-edited this with F. E. Batten and Hugh Thursfield and wrote two of the chapters.

During this early period, Dr. Garrod found time to develop his expertise in spectroscopy and examination of urinary pigments in unusual medical cases. This resulted in some 27 reports prior to his Croonian Lecture in 1908 and publication of his inborn errors of metabolism (3). Ten reports on urinary porphyrins, eight on alcaptonuria, and two on urobilin had preceded this, as well as still other reports on the technique and his approach. It was the possibility that alcaptonuria might be an inherited disorder due to genetic factors in 1897 to 1898 that led him to his main theme (4). In his Croonian lectures, Garrod had included albinism, cystinuria, and pentosuria, as well as alcaptonuria, as examples of inborn errors of metabolism. When he published his second edition of this book in 1923, he was able to add two new "errors"—congenital steatorrhea and hematoporphyria congenita (5). The genetic factors in these disorders of metabolism were a great stimulus to other workers, and Garrod did his best to encourage scientifically minded young physicians to pursue this course—a theme that was central to a dozen of his articles. This same theme was incorporated into the new plans of medical education instituted by Garrod and others at St. Barts following World War I. He had looked forward to the unit as a means of giving the opportunity and stimulus for an advance in clinical science to the next generation of physicians (6). He had advocated a closer connection with the University of London to improve the education of the medical students and to give facilities for research. The plan included a full-time director of medicine and surgery, as well as adequate staffing. When he was made the director, he threw himself wholeheartedly into the project. Thus, it was with considerable regret that he left his beloved St. Barts, when called to become the Regis Professor of Physic at Oxford, following the death of Osler. This background no doubt explains his efforts at Oxford to strengthen its scientific departments ant their connections with the Radcliffe Infirmary (7).

A secondary great interest of Garrod was rheumatism and rheumatoid arthritis. He published some 20 articles on these subjects and advocated that the arthritic form was essentially an articular disorder resulting from trophic disturbances. Altogether, his bibliography contains 145 publications, which involves neurological and many other subjects than those mentioned.

World War I had a devastating effect on Garrod. His own service in England and, later, in Malta as a consulting physician to the forces went well, but he was profoundly affected by the loss of his three sons.

He received many honors, including five honorary degrees and six honorary fellowships, and was awarded the Gold Medal of the Royal Society of Medicine in 1935. He was elected to several offices in the British Medical Association, was a member of the Medical Research Council, and an honorary member of many English and foreign foundations. He was elected to the Royal Society in 1910 and was knighted in 1919.

He delivered eight of the main lectureships of Great Britain. These mainly concerned his metabolic studies, but other themes involved the debt of science to medicine (Harverian lecture, 1924) and "Glimpses of the Higher Medicine," the Linacre lecture at Cambridge (8). His advocacy of science in medicine shown forth in both of these lectures.

Along with Sir William Osler and two other knighted physicians, Garrod joined in the formation of the Association of Physicians and served as joint editor of the Quarterly Journal of Medicine from 1909 to 1929.

Garrod epitomized that rare combination of the kindly physician and medical scientist. The case for the latter has been abundantly made in this essay and was emphasized in the obituary of Sir Frederick Gowland Hopkins (9). The case for the former was repeatedly made in several of his obituaries and perhaps was best phrased by an anonymous correspondent to the British Medical Journal, "In our earliest days we learnt, thanks to him, that medicine is not only a science, but an art and a philosophy, and he filled us all with love and enthusiasm for the work which still lies before us....But, above all, he taught us that the patient is an individual, and we came away from the ward with the knowledge that he was a good and great doctor, and was well loved by all his patients," (10).

A number of neurogenetic studies followed the lead given by Garrod. However, it was not until 1934 that Folling elaborated the enzyme defect of phenylketonuria and, in 1952, that Cori and Cori verified the fact that the first glycogen storage disease, alcaptonuria, was due to an enzymatic defect. This reflected the early limitations of biochemistry.

Aside from clinical familial studies, the next major advances in genetics, after Garrod, came with the investigations of Morgan.

THOMAS HUNT MORGAN (1855-1945)

As in the cases of Wilhelm Roentgen and Ernest Lawrence, Morgan was not a neuroscientist, and yet, like them, his contributions were so basic that they had profound effects on all that followed in his field. This was true, not only for his scientific contributions, but also in the great stimulus that his work gave to genetics.

Although lacking the medical background and connections of Garrod, Morgan, through his studies of plants, birds, Drosophila, and others, brought into focus the basic mechanisms of genetic replication with particular reference to the sex hormones, sex linkage, and the role of mutations. One of Morgan's major accomplishments was to develop an uncompartmentalized division of biological sciences at the California Institute of Technology. Here he encouraged the cross-fertilization of ideas from different biological disciplines, including biochemistry. In this respect, his setup was somewhat similar to Herbert Evans's Institute of Biological Sciences at the University of California, Berkeley, as discussed in Chapter 14. Seven Nobel prizes have been awarded to investigators, who at one time or another, worked in Morgan's laboratories. Still more became members of the National Academy of Sciences. The future of genetics depended on this type of interdisciplinary collaboration, and Morgan's influence on the revolution that followed was great indeed. This involved the recognition of DNA as the carrier of genetic information and the elucidation of its molecular structure and replication.

As in other cases, it is of interest to see the background of such a man and the molding influences that determined his career and accomplishments. Julian Huxley visited Kentucky for this purpose and concluded that "it explained a great deal in his character."

Born and raised in Kentucky, his family was well known because of an uncle, John Hunt Morgan, the famous Civil War raider, who was known as the "Thunderbolt of the Confederacy." In his youth, Morgan developed a great love of nature that probably influenced his later interest in zoology, biology, and the study of both plants and animals.

Before entering Johns Hopkins University, Morgan attended a small summer school of marine biology at Annisquam, Massachusetts, where the next year, the Marine Biological Laboratory at Woods Hole was to start. In the following year, at Hopkins, there was great emphasis on laboratory work in the Department of Biology. He highly approved of this experimental approach to science. His studies resulted in several small articles, and he qualified for the M.S. degree in 1888. Having studied experimental biology, Morgan stayed on in graduate work. At Woods Hole, he did his research for his Ph.D. thesis on the water spider. I well recall this, because one of my fellow members of the Telluride House at Cornell, Bruce Simonds, had elaborated Morgan's data on the water spider into a fascinating dinner story. Bruce was a fourflusher of the first order, but when it came to the social graces and entertainment of the university guests (as discussed in a footnote in Chapter 4), he easily outshown the other, more scholarly members of the house. It, also, was at Woods Hole that Morgan met his future bride, Lillian Sampson, a student from Bryn Mawr.

Morgan won the Bruce fellowship at Hopkins that permitted him to do further research in the West Indies and travel to Europe. In 1891, he obtained an associate professorship of biology at Bryn Mawr. On a sabbatical leave (1894 to 1895), he visited the Stazione Zoologica on the Bay of Naples in Italy. On his return to Bryn Mawr in 1895, he was promoted to the full professorship. His early studies were largely embryological on the regeneration of tadpoles, fish, and earth worms.

In 1903, he accepted the first professorship of experimental biology at Columbia University. It was here that his famous genetic work on male and female chromosomes, sex linkage, and mutations developed, using the fly Drosophila. A summary of the chromosome experiments was published in book form, *Heredity and Sex* (11). In 1915, he published his best known book, *The Mechanism of "Mendelian Heredity"* with three of his young colleagues (12). All of the Drosophila studies were summarized in this book.

The success of the Drosophila studies was soon recognized internationally and many honors followed—honorary degrees from Johns Hopkins University (L.L.D.) and the University of Kentucky (Ph.D.), several honorary awards, and membership in the National Academy of Sciences and the Royal Society. He was elected president of the Society for Experimental Biology and Medicine (1910 to 1912), of the National Academy of Science (1927 to 1928), and of the American Association for the Advancement of Science in 1929.

Morgan was a prolific writer—some 20 books in addition to his scientific articles. His first Drosophila article appeared in 1910, and 15 of his books were on genetics. *The Genetics of Drosophila* and *The Theory of the Gene* became well known and widely quoted (13,14). It was his writing and his impact on his many students that produced the early scientific revolution in genetics and that set the stage for the next generation of molecular genetics.

ASBJÖRN FÖLLING (1886-1972)

Progress came slowly in the early days of genetic advances and often from unexpected sources. So it was with phenylketonuria, an important inborn error of metabolism, which was discovered by Fölling quite independently of Garrod's approach and 11 years after Garrod's report of 1923 (5).

The unexpected aspect concerned Fölling's background and the circumstances of his discovery. He was the youngest of six children of a farmer who lived near Trondheim, Norway. By living with the family of an older married sister, Fölling was able to continue his scholarly interests beyond high school. He graduated in 1916 as a biochemist from the Trondheim technical college and then worked his way through medical school in the University of Oslo by 1922. Following 6 years of work in the University of Oslo's medical clinics, he obtained a Rockefeller Foundation travel grant. This took him to the United States, where he studied metabolic disorders at the Mayo Clinic and the medical schools of Harvard, Yale, and Johns Hopkins. He received his doctoral degree from the University of Oslo in 1929.

Although primarily a clinician and teacher at that point, he undertook laboratory work when the professor of medicine at Oslo asked him "to make some insulin" for a patient in a diabetic coma. He was promoted to be professor of nutritional medicine in 1932, but 2 years later, he accepted the position of professor of biochemistry and physiology at a new veterinary college in Oslo. It was his desire to teach and have contact with students that prompted him to make this change.

In 1932, he was consulted by a dentist who felt that his asthma was exacerbated by the peculiar odor of his two mentally retarded children. The odor was traced to their urine, and this gave a positive test for ketones. Working in a nitrogen atmosphere to prevent oxidation, Fölling extracted a compound that he eventually identified as phenylpyruvic acid.

This led to urine tests on hundreds of patients in the psychiatric clinics and homes for the mentally retarded. Nine retarded patients were found whose urine contained phenylpyruvic acid. Because two of these were siblings, like his original two, he concluded that the condition was a hereditary disorder of phenylalanine metabolism. The condition was labeled *imbecilitas phenylpyruvia*, but as in the case of Refsum's disease, the name was soon changed to Fölling's disease (15).

Further studies showed the condition to be associated with seizures, involuntary movements and postural changes, as well as mental retardation, and the name, phenylketonuria, was eventually adopted. Fölling later reported elevations of the levels of phenylalanine in the blood and brains of his patients (16).

The German occupation of Norway delayed further publications, although his laboratory remained active. With Professor O. L. Mohr and a medical student, L. Rudd, he proved that phenylketonuria was an autosomal recessive disease (17). With S. Sydnes, he showed that phenylalanine loading was excreted in carriers of phenylketonuria (18).

His laboratory, also, was active in another respect during the German occupation. Ole J. Malm perfected the invisible ink that was used by the Norwegian Resistance in its underground communications, and this went undetected by the Germans throughout their occupation.

Fölling was recalled in 1953 to the University of Oslo to reorganize its clinical laboratory. On his retirement 5 years later, he returned to his research at the Veterinary College.

He received many honors and awards, including the Order of St. Olav in Norway, the Danneborg Order in Denmark, and the Order of St. Blasius, the patron saint of veterinary students, for his teaching and friendship. He was elected to membership in the Norwegian Academy of Sciences and Letters and won the Jahre and Kennedy awards.

Fölling's research on phenylketonuria was important in at least three respects: (1) it was the first "inborn error of metabolism" that could be diagnosed prenatally by biochemical analysis; (2) it initiated the study of neurotoxic disorders caused by genetically produced enzyme deficiencies; and (3) it showed that dietary restrictions could be used therapeutically with success, providing diagnosis and treatment was started sufficiently early.

Good luck in his early training and later contacts were involved in Fölling's success, but his scholarly abilities and persistence were the determining factors. He well illustrates the aphorism that it is only the prepared mind that can grasp the opportunities that come to all of us. Probably his background explains such attributes as simplicity in person; direct, practical, and hard working in action; and yet, scholarly and thorough in his biochemical research. Certainly, his instincts for teaching and research drove him to a high, creative life of service

Going hand in hand with the early biochemical advances, the familial approach to genetics was richly extended in the early and middle decades of the 20th century.

To exemplify this aspect of neurogenetics, I have selected Sigvald Refsum. Not only did he describe a new hereditary syndrome, he was an influential leader in the field of neurogenetics, a role that was greatly strengthened by his serving for 8 years as president of the World Federation of Neurology.

SIGVALD REFSUM (1904-1991)

Refsum was a student of Monrad-Krohn in Oslo. His thesis for his doctorate degree involved the description of a family constellation characterized by a slowly progressive polyneuritis with remissions, distal muscle wasting, and paresis. This was associated with ataxia and cerebellar signs, retinitis pigmentosa in combination with hemeralopia, and a concentric constriction of the visual fields. Other findings involved pupillary abnormalities, central deafness, a dry scaly skin, electroencephalographic changes, and raised levels of cerebrospinal fluid protein. Refsum named the condition, heredopathia atactic polyneuritiformis, a name that predictably was commonly referred to as Refsum's disease (19). The genetic defect was thought to follow an autosomal recessive course, and the pathologic condition involved degenerative changes in the nuclei and tracts of the brainstem (rubrodentate and olivopontocerebellar) in addition to the polyneuritis and peripheral muscle wasting.

Various authorities, including Houston Merritt, doubted that it was a distinct neurological entity. Merritt thought it probably was a variant of the Dejerine-Sottas disease (20). Brain considered it to be a familial form of progressive hypertrophic polyneuritis (21). However, Refsum was right. In 1963, it was shown to be an inborn error of lipid metabolism with storage of 3,7,11,15-tetramethylhexadecanoic acid in the kidneys, liver, and urine (22).

I was exceedingly pleased with this turn of events, not only because it vindicated the clinical judgment of an old friend, but also because it showed that we must be more alert to genetic entities, as opposed to the idiopathic syndromes of the descriptive phase of neurology, which entrapped the erudite minds of the past.

The early approach to hereditary disorders was plagued by both clinical and genetic uncertainties. I became well aware of this when my associate, Patrick Flynn, and I suffered through these problems in describing a familial neurologic disorder, now categorized as the Flynn-Aird syndrome (23). Its dominant inheritance, determined over five generations, seemed clear, but its clinical delineation left doubts as to its being a neurological entity, largely because we could relate it to no hormonal or other neurochemical etiology. It was characterized by bilateral nerve deafness, severe myopia, ataxia, peripheral neuritis with pain, joint stiffness, and muscular wasting. Variable findings included retinitis pigmentosa, bilateral cataracts, kyphoscoliosis, skin atrophy, and blindness. Extensive clinical and laboratory findings suggested a genetically determined enzyme defect, but how much was due to an underlying genetic factor, as opposed to superimposed, environmentally conditioned changes, remained doubtful.

The efforts of Pratt and the younger generation of neurologists trained in neurogenetics is the obvious proper trend. This does not mean that neurologists must cope with all the details of neurogenetics, but it does mean that they should recognize genetic possibilities and obtain the aid of specialists in this complicated field. This is important to genetic counseling, especially, in a field that is so rapidly expanding.

My contacts with Refsum were very close when he spent 1 year with me at the University of California, San Francisco (UCSF), from November 1951 to November 1952. He came while waiting for his department at the University of Bergen to be built. His duties were twofold—to alleviate the pressures on my neurological consultations and on my electroencephalographic work. He performed admirably in both; Refsum's neurological workups were concise and yet comprehensive in their coverage of the essential factors that were involved in each case. I checked all pertinent details, especially in those patients not requiring a more complete hospital workup. It was this close neurological contact that made me aware, not only of his neurological competence, but also his tact in what for him must have been a difficult position, especially in the good rapport he invariably developed with each patient. His kindly concern and thorough study impressed the patients, as well as myself. His approach so closely tallied with my own that he seriously considered staying on. Wind of this possibility got back to Norway by way of occasional visitors, and he was finally ordered back to Norway by King Haakon VII, who sent 1,000 krone to implement his order. I had reached the opinion that he would have a brighter future in Norway than with us. Also, in the post-World War II period, the licensing of doctors from other states and, especially, foreign countries had been made almost prohibitive in California. A 2-year internship for Professor Refsum appeared ridiculous, and there was the added problem of his family.

His work in our electroencephalographic laboratory also went well. We were using a system comparable to the international 10-20 placement system. It differed, however, in stressing recordings over physiologically important cortical sites, such as the anterior temporal regions, as well as the posterior temporal area to obtain optimal recording in patients with temporal lobe epilepsy and other conditions. Following the underlying principle of the neurological examination, the system made a close analysis of the recordings obtained simultaneously from bilateral, homologous sites because it was found that slight, consistent differences of voltage, frequency, and form were of value for purposes of focal diagnosis. Refsum adapted very quickly to our system, and his analyses and reports were excellent.

On Monrad-Krohn's retirement, Refsum became professor of Neurology at Oslo and held this post from 1954 until 1978, when he retired. He was president of the World Federation of Neurology for two terms (1973 to 1981), and many honors followed, including honorary presidency of the Scandinavian Congress of Neurologists, fellowship in the Royal College of Physicians, England, and honorary membership in the Royal Society of Medicine (London) and 16 national societies of neurology. He was made a member of the Norwegian Academy of Science and Letters as early as 1956 and received the appointment of Knight First Class in the Royal Order of St. Olav in 1967.

One of his most notable public duties involved his serving as a medical consultant to the Norwegian Organization of Disabled War Veterans. In this capacity, he became an extraordinary medical diplomat for Norway, warmly welcomed by countless Norwegian veterans scattered in many countries of the world. Because of Refsum's command of several languages and exceptional cultural background, he made a fine head of the World Federation of Neurology, but in his person-to-person contacts with the Norwegian veterans, he excelled. It was an extension of the same superior patient rapport that he achieved in 1951 to 1952 when he served with us as a visiting professor of neurology.

A comment on Refsum's attitude to medical teaching may also be of interest. I have recorded elsewhere his reaction to Professor Wartenberg's dramatic teaching demonstrations (discussed in Chapter 15). He thoroughly agreed with our emphasis on bedside teaching, which held each student responsible for his workups and follow-ups on assigned patients. Fundamentally, this involved his emphasis on a thorough, comprehensive study and a close, supportive rapport with each patient.

Innumerable stories could be related about our contacts extending over nearly 40 years—our trips to Death Valley, Vancouver, and through the mountains and fjords of Norway; driving from Norway to Lisbon and the return in 1953; and our many visits both in Norway, San Francisco, and at many neurological meetings. It may be worthwhile to include one story because it showed his Norwegian pride.

Because Refsum had never driven and lived close to us in Marin County, I drove him from his home to the UCSF Medical Center and back each day. Our conversations ranged far and wide, but it soon became apparent that he took great pride in the fine records of many Norwegian-Americans. I had assumed that such men as Earl Warren and Ernest Lawrence were of English descent. Sigvald quickly corrected me on these and several others. His explanation of so many outstanding leaders of Norwegian descent involved their hereditary traits developed over centuries as a result of the rugged conditions of life in far northern Norway, which strengthened their characters and drive. In one of our good-natured and often jocular exchanges, I tried to expand his thesis to the other side of the North Sea and Scotland's splendid leaders. Refsum would hear nothing of this until one day I dilated on the wealth of songs and music of Scotland. I added that the only musician of note that I could think of from Norway was Edvard Grieg. Sigvald's face fell, and he finally admitted that even Grieg was of Scottish descent.

The account of Refsum can reasonably well portray the status of medical neurogenetics in the middle decades of the 20th century. Following the studies previously mentioned, plus the pressure of genetic counseling in medical practice, the clinical study of family lines gradually multiplied. The bulk of these involved neurological or psychiatric conditions (24). Refsum credited the report that between 3% and 5% of the population were "victims of genetic neuropsychiatric disorders." I should add that, among the many articles on genetics, Refsum's discussion of the principles of clinical genetics and their applications in clinical genealogy are perhaps the most lucid and well illustrated (24).

Family records were particularly good in Scandinavia, and this led to several other reports in addition to Refsum's disease. In America, among many others, Lawrence H. Snyder was a notable geneticist, and in a series of reports from 1926 to 1945, he dealt with the genealogical aspects of blood groups and such other conditions as polydactylism and hemophilia (25). Among those included in these essays, Von Bogaert, Holmes, Mackay, and Critchley made important contributions, along with a host of others. Lennox did early twin studies in epilepsy. Epidemiologists, such as Kurland and Kurtzke added to the field. Another large source of family records is the genealogical records of the Mormon Church, which has collected millions of family lines to encourage the Temple work of its members to save their ancestors and to enlarge their respective kingdoms in Heaven. The studies of Eldon J. Gardiner and Fayette E. Stephens were especially notable in this connection. The latter reported an autosomal dominant gene in facioscapulohumeral progressive muscular dystrophy (26). The Duchenne dystrophy of youth and important twin studies were other contributions.

The need for genetic counseling has increased as the public's awareness and expectation of medical "miracles" has increased. This need has been aided by compendiums, such as Pratt's second edition of *The Genetics of Neurological Disorders* (27). Counseling has been hampered by problems of clinical syndrome identification, lack of knowledge of the precise mode of inheritance involved, difficulties of carrier detection and prenatal diagnosis, and the resulting interpretation of risks in each individual case. Only as geneticists are consulted and further research broadens our basis of understanding of genetic disorders can these problems be minimized. The data in rare conditions may not be adequate, and the underlying enzymatic and molecular basis is only now beginning to be determined. Nevertheless, important advances are being made that give promise of early diagnosis, better counseling with respect to prevention, and possibly even therapy in some cases.

Shortly after Refsum was with us and while we were driving together from Norway to the 1953 Lisbon meeting of the International Neurological Congress and returning, Watson and Crick unraveled the double helix structure of DNA. This was important because it explained cellular replication (1). In the next major step, Nirenberg showed that 64 triplet "codons" of nucleic acid "encoded" the 20 amino acids and provided the "start" and "stop" signals of protein synthesis (28).

These and other items on the list of major advances in genetics may not be helpful to those whose biochemical background is weak. I was informed that I had led in the biochemical examination of the National Board of Medicine, but that was over 60 years ago! The pace of chemistry has been explosive, and I am now little better in understanding it than the next untutored clod. Unless one's mind is very nimble and the effort is made, the molecular chemistry of modern genetics approximates a *morass incognito*. In any case, it would be a tedious and counterproductive exercise to attempt an explanation of the technical aspects of the advances in genetic chemistry, except in its broadest terms.

The list, however, is important in its emphasis on the step-by-step progress in the biochemical aspects of modern genetics. I was reminded of this in reviewing the list with our Nobel Laureate, Michael Bishop. He immediately pointed out that the Gusella and co-workers study could not have been done, except for the genetic linkage mapping work of Botstein and associates shortly before (29), an important point

I had missed in organizing the list. It was doubly important, inasmuch as it led to the Human Genome Project (see the year 1990 on the the the list of basic genetic advances).

Still another major step was the recombinant DNA gene splicing of Boyer and Cohen (30). By using the gene splicing enzyme of Boyer, they were able to insert a eucaryotic gene into the bacterial plasmid of Cohen. This was the beginning of genetic engineering. I have selected Boyer to illustrate this advance for two reasons: (1) because Boyer was on our staff at the UCSF, I have been able to check with several other geneticists and, thus, develop some perspective of his contribution and its effects, and (2) because of his development of Genentech, which has continued much of the work he started.

HERBERT W. BOYER (1936-   )

Born in Pittsburgh, Pennsylvania, Boyer obtained his B.A. in 1958 from St. Vincent College in nearby Latrobe. He majored in biology and chemistry, and this was followed by postgraduate studies in bacteriology at the University of Pittsburgh (M.S. in 1960 and Ph.D. in 1963). He then did further work in microbiological genetics at Yale from 1963 to 1966. He moved to UCSF in 1966 as an assistant professor of microbiology. In 1971, he was advanced to the tenured position of associate professor and, in 1975, shifted to the Department of Biochemistry and Biophysics. One year later, he became director of the graduate program in genetics, a Howard Hughes investigator, and a professor in the Department of Biochemistry and Biophysics. These positions were retained until retirement in 1992.

It was in 1972 that Boyer and Cohen got together on using Boyer's splicing enzyme to transfer human genes to Cohen's bacterial DNA plasmid. Boyer approached Cohen about a joint research effort. One year of intensive research followed, conducted both at UCSF and Stanford. Their successful results led to the production of insulin, antibiotics, and growth hormone, as well as to genetic engineering with its therapeutic potential (30). The process was patented with royalties being assigned equally to the University of California and Stanford.

Cohen became head of the Stanford genetic setup, and Boyer later joined with a venture capitalist to establish Genetech, the purpose of the company being to exploit new techniques and to extend genetic research. Genetech has been successful and has been in the forefront of genetic research ever since its formation. In a limited sense, the research firm of Laborit in Paris (as discussed in Chapter 13) was an early prototype of this, but the problems of educational institutions are more involved in their patenting regulations and the standards of consultation for their full-time academic staff members. In the case of Boyer, this involved the establishment of a commercial research firm, which technically went beyond consultation. However, other than lending his name and giving limited consultations, Boyer played no role in the commercial aspects of Genetech. Even so, he has come in for some criticism from academic circles. In so far as I have been able to determine, Boyer acted entirely within the university regulations of the time. With the development of other similar firms, the problems involved have now been reasonably well defined, and the regulations accordingly adjusted. Such firms have multiplied, appear to be flourishing, and are fulfilling a useful role in society. Also, to the extent that recombinant DNA gene splicing techniques are used by such companies, both the University of California and Stanford benefit from the royalties involved.

The criticism of Boyer in some respects was similar to that suffered by Herbert Evans. In an earlier period, Evans was criticized for his introduction of the "ruthless competition" of "big science," as discussed in Chapter 17. Both men were in the forefront of transitional periods, which finally resulted in useful gains to research, universities, and society.

Boyer certainly did his share of university committee work, ad hoc reviews for national research organizations, and several scientific journals. He is a board member and consultant to several foundations and universities.

He published over 100 articles in the field of genetics. For 5 years, from 1974 through 1978, he produced from 7 to 13 articles per year. This involved several collaborators and included the year of collaboration with Cohen. Needless to say, it was this work that stimulated a second major advance in the field of genetics. This was aided by the rapid sequencing techniques of DNA base pairs that show where genes start and end (see Gilbert and Singer, 1977, on the sequential, basic advances list).

The potentials of genetic engineering in altering DNA structure to modify genetic replication may be summarized as follows:

1. To produce desired substances, such as insulin (see Rutter, et al., 1977, in the list of genetic advances).
2. To produce transgenic mice and flies, which permits a study of genetic mutations (used by Prusiner in his prion studies, as discussed in Chapter 11, and others— also see Palmitter, 1982, in the list of advances).
3. To produce enzymes to correct enzyme defects (see Friedman, 1984, in list of genetic advances).
4. Possibly to correct genetic defects, which are known to cause many genetic disorders.

Boyer has received nine awards, including the Albert Lasker, and many other honors, such as the National Medals of Technology and of Science, and an Honorary Doctor of Science degree from St. Vincents College. However, if my chart indicating the inflationary trend of honors is correct, Boyer has not reaped as many honors as might have been expected. This may reflect academic attitudes, as discussed previously.

Another important advance in genetic research was the study of oncogenes by Bishop and Varmus. Although not specifically an advance in neurogenetics, their work involved basic aspects of oncogenesis, which may be of great significance to a better understanding of tumors of the nervous system. They shared the Nobel prize in 1989 for their investigations (31). I have selected Bishop to illustrate this advance in modern genetics.

MICHAEL BISHOP (1936-   )

Bishop was a scholarly youth from the suburbs of Harrisburg, Pennsylvania, and graduated summa cum laude from Gettysburg College. His outstanding record led to his medical training at Harvard, where he graduated cum laude in 1962. His interests in research developed early, and in 1959 to 1960, he was a research fellow at the Public Health Service, after his second year at Harvard. In that same year, he was a research fellow in pathology at the Massachusetts General Hospital, where he was involved in the microanalysis of enzyme activities in hepatic tissue. In 1961 to 1962, he was a student research fellow in the Department of Bacteriology and Immunology at the Harvard Medical School. This involved biochemical studies on the replication of an RNA-containing arbovirus, and this was the start of his interests in genetics.

Bishop persevered in his medical studies and passed all three parts of the National Board of Medical Examiner's certification. He was an intern and assistant resident in internal medicine at the Massachusetts General Hospital in 1962 to 1964 and, thus, had superior clinical training, as well as considerable training in biochemistry and genetics. His military service in the post-World War II period was in the Public Health Service (1963 to 1967), where he pursued studies on the replication of poliovirus. In 1957 to 1958, he did postgraduate studies on the purification and characterization of the branched RNA molecule, "replicative intermediate" at the Heinrich-Pette Institute in Hamburg, Germany.

Bishop's first academic appointment was assistant professor of microbiology at UCSF in 1968. His research studies involved the replicative form of poliovirus and later the biochemistry of the Rous sarcoma virus. He rose rapidly through the academic ranks and became a full professor of microbiology by 1972. His primary research since 1970 has been on RNA tumor viruses—genome structure, viral replication, cellular transformation, and RNA-directed DNA synthesis (32–34). In 1981, he was made director of the George F. Hooper Research Foundation. In 1982, he became professor of biochemistry and biophysics and, in 1986, was the director of the Program in Biological Science, UCSF.

His membership on national advisory boards and committees in UCSF and other universities is astonishing (35). In addition, he has served on ten editorial boards and is an ongoing ad hoc reviewer for seven other journals concerned with cancer, genetics, biological chemistry, and so forth.

In addition to 39 review articles, he has published 249 research articles, has given presentations at 53 symposiums and conferences (published in proceedings or as chapters), and has written 3 books. He is a member of 17 societies and has excellent staffs that permit him to function well from his superstratospheric level. Honors have involved 22 awards, some 60 lectureships, and 2 honorary degrees. In 1989, he shared the Nobel prize with Harold Varmus (31).

I like to think of myself as one of those who helped to develop UCSF from its early proprietary status to a first-class medical school and Bishop as one of those who have pushed UCSF into its present outstanding status. This may be an optimistic appraisal of my past role, but certainly it is not of Dr. Bishop's. Of slight frame, his white beard and alert countenance combine to give the impression of the "eager beaver." He is this but is also much more. Many people talk big, but Bishop achieves big. His vast knowledge is buttressed by incisive depth of thought. On top of this, he is an unassuming and kindly person, whose command of the English language is exceptional.

Although Bishop's research does not explain the underlying physiopathogenesis of the different forms of brain tumor or other tumors of the nervous system, it has been concerned with the basic mechanisms of oncology at the molecular level. It is somewhat reassuring to know that able workers, such as Mark Israel, a professor of pediatrics and neurosurgery, are working on brain tumor problems at the molecular level and are aware of the work of both Bishop and Prusiner in nearby laboratories. Much of Bishop's work concerns a viral basis for tumor growth, and Prusiner has shown that prion protein subunits can be both infectious and have the power of replication.

Another geneticist more specifically involved in the field of neurogenetics is Dr. James Gusella. His accomplishments are of particular importance in documenting the basic role of science in neurology and the necessity of integrated team work in achieving neurological advances.

JAMES FRANCIS GUSELLA (1952-   )

Gusella, a Canadian, born in Ottawa, graduated from the University of Ottawa summa cum laude with honors in biology (B.S.). In 1976, he obtained a M.Sc., from the University of Toronto, and in 1980, he received a Ph.D. degree in biology from the Massachusetts Institute of Technology, Cambridge, Massachusetts. This led to his connection with Harvard, and from 1980, he advanced from an instructorship in neurology (genetics) to the full professorship of genetics in 1992. He taught and did his research in the Massachusetts General Hospital neurology genetics unit. From 1984 on, he has been the director of the molecular neurogenetics laboratory there. In addition, he holds appointments at the Massachusetts Institute of Technology, serves on the editorial boards of nine journals, and is an active member of six societies and many national advisory boards and executive committees, with special reference to those concerned with Huntington's disease.

From 1976 to 1993, he published 196 research articles and 66 reviews in symposia and as chapters of books. He was soon studying molecular linkage and, in 1983, reported a polymorphic DNA marker genetically linked to Huntington's disease (36). Many other studies followed on human chromosomes, searching for the genetic linkage of Alzheimer's dementia, von Recklinghausen's neurofibromatosis, myelogenous leukemia, neoplastic tumors of the central nervous system, Duchenne's muscular dystrophy, torsion dystonia, and many other neurological disorders. The outlines of a frenetic, genetic search of over a dozen chromosomes are documented by Gusella's bibliography with particular reference to chromosomes 21 and 4, chromosome 4 being the site of Huntington's disease (36) and chromosome

21 being the site of the familial Alzheimer's disorder (37). However, later studies suggested that the familial form of Alzheimer's disease is not a single homogeneous entity (38). A good review of Gusella'a search for the genetic linkage of Huntington's chorea was presented in the annual meeting of the Association for Research of Nervous and Mental Disease (39).

Dr. Gusella, also, well illustrates the great changes that have occurred in modern biological research and the in-depth preparation of the leaders conducting it. Whereas the early geneticists, like Garrod and Morgan, were broadly trained, the modern geneticist is a Ph.D. with a medical or medical science background who is intensely trained in molecular chemistry.

The Harvard genetic unit at the Massachusetts General Hospital, likewise, illustrates the necessity of coordinated team work in modern genetics. The highly trained molecular geneticist cannot work alone. In the case of the Huntington Disease project, it was Nancy Wexler, head of the Huntington Disease Foundation, who heard about the chromosome mapping work of Botstein, et al. (see list of basic genetic advances) and realized its possible application to Huntington's disease (25). The necessary blood samples were obtained through the National Research Register for Huntington's Disease Patients and Families at Indiana University. A Venezuelan Huntington's disease family was obtained through the Venezuelan Collaborative Huntington's Disease Project. Again, Nancy Wexler was a key figure in these arrangements. The point to be made is that, although it required a molecular biologist to head the project, he could not function without the support of a broad-based technical staff, human geneticists, and neurologists, The comprehensive team work initiated by Herbert Evans over 60 years ago (as discussed in Chapter 16) has long since become mandatory in the complex and integrated research of modern times. The early lines of genetic research (clinical study of familial disorders and biochemical approaches) have merged.

Also, much credit must be given to Dr. Joseph Martin who headed the neurological department and genetic unit of the Massachusetts General Hospital and Harvard Medical School.* His vision and practical organization of the research team and obtaining the support necessary to see the project through were basic. Six other institutions were involved in the Huntington Disease Collaborative Research Group. Again, without the continuing support of the National Institutes of Health and several paramedical societies and foundations, the project would not have been possible. Incidentally, it was Martin who was selected by the Institute of Medicine of the National Academy of Sciences to chair the committee that organized the current integrated program of mapping the human brain.

It also should be emphasized that, although the first step of being able to identify patients with Huntington's chorea is very important, the mechanisms of how the defective genes produce the cerebral pathology underlying Huntington's chorea is still unknown. In addition to the human genome phase of genetics, this is a whole

---

*Dr. Martin served as Dean of the School of Medicine, UCSF, for several years, and now is the Chancellor of UCSF.

supplementary phase that must be addressed, if the full pathophysiological picture is to be developed. Corrective measures may well depend on this.

The field of molecular genetics is obviously very complex, and this would appear to be especially true in neurogenetics. Although the field is probably still in its pioneering stage, enough has been disclosed to document its tremendous importance and promise for the future.

SUMMARY

Neurogenetics has been one of the most difficult subjects to organize in this series of essays. It has two principal facets: (1) that essential to the neurological counseling of patients and families afflicted with genetic disorders and (2) the underlying molecular chemistry of DNA and its complex clinical expression. The former was summarized in the career of Sigvald Refsum.

The biochemical aspect of genetics started with Garrod, was extended by Morgan, and progressed in a stepwise fashion as outlined in a sequential list of basic scientific advances. Boyer and Cohen started recombinant DNA gene splicing and genetic engineering. Bishop with Varmus won the Nobel prize for their basic oncogenetic studies. Utilizing the chromosome mapping technique developed by Botstein and co-workers, Gusella and his research team identified the gene responsible for Huntington's chorea on chromosome 4. This investigation was particularly important in demonstrating the cooperative teamwork that is essential in modern genetic research. It was this background that led to the Human Genome Project, which in turn gives great promise for the future of this field.

The "explosive" development of genetic research is most promising with respect to the diagnostic phase of neurogenetics and, possibly, involves some therapeutic aspects as well. It nicely illustrates the stepwise advances of science, the close integration of the clinical and biological sciences that are now required, as well as the point of this section, namely that research carries on.

REFERENCES

1. Watson, J.D., and Crick, F.H.C. Molecular structure of nucleic acids—a structure for deoxyribose nucleic acid. *Nature*, 171:737-738, 1953.
2. Pratt, R.T.C. *The Genetics of Neurological Disorders*. London, Oxford University Press, 1967.
3. Garrod, A.E. The Croonian Lectures on inborn errors of metabolism. *Lancet*, 2:1, 73, 142, 214, 1908
4. Garrod, A.E. Alkaptonuria: a simple method for the extraction of homogentisic acid from the urine. *J. Physiol.*, 23:612-614, 1988-1989.
5. Garrod, A.E. *Inborn Errors of Metabolism*. 2nd ed. London, Milford, 1923.
6. Garrod, A.E. *Science of clinical medicine*. B.M.J., 2:621-824, 1926.
7. Hopkins, F.G. *Sir Archibald Garrod*, Memoirs of the Royal Society. London, The Royal Society, 1936, pp. 12-26.
8. Garrod, A.E. Glimpses of the higher medicine. *Lancet*, 1:1091-1096, 1923.
9. Hopkins, F.G. Sir Archibald Garrod. *B.M.J.*, 1:775-779, 1936.
10. A correspondent. Comment on Sir Archibald Garrod as a teacher. *B.M.J.*, 1:732-733, 1936.
11. Morgan, T.H. *Heredity and Sex*. New York, Columbia University Press, 1913.
12. Morgan, T.H., Sturtevant, A.H., Muller, H.J., and Bridges, C.B. *The Mechanism of Mendelian Heredity*. New York, Henry Holt, 1915.

13. Morgan, T.H., Bridges, C.B., and Sturtevant, A.H. The genetics of Drosophila. *Bibliographia Genetica*, 2:1-262, 1925.
14. Morgan, T.H. *The Theory of the Gene*. New Haven, Yale University Press, 1926.
15. Fölling, A. Utskillelse av fenylpyrodruesyre i urinen som stoffskifre anormali i forbindelse med imbecilliter. *Nord. Med. Tidskr.*, 8:1054-1059, 1934.
16. Fölling, A., and Closs, K. über das Vorkommen von 1: Phenylpyruvia in Haen und Blut bei Imbecillitas phenylpyruvica. *Hoppe-Seylers Z. Physiol. Chem.*, 254:115-116, 1938.
17. Fölling, A., Mohr, O.L., and Rudd, L. *Oligophrenia Phenylpyruvica. A Recessive Syndrome in Man.*, Oslo, Det Norske Videnskap Akademi, 1945.
18. Sydnes, S., and Fölling, A. On detection of heterozygotes for phenylpyruvic oligophrenia. *Scand. J. Clin. Invest.*, 14:44-46, 1962.
19. Refsum, S. Heredopathia atactica polyneuritiformis. *Acta Scand* (suppl 38):1-303, 1946.
20. Merritt, H.H. *A Textbook of Neurology*. 3rd ed. Philadelphia, Lea & Febiger, 1963, p. 525.
21. Brain, R. *Diseases of the Nervous System*. 6th ed. London, Oxford University Press, 1962, p. 727.
22. Richterich, R., Kahlke, W., van Michelen, F., and Rosse, E. Refsum's syndrome (Heredopathia atac tica polyneuritiformis) Ein angeborener Dafaket in Lipid-Stoffwechael mit Speicherung vomt 3,7,11,15-tetramethylhexadecan saure. *Klin. Wochenschr.*, 41:800-801, 1963.
23. Flynn, P., and Aird, R.B. A neuroectodermal syndrome of dominant Inheritance. *J. Neurol. Sci.*, 2:161-182, 1965.
24. Refsum, S. Genetic aspects of neurology. In: Baker, A.B. (ed.). *Clinical Neurology*. New York, Hoeber-Harper, 1962.
25. Snyder, L.H. *Medical Genetics*. Durham, NC, Duke University Press, 1941.
26. Tyler, F.H., and Stephens, F.E. Studies in disorders of muscle: II. Clinical manifestations and inheritance of facioscapulohumeral dystrophy in a large family. *Ann. Intern. Med.*, 1950.
27. Pratt, R.T.C. *The Genetics of Neurological Disorders*. 2nd. ed. London, Oxford University Press, 1982.
28. Nirenberg, M.W., and Mattheai, H. The dependence of cell-free protein synthesis in E. coli upon naturally occurring or synthetic polyribonucleotides. *Proc. Natl. Acad. Sci.* U.S.A., 47:1588-1602, 1961.
29. Botstein, D., White, R.J., Skolnick, M., and Davis, R. Construction of a genetic linkage map in man using restriction fragment length polymorphisms. *Am. J. Human Genet.*, 32:314-331, 1980.
30. Cohen, S.N., Chang, A.C.Y., Boyer, H.W., and Helling, R.B. Construction of biologically functional bacterial plasmids *in vitro. Proc. Natl. Acad. Sci.*, U.S.A., 70:3240-3244, 1973.
31. Bishop, J.M. *Retroviruses and oncogenes*. In: *Les Prix Nobel*, 1989. Stockholm, Almqvist & Wiksell International, 1990.
32. Bishop, J.M. The molecular biology of RNA tumor viruses: a physician's guide. *N. Engl. J. Med.*, 303:675, 1980.
33. Bishop, J.M. *Viruses, genes and cancer*. Harvey Lect., 78:137, 1983-1984.
34. Bishop, J.M. The molecular genetics of cancer. *Science*, 235:305-311, 1987.
35. Bishop, J.M. Professional activities in curriculum vitae. San Francisco, University of California, San Francisco, 1992.
36. Gusella, J.F., Wexler, N.S., Conneally, P.M., Naylor, S.L., Anderson, M.A., Tanzi, R.E., Watkins, P.C., Ottina, K., Wallace, M.R., Sakaguchi, A.Y., Young, A.B., Shoulson, I., Bonilla, E., and Martin, J.B. A polymorphic DNA marker genetically linked to Huntington's disease. *Nature*, 306:234-238,1983.
37. St. George-Hyslop, P.H., Tanzi, R.E., Polinsky, R.J., Haines, J.L., Nee, L., et al. The genetic defect causing familial Alzheimer's disease maps on chromosome 21. *Science*, 235:885-890, 1987.
38. St. George-Hyslop, P.H., Haines, J.L., Farrer, L.A., Polinsky, R., Van Broeckoven, G.A., et al. Genetic linkage studies suggest that Alzheimer's disease is not a single homogeneous entity. *Nature*, 347:194-197, 1990.
39. Gusella, J.F., Wexler, N.S., and Conneally, P.M.A. molecular genetic approach to Huntington's disease. *Res. Publ. Assoc. Res. Nerv. Ment. Dis.*, 65:133-141, 1987.

CHAPTER 13

Behavioral Neurology

The use of plants and their extracts for medical use, including psychotherapy, extends back into antiquity and involved essentially all early cultures. Alcohol in its various forms has served as the tranquilizer of the ages and afforded a means of "escape" from the harrowing exigencies of past centuries. Quinine from cinchona bark, digitalis from foxglove, opium from the poppy, cocaine from coca leaves, and rauwolfia are but a few of our herbal agents, now largely superseded by the products of pharmacological chemistry in the past half century. When I led an exchange group of neurologists to China in 1981, we were told that they are doing clinically controlled studies on their herbal medicines and that chemical extraction, purification, and identification of the active ingredients were being done in selected cases. In this way, as well as in active practice, their two systems of medical practice (herbal and modern Western) are slowly being merged. However, when I asked an acupuncturist in Guangzhou, who was treating a poststroke patient, about control studies, he had no idea as to what I meant. He was comfortable with the backing of centuries of practice.

Actually, we in the West, have not been that much ahead. It is only in the past 30 to 40 years that we have utilized adequate clinical control studies. Psychopharmacology and behavioral neurology, thus, have only recently entered their flowering stages. The therapeutic myths and "snake oil" practices of the past will take another generation or more to be eradicated completely. Those interested in the exotic medical beliefs and practices of earlier ages would do well to read the *History of Psychopharmacology* by A. E. Caldwell (1).

Some of the early stirrings of scientific behavioral neurology have already been mentioned in these essays. The cessation of gastrointestinal activity with rage, the fight-or-flight reactions, sham rage, and the discovery of "sympathin" were discussed in the section on Walter Cannon (Chapter 5). The anatomical basis of emotional expression was delineated by Papez and confirmed by Kluver and Bucy, when they ablated the temporal lobe structures of an ape bilaterally (as discussed in Chapter 4). Frontal lobe lobotomy of primates by Fulton and Jacobson produced a passivity, which was capitalized on by Moniz and won him a Nobel prize (discussed subsequently).

These early threads of behavioral neurology can be summarized in large part in the career of Philip Bard.

PHILIP BARD (1898-1977)

Born in Huenera, California, Bard attended the Thacher School in nearby Ojai Valley. Except for his service in France in World War I, his entire subsequent career was in the East. He graduated from Princeton in 1923 and obtained his Ph.D. in physiology under Cannon at the Harvard Medical School in 1927. He served as a teaching fellow and instructor in physiology at Harvard from 1925 to 1928. He was my instructor in physiology in early 1927. There were four of us assigned to one of the physiological laboratory tables under his supervision. Because of his service in World War I, Bard was some 5 years older than our group, although he had still been at Princeton when my Princeton classmates were freshmen there. My Cornell background seemed to rate well with Bard. He had heard of the great Vosberg hoax at Cornell (as discussed in Chapter 5) and also the many wild hoaxes of my classmate, Hugh Troy, which had received much newspaper publicity at that time. This created a bond of sorts but not the warm attention received by my Princeton classmates.

I decided that I should work on my Princeton "credentials." In my early elementary school days, I had attended Proctor Academy, a private school in Provo, Utah, supported in part by the Congregational Church before World War I. Our teachers were from the East and Midwest, and I received an excellent grounding. Our principal was S. H. Goodman, a Princeton graduate, and we used the Princeton colors. Our joyous but very surreptitious school chant went like this:

> S. H. Goodman is a grand old man: He goes to church on Sunday: He prays to the Lord to give him strength.To rawhide the boys on Monday.

As ridiculous and farfetched as this may seem, it brought a laugh and at least showed my appreciation of Bard's beloved Princeton. Like my membership in the Southern Club of Harvard, in which I qualified by extrapolation of the Mason-Dixon line to the Pacific Ocean, the bonds of youth transcend the barriers of school and region.* In any case, Bard seemed delighted, and I was immediately taken into the extended Princeton fold. The end result in physiology was that we all developed a close working relation with Bard, and he did much to stimulate my interest in physiology.

That Bard was greatly interested in Princeton was borne out by his going there to teach as an assistant professor of biology. However, after 2 years at Princeton, he returned to Harvard as an assistant professor of physiology in 1931 to 1933. An opening at Hopkins and the support of Cannon at Harvard gained him the position of professor of physiology and director of the Department of Physiology at Johns Hopkins Medical School in 1933, where he remained for the rest of his career. He served as the dean of the faculty at Hopkins in 1953 to 1957 and became professor emeritus in 1964.

---

*Unless it was too close to the Mason-Dixon line east of the Mississippi!

His research interests were drawn to the sympathetic nervous system and rage reactions of the diencephalon as a result of Cannon's earlier investigations. His first article on this was in 1928, and he produced several more in subsequent years (2). The central representation of the sympathetic nervous system and its role in behavioral problems was explored by Bard in some seven additional studies (3-5). Early publications chiefly involved decortication and localization investigations on the diencephalon and hypothalamus and other problems, such as temperature regulation, posture, obesity, and the vascular system (6,7). Later studies involved evoked potentials to localize cutaneous tactile sensibility in the primate cerebral cortex and related problems of motion sickness (8). He wrote several chapters in texts and two excellent essays on his early mentor, Walter Cannon (9).

Bard attracted and trained such notable neurophysiologists as C. N. Woolsey, C. M. Brooke, D McK. Rioch, W. K. Marshall, H. C. Curtis, R. S. Snider, H.-T. Chang, V. B. Mountcastle, and J. W. Woods. He served as editor of several physiological texts and was on the editorial boards of the American Journal of Physiology, Physiological Reviews, and others.

Bard was a member of several prestigious national societies, including the National Academy of Sciences, and was elected president of three of them. He was an honorary member of several foreign societies, fulfilled five named lectureships, and won two awards and four honorary degrees.

Following the death of his first wife, he married Janet M. Rioch, M.D., in 1965. I knew Janet in my postgraduate period at the Strong Memorial Hospital (University of Rochester) in 1931 and helped to take care of her when she was ill on one occasion.

Bard's contributions served to extend, refine, and integrate many of the earlier, disparate studies on the behavioral responses of the central nervous system. He was one of the pioneers in this but also served as a transitional figure through the flowering period of neurophysiology and behavioral neurology.

Aside from these early phases of behavioral neurology, psychiatry went through a nebulous period of trials, claims, and counterclaims, based on anecdotal data that could not meet the strict statistical demands of science. Psychologically inclined leaders of critical scientific abilities, such as Percival Bailey, Herbert Jasper, and Raymond Adams, featured in these essays, and several others were disappointed in the lack of a scientific basis in psychiatry and pursued various careers to correct this. This does not mean to imply that psychiatry was a sham and delusion. It had great supportive value to emotionally disturbed patients and individually aided them in sorting out their problems and improving their interpersonal relations. This supportive aspect of psychiatry should not be underestimated, as was strikingly shown in a patient who developed a right frontal brain tumor during a period of well over 1 year while under the hospitalized care of psychiatrists. Only after he complained of visual impairment was I asked to see him. His choked discs and neurological findings clearly pointed to the diagnosis, and following neurosurgery, he made a good recovery, including his depression for which he had been originally hospitalized. Nevertheless, he was enthusiastic about the care he had received over the previous year and emphasized his better understanding of himself and improved relations with others. The psychiatric team had done a wonderful job from a functional psychiatric standpoint, but they failed miserably as doctors of medicine. His failure to relate his depression to his tumor was fortunate in this litigious age but also perhaps raises questions as to his insight.

At a higher level, psychiatrists have attempted to classify the various behavioral disorders on a clinical basis. However, the overlap of excitatory, depressive, neurotic, manic, paranoid, and schizoid states has produced a confused picture that has made strict classification difficult. Some early psychiatrists believed that all behavioral disorders not associated with neuropathology must be psychiatric and amenable to psychotherapy. This approach failed to consider pathophysiological and biochemical syndromes, such as hyperthyroidism and myasthenia gravis, which were finally sorted out and removed from the psychiatric field. When do pathophysiologic disorders produce pathology, and do not all such disorders, whether associated with known pathological conditions or not, produce anxiety and psychosomatic reactions? This applies to all disorders, whether caused by pathophysiological conditions, such as epilepsy and other medical conditions, or environmental circumstances that produce critical stresses in the individual. How often are medically related anxieties treated for long periods by psychological therapists? As the neurologic consultant to the Langley Porter Clinic (University of California, San Francisco), I saw this happen repeatedly, even with medically trained psychiatrists. It is still a confused field and will remain so until its various disorders can be related more definitely to underlying neurophysiological and neurochemical processes as opposed to secondary anxiety reactions. In some conditions, such as epilepsy, the psychosocial problems may transcend the medical in importance. Personality characteristics, intellectual levels, and the emotional maturity of the patient are factors that determine the individual ability to cope with the environment and to make social adjustments. These must be considered by the neurologist and other physicians in handling medical problems. This is part of the art of medicine (as discussed in Chapter 14), but when the patient's reactions exceed the levels of normal anxiety, consultation with medical psychologists and psychiatrists is important.

Psychosomatic disorders related to diseases of unknown origin, such as colitis, rheumatoid arthritis, disturbances of menstruation, dysuria, and hypertension, seem to be distinct from the psychoneuroses. More distinct still are those behavioral disorders that respond to organic forms of therapy, such as shock treatment and psychopharmacological agents. Some of these have suggestive or more definite genetic backgrounds and, because of their more distinctive clinical character, are probably medical diseases. Such are the manic, depressive, paranoid, and schizophrenic states. The fact that their underlying etiological mechanisms remain obscure reflects the "functional" nature of their neuropathophysiology and biochemistry. So far, it has been like "hunting for a needle in a haystack." This analogy, however, is probably poor, because the brain is far more complex than a haystack. In any case, it seems likely that these disorders will eventually fit into the "organic" phase of the broad spectrum of behavioral disorders. Also, like all other disorders, they probably are subject to secondary, environmentally conditioned, behavioral reactions, as suggested by their precipitating mechanisms, the negative reactions of the catatonic form of schizophrenia, and others.

It may be worthwhile to present one or two examples to illustrate these points, inasmuch as it remains a confused subject, still much debated.

Mr. A, a 22-year-old white man, was referred for study 32 years ago. His failure in college courses 1 year earlier had led to his withdrawing from college and later joining the Navy. He had done poorly in naval training, had been hospitalized for bizarre behavior and given a diagnosis of schizophrenia, and finally, had been discharged.

Examination showed disorganized speech, punctuated by inappropriate bursts of laughter, inability to hold to a sequential line of thought, faulty recall, and impaired abstract intellectual functioning. Mr. A appeared withdrawn, and his affect was quite flat. He reported depressive moods, detached periods in which everything seemed strange and unreal, déja vu, and occasional hallucinations of hearing voices. There was no paranoia, nor did he have delusions of control.

His personal and family histories were not notable, except for considerable conflict between his divorced parents and their families. His physical and neurological examinations were normal.

An electroencephalogram showed a right temporal and adjacent low frontal focus. Pneumoencephalographic studies showed dilatation of the right lateral ventricle and shift of the midline to the left. On repeated trials, the gas could not be dislodged from the dilated ventricle, and follow-up studies suggested its progressive dilatation.

Mr. A's neurological diagnosis was temporal lobe syndrome associated with a dilated right lateral ventricle and shift of the midline to the left, caused by an unidentified ballvalve block of the right foramen of Monroe. His psychiatric diagnosis was schizophrenia, acute and undifferentiated.

Neurosurgical exploration showed an enlarged choroid plexus, attached by pedicle to the ventricular wall, that blocked the foramen of Monroe. Following successful corrective surgery, Mr. A rapidly improved and has lived a successful life in a competitive field without recurrence of his illness over a follow-up period of 32 years.

Although Mr. A's clinical diagnosis of schizophrenia well preceded the present more rigid criteria of the current classification system, schizophrenia was independently diagnosed by two distinguished and nationally known psychiatrists. The case is unique in that it involved a discrete ventricular block mechanism but no intrinsic cerebral pathology, aside from a possible secondary periventricular atrophy. The implications for modern studies that have identified periventricular abnormalities in schizophrenia are highly suggestive (10).

Another case report, which involved a very different clinical picture but also showed the overlap of organic and functional findings, was that of P.T.

P.T., a young woman artist, 32 years of age, was referred by a psychiatrist for treatment of her severe epilepsy. Her spells had started 2 years after a severe head injury involving her right frontotemporal region, 16 years before. She was a high-strung, sensitive person, who had developed schizophrenic symptoms 3 to 4 years after her spells had started. At least for 10 years, her epilepsy and schizoid state had shown a distinct alternate pattern.

The psychiatrist reported prolonged periods of confused thought, disorganized speech, poor memory, and impaired abstract thinking, inappropriate affect, impaired insight, and occasional auditory hallucinations were said to accompany her episodes.

My examination showed none of these findings, and her physical and neurological examinations were essentially normal, aside from a left lower facial underaction and suggestive increased deep reflexes on the left.

She exhibited considerable anxiety about her condition, verified the psychiatrist's report and added that she had depressive moods, associated with detachment. Glimpses of her psychiatric problems eventually appeared and were interwoven with her temporal lobe syndrome. She also reported that her spells were preceded by déja vu and a sense of fear and that sometimes these symptoms occurred with confusional periods, in which she could not understand what she read or heard but did not develop into her usual generalized seizures.

Previous treatment had consisted of phenobarbital 60 mg three times a day. Phenytoin 100 mg three times a day and phenobarbital 30 mg three times a day controlled her spells, but both the patient and the psychiatrist reported that her schizophrenia-like state was worse. When she stopped receiving phenytoin, her spells recurred, and following this, her schizoid state cleared. Various regimens were tried over a period of 2 years, but the alternate pattern of spells or schizophrenic-like state persisted. Her insight at times caused her to dread the schizoid states more than her spells, and it was impossible to maintain her on an adequate antiepileptic schedule, which included a low fluid and salt regimen. She finally committed suicide.

These cases, including the right frontal tumor depression, emphasize the close interrelationships between behavioral disorders and organic mechanisms, and it was primarily in this area that major advances in psychiatry have occurred. This has involved a series of therapeutic measures that can be illustrated by the careers of those who introduced them.

The first important turn in psychiatry developed with the introduction of insulin shock therapy. Sakel's approach to this well illustrates the limited and confused conceptualization of behavioral disorders in the early 1930s.

MANFRED SAKEL (1900-1957)

Of Jewish origin in Poland at the time Nadworna was part of the Austro-Hungarian Empire, he matured in the period between the wars when anti-Semitism was growing in Central Europe. His reaction was one of pride in withstanding the oppression of a minority, ethnic group. He graduated from the First State College of Brno, Czechoslovakia, and obtained his medical education in Vienna (1920 to 1925). A research fellowship in Berlin followed, and in 1927, he became the chief physician to the Lichterfelde Hospital in Berlin. This was a private hospital in which morphine addiction was frequently treated. Sakel was impressed by the stormy withdrawal symptoms of morphine, which he related to thyrotoxicosis. Because insulin had recently been shown to have an antagonistic effect to the thyroid, he tried it in the withdrawal phase of the treatment of morphinism. This proved beneficial, and after animal experiments that showed hypoglycemic insulin shock could be administered safely, he tried it in other types of psychiatric excitement, including schizophrenia.

Thoroughly convinced of the beneficial effects of insulin shock therapy, he returned to Vienna and worked as a volunteer in the university psychiatric service, then under Professor Poetzl. He was able to employ insulin shock in patients exhibiting abnormal states of excitement. Professor Poetzl became convinced of its efficacy, and in spite of a stormy period of claims and counterclaims, Poetzl vouched for the benefits of Sakel's insulin shock therapy. This led to its trial by several leading psychiatrists, who became advocates of insulin shock therapy, particularly in schizophrenia. Its value soon spread to other centers in Europe. Sakel's main publication was on insulin shock therapy for schizophrenia (11), but his opus on schizophrenia was delayed for another 20 years (12).

Sakel was invited to the United States to treat a patient, and through the influence of Dr. A. A. Brill and Frederick Parsons, the New York State Commissioner of Mental Hygiene, training programs were established under Sakel's direction in the New York mental hospitals. Sakel stayed on in America and was in much demand as a speaker and for private consultations. He received an honorary degree from Colgate University in 1936 and turned down a professorial opening. The latter was probably just as well because his background was limited. In his obituary, Joseph Wortis, M.D., refers to some of his scientific utterances" as being "surprisingly naive." However, Wortis gave high marks to Sakel for his powers of keen observation, his insight, and his "courage and tenacious persistence" (13).

Sakel became a private practitioner and eventually was ignored by academic circles. However, in his defense, I should mention that he maintained a large free practice, lived very simply, contributed extensively to charitable causes, and developed great interest in the work of the Friends (Quakers). A serious heart attack in 1948 forced him to limit his activities, and following this, he lost contact with essentially all scientific and academic groups. His death was due to a recurrent heart attack 9 years later.

Sakel was an innovator and his emphasis on the pathophysiological nature of major psychiatric disorders was important in setting the stage for the second principal step in shock therapy. This involved electroshock therapy (EST) introduced by Ugo Cerletti in 1938. The background and results of this can best be presented by a brief account of Cerletti's career.

UGO CERLETTI (1877-1963)

Cerletti was born in Conegliano, a village in the northeastern part of Italy. His medical training was at Rome and Turin, and he had postgraduate training in psychiatry with Kraepelin at Heidelberg and also in Munich. He studied neurology and neuropathology with Pierre Marie and Dupré in Paris. He also worked with Nissl and Alzheimer.

His early career was in Rome, where he did neuropathology and research. Following World War I, he was the director of research at Monbello, a mental hospital near Milan. His research mainly involved the neuroglia, the nerve networks of the cerebral vessels, and cerebral senile plaques.

In 1925, he accepted the chair of neuropsychiatry at the University of Bard, and 3 years later, he founded the Neuropsychiatric Clinic at the University of Genoa. In 1935, he became director of the Neuropsychiatric Clinic in Rome, where he remained until retirement in 1948.

While in Genoa, his research was on the parameters of EST on dogs, and this was followed by studies in Rome, which showed a considerable safety factor between the electric currents needed for producing convulsions as opposed to those that were fatal. This was done on pigs that were to be killed anyway at the slaughter house of Rome. With this background and using precise electroshock equipment made by his associate, Lucio Bini, the first trial was made on a schizophrenic patient in April 1938. After 11 EST treatments, the patient was discharged home markedly improved. EST was noted to be effective in depressive states as well as in schizophrenia (14).

Aside from some confusion due to the isolation of Italy in World War II, EST soon gained wide acceptance and was hailed for its low cost in comparison with insulin shock therapy. By the time that Kalinowsky and Hoch made their comprehensive study of EST, they were able to make the statement that it was "the most widely used shock therapy in psychiatry prior to the introduction of new drugs in the 1950s" (15).

Cerletti won international fame for his introduction of EST. He was elected to be President of the Italian Psychiatric Association and Honorary President of the Italian Neurological Society, and he received a special award from the Academy of Italy. Honorary degrees were received from four foreign universities.

As a man, Cerletti was well known for his keen intellect and personal modesty. He was a lover of the arts and was said to be an excellent draftsman. His association with Lucio Bini was close and supportive.*

Cerletti's discovery of EST and his relations with Bini are fully covered in an interesting article in the American Journal of Psychiatry in 1950 (17).

The technique of EST was followed by a surprising development, psychosurgery, which was more striking in some respects than practical. However, it verified the earlier neurophysiological observations of Fulton and Jacobson (discussed subsequently) and validated still another aspect of the organic approach to the severe psychopathological disorders. The story is an interesting one and largely dependent on the career of Egas Moniz.

EGAS MONIZ (ANTONIO COSTANO DEALBREA FREIRE) (1875-1955)

Although Moniz dates back into an earlier period of neurology, he had two careers, and in his second, starting at the age of 55, he had a profound effect on both neurology and psychiatry. His fascinating story can only be understood in the context of his time and place.

He was born on a farm near Avanca in northern Portugal that had belonged to his ancestors for some five centuries. At his christening, his godfather added the name, Egas Moniz, to an already complicated name. Egas Moniz had been a hero in the resistance of the Portuguese to the Moors in the middle ages, and Antonio adopted it later, at first as a nom de plume in his early political writing and later in his medical career.

Moniz graduated in medicine from the University of Coimbra in 1899. Graduate studies in neurology at Bordeaux and Paris followed, and on his return to Coimbra, he was appointed to the chair of neurology. Later, he was made a professor of neu-

---

*Bini was an outstanding psychiatrist in his own right. In 1956, he was made chief of neurology of hospitals in Rome and established an excellent neuropsychiatric center at the Hospital San Camillo. It was Bini who constructed the EST equipment, handled the shock treatments, and collaborated with Cerletti on the original report. He also established the indications for EST (16). With Bazzi, Bini wrote the only modern Italian textbook of psychiatry.

rology at the University of Lisbon, a position that allowed him to exploit his earlier, antimonarchist political beliefs. With the overthrow of the monarchy, he became Minister of Foreign Affairs and, later, Ambassador to Spain. He represented Portugal at the Treaty of Versailles at the end of World War I.

His political fortunes turned with the restoration of the monarchy, following which he resumed his medical career as a professor of neurology at Lisbon. In 1927, he conceived the idea of visualizing the arteries of the brain by means of x-rays, following the intravenous injection of radiopaque substances. After much experimentation on animals, he reported carotid angiography with the use of sodium iodide (18). Following a later report from Germany, he switched to thorium dioxide, a well-tolerated colloidal substance that was more opaque and with which he could better visualize vascular abnormalities of the brain. However, thorium dioxide was later shown to have carcinogenic properties, and the new technique did not gain general acceptance until Swedish radiologists, using a nonirritating iodine compound, popularized the technique.

Moniz developed his second revolutionary concept in 1935 as the result of attending the Second International Congress of Neurology in London. Fulton and Jacobson reported docile responses in chimpanzees following bilateral frontal lobotomy (19). Realizing the possible significance of this for disturbed psychiatric patients, he convinced his neurosurgical colleague, Alomeid Lima, to devise a leukotome for prefrontal lobotomy in selected patients. This human experiment, which probably could have been done only under the special circumstances in Lisbon, was startlingly successful. Not only was it successful clinically, but it profoundly jolted the prevailing psychiatric thought that the psyche could be altered by surgical means. This indeed was an organic approach! Great opposition developed, in spite of which Moniz was able to report 100 lobotomized patients (20). It was widely used elsewhere, even though the opposition continued. Moniz was awarded the Nobel prize in 1949.

This dramatic development, the suggestion by Papez of an anatomical basis for emotional expression, as discussed in Chapter 4, the success of the earlier insulin shock treatment, and EST in schizophrenia and depression slowly forced the psychiatric acceptance of organic therapeutic mechanisms. To this should be added the behavioral effects of sedative and stimulant drugs, D-lysergic acid diethylamide, the antihistamines (synthesized by my friend Gordon Alles in 1927 and later used in depressive states*) and lithium carbonate (introduced by Cade in 1949 for manic-depressive disorders**

In 1940, Moniz was critically wounded by a gun shot from one of his schizophrenic patients. He made a full recovery from this and did not retire until the age

---

*A building is named in his honor at the California Institute of Technology.

**The famous neuropsychiatrist, Weir Mitchell, had tried lithium bromide in 1870 for the epilepsies, hemicrania, and insomnia. Although his results were excellent, his study was centered around the bromides and was not applied to manic-depressive conditions.

I tried lithium chloride to enhance dehydration in epilepsy. Like Mitchell, I "missed the boat" because it was never tried in severe behavior.

of 69 in 1944. He continued to write and welcomed the International Congress of Psychosurgery in 1948. The Centro dos Estudos Egas Moniz was established in Lisbon in his honor.

It was largely on the basis of these developments and the Nobel prize in 1949 that the Fifth International Congress of Neurology met in Lisbon in 1953. Portugal had bestirred itself after the decision was made in 1949, and although the new medical school of the University of Lisbon was still not complete, the Congress successfully met in the new quarters. What a triumphant conclusion to a stormy career, or one might say to his two careers.

Personally, Moniz was said to be a genial and even convivial person. His physique seemed typical of Portugal to me, but there was no question about the alert mentality and dignity of the man. There was no chance for personal contact at the 1953 Congress, aside from limited formal introductions. He died at his estate in Avanca on December 18, 1955.

The fourth therapeutic "organic" approach to psychiatric conditions developed with psychopharmacology. This was by no means a new approach, but one that had floundered for centuries because of its lack of success. The lack of definition of some psychiatric disorders, their overlap, and the failure to differentiate sedative effects from ataraxy (as discussed under Laborit) in combination with the supportive and remunerative aspects of traditional psychotherapy served to delay progress for many years. With the development of chlorpromazine in 1953, the breakthrough of psychopharmacology finally took off (1). This is a complex story, which can best be conveyed by the career of Dr. Henri Laborit, a French surgeon. His story is a very unusual one, and his "neurolytic cocktail" is basic to the development of the modern era of psychopharmacology.

HENRI LABORIT (1914-   )

Born in Hanoi, the son of a French army surgeon in Indochina, Henri's early life was unusually turbulent. This and his ethnic background (Chouans of the Vendel region of France, who fought the revolutionary government of France in 1793 but who were finally subdued by Napoleon) may have nurtured his independent and questioning mind. His father died of tetanus in the leper colony of French Guiana, and it was this tragic event that turned young Henri to medicine.

His early schooling was in Paris, and he studied medicine in his father's alma mater, the Health Service of the Navy and Colonial Troops in Bordeaux. His mother influenced him to choose the Navy, rather than the dreaded colonial army service.

When World War II broke out in 1939, his ship, the destroyer, Sirocco, fought in the North Sea battle with the German fleet and later aided in the English Channel evacuation at Dunkirk. His ship was torpedoed while evacuating 800 men. Only 80 survived, but Laborit, a good swimmer, was one of them. He then was assigned a post in Togoland on the Ivory Coast of Western Africa and served as a surgeon in a hospital at Dakar. Following the Allied advance in North Africa (1942), he was assigned to a hospital in Oran, and later, as a surgeon on a French cruiser, he participated in the Anzio landing in Italy.

Posts followed in Toulon, Lorient, and Bizerta (Tunis). His career changed while in Toulon, where he met the distinguished biologist-chemist, Pierre Morand. Laborit had become interested in traumatic shock as a result of his surgical experiences. He envisioned pharmacology as a method of reducing sensory input to the autonomic nervous system, at that time postulated as the center of origin of shock. He worked for several years at the physiological laboratory of the French Army trying to block sensory input at the synaptic level of the sympathetic ganglia. His studies included cholinesterase and curare. The use of the latter finally found acceptance in obstetrics and, later, as a surgical technique to reduce muscle tension and, thus, relieve the necessity of deep anesthesia. With the use of tetraethyl ammonium, a new ganglionic blocker, American and British surgeons confirmed Laborit's thesis and approach. This was the basis of his "potentiated anesthesia." However, Laborit's presurgical "lytic cocktail" contained a combination of drugs of low toxicity, which acted both centrally and peripherally on the autonomic nervous system. Among these agents were promethazine and mesopyramine, recently developed by the French biochemist, Paul Charpentier. They were used as antihistamines, the central effects of which were thought to have a cortical sedative and "hypnotic" reaction (21).

Laborit next sought even stronger, centrally acting neuropharmacological measures to inhibit the overreactions of the autonomic nervous system to shock. His reasoning in this was to reduce the sensory input and metabolism of the central nervous system (the milieu intérieur of Claude Bernard and homeostasis of Walter Cannon) to levels comparable to the hibernation of animals. By using a number of blocking agents in his lytic cocktail in combination with ice packs, he achieved his "artificial hibernation" (22).

As a result of his comparative use of different agents in his cocktails and his keen powers of observation, Laborit detected the fact that the phenothiazines produced a different reaction than the sedatives. This difference was especially prominent when chlorpromazine was used. The effect involved a state of serenity, in which patients no longer suffered anxiety in the preoperative period and continued in a painless somnolence postoperatively. Thus, the phenothiazines replaced the barbiturates preoperatively and morphine postoperatively. Laborit termed it an autonomic effect, but it required several more years before this important distinction was widely recognized. The new serene effect was eventually termed ataraxy by my friend, Howard D. Fabing, with the aid of a Greek scholar.

So striking was the effect of chlorpromazine, Laborit investigated its use alone, wrote several articles on its potential in psychiatry, and urged psychiatrists to try it (1). Psychiatrists had tried promethazine in mental patients earlier but were not enthusiastic. Many had become drug shy as a result of poor results and toxic side effects.

In 1950, a striking "calming" effect in schizophrenic patients had been noted with a phenothiazine developed by the Geigy pharmaceutical company, but there had been no follow-up on this. Thus, it remained for Laborit to cajol his psychiatric colleagues in the Val-de-Grâce Hospital of Paris to try chlorpromazine (1). A host of reports followed, and various pharmaceutical firms quickly entered the field. This in turn led to a strong development of psychopharmacology. In the review article written by Joseph Wortis in 1964, 10 "familiar" drugs, 23 new ones, and 13 other psychopharmacological agents were discussed (23). The revolution in psychiatry had occurred; actually, this had started considerably earlier. In the planning phase of the Langley Porter Clinic in the late 1930s, the argument for state funds had turned on the good effects of Sakel's insulin shock treatment. The promising picture was painted of greatly reducing the numbers of patients requiring endless custodial care and the tremendous tax savings that would ensue. The example of Sakel's training in the New York mental hospitals was cited, and insulin shock therapy became one of the mainstays in the Langley Porter Clinic. However, the early dream did not actually materialize until the introduction of chlorpromazine and the psychophar-macological revolution that followed. Problems of outpatient supervision were not envisioned, but in spite of this, there is no question of the profound impact of psy-chopharmacology.

The role of Laborit in all this involved several basic aspects. His methods of study with his lytic cocktail and his development of potentiated anesthesia and artificial hibernation overlapped in several respects with the field of psychiatry. He was the first to note ataraxy and to differentiate it from the prevailing idea of a cortical sedative-hypnotic effect. He was the one to urge the development of a stronger, centrally acting "autonomic" inhibitor, which led to the development of chlorpro-mazine. More specifically, it was Laborit's work that triggered the pharmaceutical company, Specia, to produce chlorpromazine (1), and finally, it was his articles and personal urging that led to the first trial of chlorpromazine in psychiatric patients.

Still later, Laborit conceived the idea that shock might involve metabolism at the cellular level (22). This required biophysical studies on the permeability of the cell membrane, and he even dealt with the problems of neurophysiological feedback and cybernetics (as discussed under McCulloch in Chapter 17). He also investigat-ed the possible role of serotonin in the activity of Evan's somatotropin growth hor-mone (as discussed in Chapter 16). Thus, the naval surgeon progressed from an interest in anesthesiology through neurophysiology, neurochemistry, neuropharma-cology, biophysics, and cybernetic theory.

His success and research eventually led to his becoming director of a laboratory Centre d'Etudes Expérimentales et Cliniques de Physiologie, de Pharmacologie, et d'Entomologie" at the Boucicaut Hospital in Paris. It is a private nonprofit organi-zation, supported by royalties from patents developed by Dr. Laborit and his research colleagues. In all this, Laborit was the one whose theories stimulated many lines of neurochemical and neurophysiological research. Much of this was summa-rized in Les Régulations Metaboliques (24).

His publications involve some 15 books in addition to many monographs and sci-entific articles. In 1959, he started a journal called *Agressologic* devoted to those aspects of physiology that are involved in human problems of aggression. In addi-tion, he has organized several conferences, *Journées de l'Agressologic*, at the Val-de-Grâce hospital.

Laborit has received a number of honors, the highest that I have been able to verify being the Albert Lasker award in 1957.

The organic approaches to behavioral disorders extended from 1931 to 1953, and they have been continued, amplified, and refined over the past several decades. This has led to two important developments: (1) a reevaluation of the neuroanatomical, neurophysiological, neurochemical, neuropsychological, and clinical data, which might throw light on the etiological mechanisms underlying behavioral disorders, and (2) the training of young neuroscientists in the field of psychiatry, whose research we hope will unravel its complexities.

The first approach has been led by Dr. Norman Geschwind of Harvard, and a review of his work in the behavioral sciences makes a fitting close to this chapter.

NORMAN GESCHWIND (1926-1984)

Born in New York City, Geschwind grew up in Brooklyn and obtained a solid grounding at the Boys High School (25). Through the influence of one of his teachers, Mr. Mann, he went to Harvard. World War II interrupted his academic career, and he served in Germany, Czechoslovakia, and finally, in the occupation force of Japan. He returned to Harvard and graduated magna cum laude in 1946. His period at the Harvard Medical School was also distinguished. He graduated in 1951 cum laude and, then, took his internship at the Beth Israel Hospital in Boston. In 1952, he obtained a Mosley Fellowship at the National Hospital, Queen Square, London, and worked under Sir Charles Symonds. He obtained Public Health Service Fellowships for 2 more years, working with Arnold Carmichael and Godwin Greenfield at the National Hospital, Queen Square, London. On his return to America, he served as Chief Resident on the neurological service under Denny-Brown at the Boston City Hospital (as discussed in Chapter 15). Two years of research in neurophysiology followed at the Massachusetts Institute of Technology. In 1958, he joined Dr. Quadfasel's neurology service at the Boston Veterans Administration Hospital (affiliated with Boston University). Five years later, when Quadfasel moved to Washington, D.C., Geschwind became chief of the neurology service, and in 1965, he was made the chair of the Department of Neurology at Boston University.

It was at the Veterans Administration Hospital that his interests in the higher functions of the brain blossomed and where his first case of the disconnection syndrome was reported (26). With support from the National Institutes of Health, he started the Aphasia Research Center. This led to an intensive period of clinical investigation, anatomical research, and writing on aphasia, language-induced epilepsy, the anatomical asymmetries of the brain, dominance, laterality, isolation of the speech area, the apraxias, and agnosias.

In 1969, he transferred to Harvard when he received the appointment of the James Jackson Putnam chair of neurology. He succeeded Dr. Denny-Brown in this and his service at the Boston City Hospital. However, Harvard discontinued its service at the Boston City Hospital, and Geschwind's service was transferred to the Beth Israel Hospital in 1975. In 1978, he accepted a joint appointment at the Massachusetts Institute of Technology as a professor of psychology and regularly attended rounds, not only on his service at the Beth Israel Hospital, but also at the Massachusetts Institute of Technology and the Aphasia Research Center.

His disconnection syndromes, which initiated the modern trend in behavioral neurology, also led to many studies on anatomical brain asymmetries (27,28). Following the lead of Percival Bailey and others (as discussed in Chapter 8), Geschwind thought of temporal lobe epilepsy as a useful bridge between neurology and psychiatry, and he published several articles on this subject, which we discussed on occasion (29). Another and final area of interest concerned the pathophysiology of cerebral dominance and handedness (30). Published following his death were three comprehensive articles on "Cerebral lateralization: Biological mechanisms, associations, and pathology: A hypothesis and a program for research" (31-33). The wealth of data (653 references), its diverse sources, and integration into plausible hypotheses for research are astounding and probably will stimulate research for years to come.

Geschwind was a unique person and I very much regretted his passing, especially at such a young age before his work was finished. Considering his family history, one may wonder about a genetic factor. His older brother, who was a distinguished professor of endocrinology at the University of California, Berkeley, died at the age of 54. His father died when Dr. Geschwind was 4 years old. I had known him for years, and he came to us as the Aird Visiting Professor of Neurology in 1974. We met at various meetings and Harvard reunions. He had the "gift of gab" and was a popular speaker with a keen sense of humor. His brilliance, breadth of knowledge, and linguistic ability were daunting, in spite of which he was very modest and kindly.

Despite his early death, many honors came his way—three honorary degrees, two awards, and several honorary memberships and visiting lectureships. He was elected president of the Boston Society of Neurology and Psychiatry and of the American Association of University Professors of Neurology. Except for his early death, he would have received many more honors. As the leader in the field of behavioral neurology, he makes a fitting, final addition to this essay. Will the research he advocated involve the pathophysiology of the vast network of cerebral nuclei and tracts, perhaps imbalanced by the disconnections and other mechanisms envisioned by Geschwind, or are neurochemical disorders of the cerebral neurotransmitters at work, secondary to enzymatic defects of either primary genetic or secondary environmental origin? Anatomical asymmetries suggest structural changes comparable to pathology but, possibly, caused by genetic or secondary factors. It seems likely that both are involved and constitute a complex that will produce many Nobel prize winners in the future.

SUMMARY

Although the roots of psychotherapy can be traced back to the ancient days of tutelary gods and the exorcism of demons from those "possessed," modern psychiatry could not develop rational forms of therapy until the advances of science permitted. Nevertheless, psychiatry, when offered a remunerative form of therapy, as in the case of neurosurgery, assumed the stature of an independent medical discipline 20 to 30 years before the flowering of both neurology and pediatric neurology.

However, because psychotherapy had its limitations, the true flowering of psychiatry had to await the development of behavioral neurology and, especially, the development of psychopharmacology. Its true flowering, thus, coincides with the flowering of neurology.

The stirring of modern psychiatry developed in the early decades of the 20th century as the advances of neuroanatomy and neurophysiology slowly pointed the way. These occurred as the result of the studies of Papez, Cannon, and others and have been summarized in the transitional career of Philip Bard. The physical shock methods of insulin (Sakel), EST (Cerletti), psychosurgery (Moniz), and finally, psychopharmacology (Laborit and the development of chlorpromazine) revolutionized the field. Many other agents (e.g., lithium for manic-depression) and the development of medical psychology aided in the advances made. Now the bulk of psychiatric patients can be treated in the office, and psychological therapists handle the mass of marginal patients, whose anxieties are secondary to physical, mental, and environmental stresses.

All this, however, is just a start, as shown by the behavioral neurological studies of Geschwind. It seems safe to say that only as the modern psychiatrists and others, trained in the basic neurosciences and clinical psychology, are able to advance our understanding of the cerebral basis of emotional activity, can better techniques of psychiatric prevention and therapy be achieved.

REFERENCES

1. Caldwell, A.E. *History of psychopharmacology.* In: Clark, W.G., and del Giudice, J. Principles of Psychopharmacology. New York Academic Press, 1979.
2. Bard, P., A diencephalic for the expression of rage with special reference to the sympathetic nervous system. *Am. J. Physiol.*, 84:490-515, 1928.
3. Bard, P. *The central representation of the sympathetic nervous system as indicated by certain physiological findings.* In: The Vegetative Nervous System, Proceedings of the Association for Research in Nervous and Mental Disease. 1930, pp. 67-91.
4. Bard, P. On emotional expression after decortication with some remarks on certain theoretical views: Part I. *Psychol. Rev.*, 41:309-329, 1934.
5. Bard, P. On emotional expression after decortication with some remarks on certain theoretical views: Part II. *Psychol. Rev.*, 41:424-449, 1934.
6. Pinkston, J.O., Bard, P., and Rioch, D.Mck. The responses to changes in environmental temperature after removal of portions of the forebrain. *Am. J. Physiol.*, 109:515-531, 1934.
7. Chandler, McC., Brooks, E.F., Lambert, E.F., and Bard, P. Experimental production of obesity in the monkey (Macaca mulatta). *Fed. Proc.*, 1:11, 1942.
8. Bard, P., Woolsey, C.N., Snider, R.S., Mountcastle, V.B., and Bromiley, R.B. Delimitation of central nervous mechanisms involved in motion sickness. Fed. Proc., 5:7, 1947.
9. Bard, P. *Walter Bradford Cannon's Contributions to Physiology.* In: Walter Bradford Cannon (1871-1945): A Memorial Exercise Held at the Harvard Medical School, November 5, 1945. Cambridge, Harvard University Press, 1945.
10. Aird, R.B. Neurological aspects of schizophrenia. *Am. J. Psychiatry*, 144:10, 1987.
11. Sakel, M. The pharmacological Shock Treatment of *Schizophrenia*. Translated by Joseph Wortis, M.D. New York, Nervous and Mental Disease Publishing, 1938.
12. Sakel, M. *Schizophrenia*. New York, Philosophical Library, 1958.
13. Wortis, J. In memorium, Manfred Sakel, M.D., 1900-1957. Am. J. Psychiatry, 115:287-288, 1958.
14. Cerletti, U., and Bini, L. Le alterazioni istoptologiche del sistema nervoso in seguito all'E.S. Riv. Sper. Freniat., 64:136, 1940.
15. Kalinowsky, L.R., and Hoch, P.H. *Somatic Treatment in Psychiatry.* New York, Grune & Stratton, 1961.

16. Bini, L. Electric convulsive therapy. *Am. J. Psychiatry*, 94:172, 1938.
17. Cerletti, U. Old and new information about electroshock. *Am. J. Psychiatry*, 107:87-94, 1950.
18. Moniz, E. Injections intracorotidiennes et substances injectables opaque avec rayons X. Press. Med., 35:969-971, 1927.
19. Fulton, J.F., and Jacobson, C.F. The function of the frontal lobes. A comparative study in monkeys. In: *Abstracts of the Second International Congress of Neurology*. 1935.
20. Moniz, E. Die prafrontale leukotomie. *Arch. fur Psychiatrie*, 181:591-602, 1949.
21. Laborit, H., Huguenard, P., and Alluaume, R. Un nouveau stabilisateur vegetatif (le 4560 R.P.). *Press. Med.*, 60:206-208, 1952.
22. Editorial Staff. Dr. Henri Laborit of France. In: Around the World in 80 Doctors. M. L. *Med. Newsmagazine*, 11:271-278, 1969.
23. Wortis, J. Psychopharmacology and physiological treatment. In: Review of psychiatric progress, 1964. *Am. J. Psychiatry*, 121:648-652, 1965.
24. Laborit, H. *Les Régulations Metaboliques*. Paris, Masson, 1965.
25. Damasio, A.R., and Galaburda, A.M. Norman Geschwind. Arch. *Neurol.*, 42:500-504, 1985.
26. Geschwind, N., and Kaplan, E. A human cerebral deconnection syndrome. A preliminary report. *Neurology*, 12:675-685, 1962.
27. Geschwind, N., and Levitsky, W. Human brain left-right asymmetries in temporal speech region. *Science,* 161:186-187, 1968.
28. Galaburda, A.M., Sanides, F., and Geschwind, N. Human brain: cytoarchitectonic left-right asymmetries in the temporal speech region. *Arch. Neurol.*, 35:812-817, 1978.
29. Waxman, S.G., and Geschwind, N. The interictal behavior syndrome of temporal lobe epilepsy. *Arch. Gen. Psychiatry*, 32:1580-1586, 1975.
30. Heilman, K.M., Coyle, J.M., Gonyea, E.F., et al. Apraxia and agraphia in a left hander. *Brain*, 96:21-28, 1973.
31. Geschwind, N., and Galaburda, A.M. Cerebral lateralization. Biological mechanisms, associations, pathology: a hypothesis and a program for research. Part I. *Arch. Neurol.*, 42:428-459, 1985.
32. Geschwind, N., and Galaburda, A. M. Cerebral lateralization. Biological mechanisms, associations, pathology: a hypothesis and a program for research. Part II. *Arch. Neurol.*, 42:521-552, 1985.
33. Geschwind, N., and Galaburda, A. M. Cerebral lateralization. Biological mechanisms, associations, pathology: a hypothesis and a program for research. Part III. *Arch. Neurol.*, 42:634-654, 1985.

The Art of Medicine in Neurology

I have gone to considerable length in these essays to emphasize the significance of the technical advances of science that have revolutionized neurology and established it in its present, modern form. Nevertheless, it is important to remember that the art of medicine is still vital to the successful practice of neurology. Because of the obvious important role of the nervous system and its research challenges, neurology has attracted physicians of the highest intellectual caliber. As the integrating mechanism for the body as a whole, the nervous system plays an indispensable role. Beyond this, are the challenging mysteries of the mind–brain interrelationship and the disorders of emotional expression. No other field demands the breadth of perception and understanding in treating the patient as a whole. It overlaps with almost all other specialties—especially with internal medicine, pediatrics, psychiatry, neurological surgery, ophthalmology, orthopedic surgery, and such disciplines as endocrinology, rhinolaryngology, and radiology. For all these reasons, neurology requires physicians, not only with high intellect, but also with the ability to deal with human problems in depth and with all the finesse that is termed the "art of medicine."

By the same token, neurology is not a "keyhole" specialty if properly practiced. Time and thought are required if the patient's problems are to be fully understood and if proper direction is to be given to specialty referral, preventive measures, rehabilitation, and adequate follow-up care. Frequently, only the neurologist will have the knowledge and expertise to aid and integrate the care of the referring physician properly with the support of family members to ensure the mobilization of the community resources for the benefit of the patient. This does not mean that the neurologist must handle all the details, but in some instances, it does involve personal inquiry and advice with respect to a comprehensive regimen of follow-up care. This is by no means unique to neurology, of course, but because of the nature of neurological problems, few other specialties are more demanding in this respect.

I had heard much of the doctor–patient relationship as a student at Harvard and was privileged to hear the original lecture of Francis Peabody on the "Care of Patient" (1). I had glibly accepted it, and yet I did not grasp the full significance of

Peabody's message until I later became actively engaged in clinical work. There is no question in my mind but that the art of medicine is an aspect of neurology that often is more vital than its technical and scientific aspects. It was this phase of medicine on which essentially all earlier practitioners depended. The object of this section is to illustrate this point with examples of a few outstanding neurologists.

The selection of physicians who have exemplified the art of medicine in the clinical practice of neurology, however, has not been easy. Subjective values are involved in the selection process as well as consideration of objective evidence. Neurological consultations too often involve limited keyhole reports that fail to consider the overall problem of the patient. They often are strong on diagnosis but weak on therapeutic suggestions for effective follow-up care. Therapeutic consultations can be as important as diagnostic consultations. Numerous other factors may influence and limit the quality of practice, such as the pressures of time, the background of the neurologist, and his or her ability to elicit the cooperation of the patient in both the studies undertaken and recommendations for care. Many factors are involved in this phase of medical practice, which includes the specialist as well as the referring doctor. Again, the degree of success achieved may vary from patient to patient, or from time to time. My object, however, is to illustrate the optimal situation. I have limited my selections to outstanding examples whom I have personally encountered and who were top-flight neurologists.

SWITHIN PINDER MEADOWS (1902-1993)

Of all the staff at the National Hospital, Queen Square, London, whom I knew, Dr. Meadows was the one who best exemplified the art of medicine in his dealing with patients. His hearty and open manner quickly captivated all, which included the staff and other workers in the hospital as well as the patients. He never displayed the bearing or disposition of a prima donna, as so many of his colleagues did. He was the acme of simplicity and sincerity. When the Meadows put on a reception for Mrs. Aird and myself in 1957 at their Highgate home, it was attended by essentially all the staff of the National Hospital. Two different physicians quietly informed me that several present scarcely ever spoke to each other and that Meadows was the only one who was on good terms with everyone and who could swing such an event. As I became better acquainted with the staff over the years, I gained a better appreciation of what my two informants meant and of the remarkable qualities of Meadows's character that achieved this miracle. The same qualities were implicit in his excellent rapport with patients.

Once, while visiting his country estate, Lane's End, in the Sussex Downs, I decided to rest instead of taking a walk with the others. This was very unusual for me, and on the return of the hikers, Meadows insisted on taking my temperature. Much to everyone's surprise, it was 102°F. I slept on the return drive to London, and Meadows immediately took charge. His knowledge of general medicine surprised me, and his care was most exemplary. Antibiotics brought me around within 2 to 3 days, which was fortunate inasmuch as I was scheduled for a lecture at the National Hospital. Meadows has been my physician while abroad ever since.

The background of this splendid chap is pertinent to my account. Born and raised in Wigan, Lancashire, Meadows was fortunate in his favorable early home life. His father, Thomas Meadows, was a journalist, writer, and editor for over 20 years of the *Wigan Observer*, the local newspaper. His mother, Florence, was an accomplished watercolor artist and pianist. Ten years of piano lessons resulted in Meadows becoming an accomplished musician; the piano has remained his hobby.

At the University of Liverpool, he won his Bachelor of Science degree in physiology with first-class honors in 1924 and his Bachelor of Medicine and Surgery degree in 1927, again with first-class honors. In that same year, he won the M.B. and B.S. degrees at the University of London and also M.R.C.S. in the London Royal College of Physicians. He obtained his M.D. degree at the University of London in 1930 and was appointed a Fellow in 1941.

His expertise in general medicine was gained at the Royal Infirmary of Liverpool, where he served as both House Physician in Medicine and Surgery in 1927 and 1928. Also, he was House Physician at the Royal Children's Hospital in Liverpool.

He transferred to London on winning the appointment as Medical Registrar at St. Thomas Hospital in 1929. This provided another year in general medicine, followed by 18 months in neurology. His training at the National Hospital, Queen Square, for a period of nearly 3 years, involved his working with 11 of the leading neurologists of London. He then became Medical First Assistant in the Neurological Department of the London Hospital and was the first Neurological Registrar of this hospital under George Riddoch and later Russell Brain. In 1937, he was appointed Physician to the Moorfields Eye Hospital. His appointment to the Westminster and Maida Vale Hospitals in London followed in 1938. His appointment to the staff of the National Hospital was in 1946, and many honors followed, such as Examiner in both Medicine and Neurology, Royal Society of Medicine, the Hunterian Professor, Royal College of Surgeons, President of the Section of Neurology, Royal Society of Medicine, and others.

The usual practice on the teaching wards of the London hospitals was to take histories and do examinations in the wards. It was Meadows, who fought for and obtained a side room where these basic clinical studies could be done in a more intimate, quiet, and private setting. This reflected his respect for privacy and his understanding of its importance to patient morale. It also enhanced the patient–doctor relationship and aided in attaining a greater in-depth understanding of the problems of his patients. This was not a dawdling exercise, one can be sure, because of his intense activity. In addition to consulting work to make a living, he attended three London hospitals, the London, Windsor, and St. Albans hospitals, and took his turn every 5 days for 24-hour call-outs in the Whitehall and Westminster areas. His follow-up on patients was meticulous but varied widely depending on their needs; this sometimes continued for years.

Meadows started a private consulting practice in 1938, and because of his superior training and outstanding natural abilities as a clinician, his consulting practice soon thrived. It is of considerable interest in this connection that his entire family developed and flourished in the medical field. In 1934, he married D.S. (Anne) Noble, who had been a nurse. Aside from the oldest son, who became a professor of marine biology at the University of Glasgow, the other three directly or by marriage were neurologist, neurosurgeon and cardiologist. For decades, Meadows has presided over this medical clan with love and affection while maintaining their keenness and standards at the highest levels.

Meadows's writings, as might be expected, have been of a clinical nature, but these have been recognized for their insight and sound judgment. With Sir Charles Symonds, he wrote an article on high compressions of the spinal cord (2). Cerebrovascular aneurysm was a favorite subject. Perhaps the most notable study on this involved the internal carotid artery (3). When president of the Neurological Section of the Royal Society of Medicine, his presidential address was on temporal or giant cell arteritis (4).

Meadows served with us as a Visiting Professor of Neurology for six weeks in 1957. We immediately "hit it off" and remained close friends for the next thirty-six years. Because of his broad background in general medicine, as well as in neurology, plus his sensitivity to the needs of patients and his remarkable rapport with them, Meadows transcended the limitations of consultative practice.

A stroke in July 1992 preceded his death on May 1, 1993. As Ross Russell wrote, "Swithin Meadows may not have matched the literary brilliance of Walshe, the originality of Symonds, or the sophistication of Macdonald Critchley, but for many of today's neurologists he was the finest physician of them all."

ROLAND PARKS MACKAY (1900-1968)

Due to his wit, good humor, and excellent training, Dr. Mackay became one of America's great neurologists. Although he was an excellent teacher, I have included him here because of his remarkable sensitivity and perceptiveness, which made him such an outstanding practitioner of the art of medicine.

His father was a Methodist minister, and because of many assignments in Georgia, Mackay described his boyhood as being raised "in all the small towns of Georgia." He obtained his B.S. from Emery University in 1920. When his father had a parish in Ontario, Canada, Mackay worked his way through the University of Toronto and graduated second in his class, only Charles Best of insulin fame being ahead of him. Following an internship at the Henry Ford Hospital, he trained in neurology under Dr. Henry Woltman of the Mayo Clinic. He moved to Chicago in 1929 and successively served on the faculties of Rush Medical College (1929 to 1934), University of Illinois College of Medicine (1934 to 1961), and Northwestern University Medical School (1961 to 1968).

Although he was not the showman that Macdonald Critchley and Henry Miller were and although he lacked the encyclopedic knowledge of Ray Adams as a teacher, Mackay made up for it by his charm with patients and his bantering and good humor with his students, which kept them on their toes and his faithful slaves. His analysis of problems and, especially, the psychological aspects of patients was keen and always ended up with a practical summary of the condition and what had to be done. He did extremely well as a visiting professor at the University of California, San Francisco (UCSF), in 1962, and I have been informed that he was a popular consultant in his practice in Chicago.

Dr. Mackay's sensitivity to psychological factors was shown in his handling of a patient presented to him when he visited UCSF in 1962. The patient was a married woman of 28 years of age who was referred for a suspected epileptic condition that had not responded to treatment. Mackay's examination, done at the same time as he reviewed her history, kept the patient very busy. His kindly and cheerful manner quickly won her cooperation, and he elicited a long history of problems and complaints. Her spells were of an ill-defined type with muscle spasms of her neck and back, lasting less than 1 minute. Her attacks came in repeated bouts and were associated with periods of nervous tension but were not associated with loss of consciousness. In spite of hundreds of such attacks, she had never fallen, injured herself, or been incontinent. Various antiepileptic regimens had not modified her attacks.

Her history involved repeated hospitalizations since childhood. Gastrointestinal symptoms had suggested ulcers on one occasion and colitis on another. Surgical results, however, had not been conclusive. She had been treated for hypothyroidism and "coronary occlusion," the latter being associated with typical pain radiation to her left shoulder but not associated with exertion.

Her family history was of interest mainly in two respects: (1) her siblings resented her many illnesses and believed that she used her "ill health" to avoid work and responsibility and (2) she had married a divorced man with three children. He had become exasperated by her recurrent chest pains and demanded a "thorough study."

Mackay suspected hysteria, and the possibility of a seizure state was ruled out by negative electroencephalographic (EEG) findings obtained during two of her attacks. Mackay recommended referral to a psychiatrist adept at handling hysterical conditions and, on a return visit to the patient, quickly convinced her that this was what she should do, in spite of the fact that she had resisted such care at least on one previous occasion.

In spite of repeated study over many years, no one had obtained the comprehensive history that Mackay obtained in 0.5 hours. The amazing thing was that this was deftly done with the happy cooperation of the patient.

Follow-up over a period of 8 years showed the wisdom of Mackay's diagnosis and direction. She slowly improved with supportive care, using only aspirin for occasional muscle spasms. Her spells stopped, and her family problems eventually improved. Mackay's psychological perceptiveness, combined with his charm and skill, proved to be the turning point in this patient's difficult problem.

Going hand in hand with Mackay's skill as a physician was his keen sense of public service. He served in innumerable capacities in welfare and health organizations. These activities culminated in his service as president of the National Multiple Sclerosis Society, Muscular Dystrophy Association of America, and the National Foundation for Infantile Paralysis. He also served as a member of the Advisory Council of the National Institute of Neurological Diseases and Blindness from 1953 to

1957. He served as editor of the Year Book of Neurology, Psychiatry and Neurosurgery and was an associate editor of *Neurology* and the *Archives of Psychiatry and Neurology*. He received many honors. He was president of the American Neurological Association, the American Epilepsy Society, and Society for Biological Psychiatry. He was an honorary member of four medical societies, including the Association of British Neurologists and Société Francaise de Neurologie.

One of his contributions to American neurology was his convincing the trustees of the American Medical Association in 1958 to continue with the publication of *Archives of Neurology* as well as *Archives of Psychiatry*. In this, he was ably assisted by Dr. Paul Bucy, as a representative of neurosurgery. Mackay subsequently served as an associate editor of the *Archives of Neurology*.

Mackay's research was of a clinical type and included articles such as "Toward a Neurology of Behavior" (5). I was especially aware of his studies on amyotrophic lateral sclerosis (ALS). These patients were dying in our arms, and one of the possibilities was that ALS might have an extraneous toxic origin. If so, it was conceivable that the supravital dyes, which I had shown lowered the permeability of the blood–brain barrier, might have a protective effect (6). An initial group seemed to benefit. Aside from the psychological effect of doing something for them, their muscle fibrillations subsided, which earlier had been considered an indicator of the severity of the disorder. An initial preliminary report served the purpose of obtaining referrals from all over the country (7). Further experience proved that the effect on muscle fibrillation was not a reliable indicator of the disease's activity. Although a few patients showed evidence of improvement, the great majority eventually did not, and I finally abandoned the study. Because I eventually had some 120 patients, I began summarizing the types of motor neuron disease seen and the course of the disorder. I was well along in my review when Mackay's article on this subject appeared (8). His analysis so closely corresponded with my own that I discontinued the project, being at the time extremely busy with other activities.

Mackay has been described by one of his colleagues as a "fierce Scot, proud and determined," and "He was also a stubborn Scot. All who knew him loved and admired him" (9). When properly interpreted, these statements mean that he had a keen sense of values and was loyal to his convictions of what he considered to be right. In all other aspects, he was a polished gentleman of a most genial and kindly spirit.

EDWARD GRAEME ROBERTSON (1902-1975)

I have always thought of Robertson as the absent-minded professor of neurology, but this is a cliché that touches on only one unique facet of the man and does not do him justice. When absorbed in his hobby of photography and collecting photographic material for his books on decorative cast iron banisters, gates, and fences, he indeed lived in another world. Dr. Critchley's story of this facet is worth quoting.

"Once I ran into him in New Orleans, where he was busy photographing the cast-iron work so characteristic of the French Quarter. He had set up his camera with great deliberation in the rue Royale, taken photometric readings, put his light-meter down beside him on the curb and buried his head beneath the cloth. When he emerged, the picture taken, the apparatus had disappeared. At great expense he bought a replacement in Chicago. A few days later we were both in Greenwich Village—I in search of antiquarian bookshops, he looking for cast-iron verandas. The scenario repeated itself. The camera on its stand, the light-meter on the pavement, his eyes busy focusing. A successful photograph was taken, and so was his light-meter."(10).

I have seen only three of his books, but the one entitled Sydney Lace has become well known and well justifies his antiquarian interests and fine photography.

The real Robertson was an excellent neurologist, superbly trained, and the leader in the development of modern neurology in Australia and New Zealand. His story is unusual in some respects and well worthy of review.

Aside from his postgraduate training in England, his entire career was centered in Melbourne, Australia. His education in Melbourne culminated with his graduation in medicine from the University of Melbourne with honors in 1927. Following hospital training in Melbourne, he went to London for training in neurology, which he obtained at both the National Hospital and the Post-Graduate Hospital at Hammersmith. During this period, he collaborated in studies with such celebrities as Denny-Brown (epilepsy and bladder function), F. M. R. Walshe (grasp reflex), and Godwin Greenfield (oligodendrogliomas).

In 1935, he returned to Melbourne where he practiced as a neurological consultant and was neurologist to the Melbourne Hospital and, after 1940, to the Children's Hospital as well. It was to the service at the Children's Hospital that he took me on my visit in 1962. He taught neurology at the medical school until his retirement in 1963. Most notable was that his hospital consulting and teaching services were done entirely on a voluntary basis. He made his living in private practice. I well recall on one of his visits to San Francisco (1951), after showing him our departmental clinical, teaching, and research facilities and answering his questions about staff and budgets, he wept. He had worked hard in Melbourne for 16 years, and aside from some clinical research, he had obtained very little support in the way of facilities—and no recompense at all. He explained his situation in terms of the British tradition.

It is difficult to explain some of the nebulous factors involved in the art of medicine, and this was particularly true in the case of Robertson. Perhaps the reactions of one patient to Robertson are worth while recounting because they showed the favorable supporting impact that he had on patients faced with the crucial problems of their devastating disorders.

When Robertson came to visit us at UCSF in August 1951, Dr. David Zealear and I had completed a study on the absorption of ethylene gas following its use in pneumoencephalography (11). The article had been accepted for publication by the Archives of Neurology and Psychiatry, but it did not appear until 2 months later. Because Robertson was absorbed in his own pneumoencephalographic studies and had come to present his modified technique (published in monographic form 6 years later), I thought he might be interested in our study on the dynamics of cerebrospinal fluid absorption. It so happened that one of the patients from the study had returned for a follow-up examination in the neurology clinic and for renewal of his medication.

The patient was a man 56 years of age, who told a story of progressive jacksonian seizures of his right leg, starting 10 months before his surgery. A left frontal parasaggital meningioma had been found, and he now was making a good postoperative recovery. Antiepileptic therapy started before surgery had been continued, but was slowly being discontinued as his clinical and EEG follow-up appeared to warrant.

Robertson was fascinated with the patient's pneumoencephalograms, done before surgery and a second study done 3 months later. The initial study showed no filling of the supracortical subarachnoid spaces, due to their obliteration by the pressure of his expanding tumor. The second, postoperative study showed the subarachnoid spaces to be suggestively dilated. Going hand in hand with these findings, the initial ethylene absorption rate had been reduced 35%, whereas the second study showed the absorption rate to be within the limits of normal. This was explained by the blockage of the arachnoidal absorptive bed in the preoperative study, which was relieved by the surgery. It was with great interest that Robertson reviewed our other illustrative cases prepared for the article.

With this background, Robertson took great interest in quizzing and examining the patient in the clinic. Unfortunately, I was called away during his examination, but on my return, the somewhat drab, postoperative patient seemed to be transformed. He was almost in a euphoric state, and his smiling cooperation with Robertson was something to behold. Perhaps Robertson's heightened state of interest had something to do with it, but his contact had certainly "electrified" the patient. I gathered that Robertson had conveyed the idea of how fortunate the patient was and gave him hope. The patient's earlier complaints now disappeared, and his cooperation in further follow-up visits was greatly improved. The patient repeatedly inquired about the "wonderful foreign doctor."

Robertson had developed a fine reputation and, in the next several years, was influential in establishing neurology on a firm basis in Australia. He played a key role in the founding of the Australian Association of Neurologists in 1950. On another trip that I made to Australia in 1967, he was serving as the president of the Asian and Oceanic Neurological Congress. He had asked me to attend this congress in 1965 when I saw him at the World Federation of Neurology Congress in Vienna, and he was particularly anxious to obtain American articles and support. I managed to get ten American doctors to attend the meetings. John Game and Robertson were most hospitable. The meetings were of good quality, and the side events were excellent.

Robertson's clinical research involved infectious conditions (poliomyelitis and encephalitis), toxoplasmosis, and aneurysms. As previously mentioned, he had developed a special interest in pneumoencephalography, and his technique of visualizing the structures of the posterior fossa gained wide acceptance (12).

Denny-Brown, Walshe, and Game (personal communications) have borne out my impressions of Robertson as an unusually perceptive neurologist who was sensitive to the plight of his patients and went out of his way to play a supportive role for the family, as well as the patient. His quiet, unassuming and friendly manner, coupled with his obvious intelligence and thoroughness, combined to make him an outstanding example of a neurologist who actively pursued the art of medicine in his practice.

TORVALD DALSGAARD-NIELSEN (1896-1975)

I first heard of Dalsgaard-Nielsen through Professor Sigvald Refsum, who spent 1 year with me from 1951 to 1952. At every dinner in which he was a guest, Refsum proposed a toast to Dalsgaard-Nielsen. Dalsgaard-Nielsen was a neurologist in Copenhagen who, during the German occupation of Denmark and Norway, had sent weekly packages of food to the Refsums to aid the growth of their three young sons. German rationing was tight and very restrictive, and according to Refsum, the weekly gifts from the Dalsgaard-Nielsens had helped a great deal.

Through the Refsums, Mrs. Aird and I later met the Dalsgaard-Nielsens. They were a wonderful couple with whom we immediately became friendly—a friendship that grew over the next 22 years, from 1953 to 1975. Esther was a beautiful woman, who had qualified in ophthalmology. During the period we knew her, she was a professor of ophthalmology in the University of Copenhagen. Dalsgaard-Nielsen was chief of the neurological department of the Frederiksberg Hospital, Frederiksberg being a separate city in the heart of Copenhagen. Although astute and very capable, Dalsgaard-Nielsen also exuded a friendly empathy, which his colleagues recognized as sincere and which served as an extra form of supportive therapy for his patients. One had the feeling that he would take his shirt off and give it to you if he felt that this would help. His perceptiveness and understanding of the psychological aspects of his patient's problems, as well as their physical and neurological conditions, was keen and seldom failed to win the cooperation and admiration of his patients (Muller, R., personal communications, 1960-1990). As a result of this and quite apart from the Refsum's initial influence, we have continued to toast Dalsgaard-Nielsen ever since.

Kindly consideration, usually referred to as empathy, and thoroughness of study are the usual factors involved in winning the confidence and cooperation of patients. However, skill in history taking and examination, plus keenness of observation on the part of the physician, as shown in the case of Dr. Mackay, are important added attributes that contribute to success. Dalsgaard-Nielsen's former receptionist and physical therapist, Rosa Muller, was filled with stories of his kindly handling of patients and his success in their care. The spontaneous smiles and greetings of his patients and also the nurses on ward rounds at the Frederiksberg Hospital amply confirmed this, but it can also be illustrated by a patient study on his visit to UCSF in 1964.

I showed him a hospitalized man 30 years of age, whose complaint of seizures of the generalized tonic-clonic type had resisted treatment over the previous 5 years. A total of eight seizures were reported, all brief without aura, and coming only on arising in the morning.

The personal and family histories were noncontributory, and his physical and neurological examination findings were normal.

Dalsgaard-Nielsen's contact with the patient was excellent. This may have been helped by his introduction as a distinguished neurologist from Copenhagen, but there was more to it than that. The patient quickly sensed his kindly understanding and responded to his questions. Whereas the resident had obtained a history of no excess alcohol consumption, which was true on a regular basis, the patient now admitted that, on occasions of great stress in his work, he drank four or five beers or three or four cocktails in the evenings before his spells. The result was that Dalsgaard-Nielsen suspected seizure conditioning mechanisms, such as nervous tension, sleep deprivation, and preceding alcoholic sprees, the spells finally being precipitated by morning arousal. The EEG activation studies showed marked responses to both sleep deprivation and hydration.

The precipitating mechanisms were explained to the patient, and he was thoroughly convinced by the changes found in his EEG studies. His same antiepileptic medication was continued but now was buttressed by control of his fluid intake, avoidance of alcohol and sleep deprivation, and a more mature response to his work frustrations.

No further spells were reported over a follow-up period of 6 years. On every return visit (referred by his local physician on the patient's request), he always asked news of Dalsgaard-Nielsen and attributed his excellent response to this physician's understanding and remarkable skill.

Rosa Muller later married a Bechtel engineer and came to live in the Bay Area. Over the years since World War II, I saw both Rosa and her husband, Axel, in consultation and learned much further about Dalsgaard-Nielsen from this source. She thoroughly agreed with the opinions of Drs. Jorgen Marquardsen and Erik Skinshaj that the reason for Dalsgaard-Nielsen's neurological reputation and excellent consultative practice "was not only his undisputed professional competence, but above all his personal abilities...and was able, with unfalteringly sure psychological flair, to establish a condition of trust with even the most difficult patients, who had often gone from one doctor to another before. He became the great therapist without abandoning his personal, critically scientific basic attitude. Only a few have, as him, been able to combine medical art with medical science" (translation of reference 13).

These same qualities carried over into his administrative duties. The day-to-day business of the hospital was conducted with "benevolent authority," and "he understood the art of delegating problems and to inspire his coworkers to produce the best of their abilities, and he was renowned for his ability to create "well-being" in the workplace many years before this slogan, now entirely outworn, had become commonplace" (13). He also was "an astute tactician and able negotiator," who for years, played a central role in maintaining cooperation between the hospital administration and the chief physicians of the hospital. In addition, he was involved in the long-range planning of the hospital. These same qualities assured him a leading role in medical societies. He was president of the Danish Neurological Association, consultant to the Danish Board of Health and Welfare, chair of the Danish Association of Gerontology, and founder and president of the Scandinavian Society against Hemicrania. He filled various other offices at an international level (e.g., World Federation of Neurology, National Multiple Society, and others).

On one occasion, I was able to refer the Minister of Oil of Saudi Arabia to

Dalsgaard-Nielsen. His Excellency had a severe migraine problem, which obviously was closely related to his tension and overwork. Dalsgaard-Nielsen was the obvious referral, and this worked out so well that he was invited twice to Saudi Arabia, where he met the king and was given handsome presents. On one occasion, when we were invited to dinner, Dalsgaard-Nielsen met us dressed in a beautiful, formal Arabian costume and carried the evening off in gala style.

The background of Dalsgaard-Nielsen can be summarized briefly as follows. Born and raised in Jutland, he graduated in medicine at the University of Arrhus in 1924. He married Esther Kristensen, a classmate, and they practiced in the rural community of Hellevad from 1924 to 1933. At the age of 37, they moved to Copenhagen to do graduate specialization studies. Esther pursued ophthalmology and, eventually, became a professor in the University of Copenhagen. Dalsgaard-Nielsen trained in neurology. In 1935, he went to Jena, Germany, studied with Hans Berger and developed the first EEG apparatus and clinic in Denmark.

He was made chief of neurology at the Frederiksberg Hospital in 1940, where he developed an active service with special interests in cerebrovascular and posttraumatic head injuries. His rehabilitation care of these patients opened a new field in Danish neurology. During World War II, he served in the Danish underground movement. He was arrested and imprisoned for over 3 weeks in December 1944. He had a bleeding gastric ulcer and lost 20 pounds while in prison. The tales of his underground experiences touch on the heroic (Muller, R., personal communications, 1960-1990).

Later, he developed a special interest in migraine and other headache problems. His studies on allergic forms of headache, diagnostic tests, and therapy with antihistamines were particularly notable (14). It has always been my impression that Dalsgaard-Nielsen's great success as a therapist was based on three factors: (1) his thorough training in general medicine, which he practiced for 9 years, as well as his later training in neurology; (2) his tests and experimental therapies, which must have impressed many of his patients; and (3) his great empathy and supportive role in practicing the art of medicine. Good common sense, in addition to great skill developed from his specialty training and experience, were effectively amplified by his unusual abilities in the art of medicine. He was a true example of James MacKenzie's "Beloved Physician." So great was his impact, he was the first physician without the advanced degree of Doctor to be awarded an honorary degree of medicine by the University of Copenhagen.

RUSSELL NELSON DEJONG (1907-1990)

As a result of seeing Dr. DeJong in action while he was a visiting professor with us in April 1961, I confidently have included him in this essay as an outstanding example of a leading neurologist who also exemplified the art of medicine. Although he had a certain dignified reserve, it was not a cool or forbidding aloofness, and patients invariably sensed his underlying kindness and efforts to understand their problems. One patient wrote "he always treated me with the utmost respect and consideration...I didn't appreciate his wonderful qualities until later, when further experience taught me that he was the exception, not the rule" (Obuchowski, M., personal communication, 1992). While with us, he elicited respect and cooperation—this included the house staff and senior staff, as well as the nurses and patients.

Born in Iowa, he was the son of a physician–surgeon and was of Dutch stock on both sides. The family moved to Michigan in 1915 where he remained for his entire career. His higher education was at the University of Michigan, where he received his M.D. in 1932. He was an outstanding student and received the usual honors of Alpha Omega Alpha and Sigma Xi. His mentor in neurology was Dr. C. D. Camp, but neurology did not gain autonomous departmental status until 1950 under his leadership. He was certified in both neurology and psychiatry in 1939.

DeJong was not a flamboyant showman in his clinical work or teaching. He was meticulous and thorough in his examinations and cautiously discussed differential diagnostic possibilities. I am sure he suffered in comparison with some of our other visiting professors, but in the end, he won the respect of our staff. At the undergraduate level, he was particularly good, where thoroughness of examination and careful diagnostic analysis were stressed.

His department was greatly augmented when the National Institutes of Health (NIH) training grants became available in the early 1950s. Dr. DeJong had the reputation of a kind administrator, and he was as supportive of his staff as they were of him.

His research was of the usual clinical type on multiple sclerosis, epilepsy, migraine, Parkinson's disease, and many other conditions. He was interested in the neurologic complications of system disease, and his book, *The Neurological Examination*, has been well received and reflects his great thoroughness (15,16).

He was one of the founding members of the American Academy of Neurology. One of his most noteworthy contributions was to serve as editor-in-chief of the society's journal, Neurology, starting in 1950.

DeJong served in innumerable capacities in a multitude of neurological societies, as a consultant to the NIH and various governmental agencies, and as an examiner and president of the American Board of Psychiatry and Neurology (1958 to 1959). He was an honorary member of several neurological societies and served as president of the American Neurological Association from 1964 to 1965.

In spite of his busy career as administrator, teacher, researcher, editor, consultant, and organization worker, DeJong maintained his simple, unassuming self with a primary interest in patient care.

SUMMARY

If clinical neurology is to hold the respect of patients and the public, as well as the respect of colleagues in other medical disciplines, the art of medicine must play an equal role with its scientific aspects. The qualities of character that typify those who have been selected to illustrate this aspect of neurology may be listed as follows. First, they exhibited a kindly thoughtfulness in their patient contacts, which

not only was important to win patient respect, but also to win full patient cooperation in history taking, examination, and care. Second, they were especially sensitive
to not only physical disabilities but also the psychological, emotional, and intellectual disorders that often accompany neurological problems. Third, they were superb
clinicians, which was reflected in their clinical research—its comprehensiveness
and the sound judgment it required.

Many others might have been included in this category, such as Critchley in Great
Britain, Raymond Garcin in Paris, Wohlfart and Refsum in Scandinavia, and
Masland in America. However, the five selected well serve to illustrate the different
aspects of this important subject.

REFERENCES

1. Peabody, F.W. Care of patient. *J.A.M.A.*, 88:877-882, 1927.
2. Symonds, C.P., and Meadows, S.P. Compression of spinal cord in neighborhood of foramen magnum. *Brain*, 60:52-84, 1937.
3. Meadows, S.P. Intracavernous aneurysms of the internal carotid artery. *Arch. Ophthalmol.*, 62:566-574, 1959.
4. Meadows, S.P. Temporal or giant cell arteritis. *Proc. R. Soc. Med.*, 59:329-333, 1966.
5. Mackay, R.P. Toward a neurology of behavior. *Neurology*, 4:894-901, 1954.
6. Aird, R.B. The role of tissue permeability of the blood-brain barrier in diseases of the central nervous system. *Calif. Med.*, 69:360-363, 1948.
7. Aird, R.B. Trypan red therapy of amyotrophic lateral sclerosis: preliminary report. *Arch. Neurol. Psychiatry*, 59: 779-789, 1948.
8. Mackay, R.P. Course and prognosis in amyotrophic lateral sclerosis. *Arch. Neurol.*, 8:117-127, 1963.
9. Bucy, P.C. Roland Parks Mackay, Centennial Anniversary *Volume of the American Neurological Association.* New York, Springer Publishing, 1975.
10. Critchley, M.E. The Ventricle of Memory. New York, *Raven Press,* 1990.
11. Aird, R.B. The absorption of ethylene gas following encephalography with a clinical correlation in 164 cases. *Radiology*, 30:320-336, 1938.
12. Robertson, E.G. *Pneumoencephalography.* Springfield, IL, Charles C. Thomas, 1957.
13. Marquardsen, J., and E. Skinskaj. *Danish Weekly Medical Publication*, Nov. 24, 1975.
14. Dalsgaard-Nielsen, T. Histamine headache. Ugeskr. Laeger., 107:377-378, 1945.
15. DeJong, R.N. *The Neurological Examination.* New York, Hoeber, 1950. revised 1958, 1967, and 1979.
16. DeJong, R.N. Nervous system complications of diabetes mellitus with specific reference to cerebrovascular changes. *J. Nerv. Ment. Dis.*, 111:181-206, 1950.

CHAPTER
15

Traditions of Neurological Teaching

The classic teaching of the 19th century involved much didactic instruction by means of large group lectures. Because of the vital and very practical nature of medicine, however, teaching by demonstration had been introduced centuries earlier. The German and French schools were the two principal exponents of large teaching demonstrations in medicine, and this, of course, included neurology. From this same background, the British school eventually added small group teaching at the bedside, a distinction that finally became traditional. The Scandinavian countries initially followed the German system but, later, gravitated toward the British approach. As might be expected, Great Britain's colonies followed the teaching traditions of the mother country, and this initially applied to its rebellious American colonies. As the United States grew, however, and as the scientific aspects of modern neurology developed, it borrowed from all the other systems and, eventually, developed new and independent approaches. The differences involved are interesting and afford insight into important aspects of medical teaching. They can be summarized by considering the careers of those neurological leaders of each school who implemented significant changes, which now are merging into what eventually may be an international approach to neurological training.

THE GERMAN TRADITION

I came in close contact with the early flamboyant neurological demonstrations of the German school through Robert Wartenberg, as discussed in Chapter 3. He was one of the refugees from the Hitler period in the mid-1930s. His approach, superimposed on our American system, forced us all at the University of California, San Francisco (UCSF), to evaluate the essentials of neurological instruction.

One of the widely heralded features of German medical teaching involved the possibility of students transferring from school to school to study under professors who were outstanding in the student's developing fields of interest. This system of tutelage involved student fees that went directly to the German professor. The result

223

was that many of the German professors became showmen, whose lectures and demonstrations, in vying for attention, were featured by much declamation, sometimes to the point of bombast. Their air of authority proved inimical to a proper doctor–patient relationship and too often reduced their demonstrations to little more than text book pictures of disease processes. Diagnosis was the emphasis, inasmuch as, in that former period, therapy was very limited and still largely palliative and symptomatic.

This earlier system of medical instruction, thus, although very striking with its prima donnas, failed in comparison with the personal patient contact and understanding developed as a result of bedside teaching, or individual laboratory instruction as afforded by James Papez (discussed subsequently under Neurological Instruction in the United States). It also lacked the more realistic experience of patient workups and follow through with their complex problems. I became very conscious of this difference with the teaching of Robert Wartenberg at UCSF from 1947 to 1956 (1). His dramatic demonstrations attracted considerable attention and were loved by the undergraduate students because they presented the textbook pictures they thought they needed as beginners. Although useful in that respect, my concern was that this did not fully present neurology as it should be taught. It ignored the many facets and complications of disease processes that are of importance to the patient and to proper patient care. In some instances, simplistic portrayals were presented that involved the essentials that Dr. Wartenberg wanted to discuss but actually were not the real diagnosis at all. This distortion was illustrated in the story that Professor Sigvald Refsum of Norway delighted telling from his year with us in 1951 to 1952 (2). Professor Wartenberg was lecturing on double athetosis and drew attention in his demonstration to the patient's jaw movements that he likened to gum chewing. At this point, the patient, with a big grin, stopped his chewing and drew a huge mass of gum from his mouth. The quick-witted Wartenberg, not to be outdone, struck a masterful pose and exclaimed, "Gentlemen, you have seen a most remarkable condition—a case of double-double athetosis." This brought the house down and saved the day for Wartenberg.

The efforts of our neurological staff had to be doubled to ensure that sound bedside teaching was primary and not supplemental to Wartenberg's popular demonstrations. Although his review of textbook conditions had its place in the overall teaching, the students, in addition, worked up assigned patients in the clinic and hospital and were held to thorough history taking and examinations, which were reviewed in detail. The end result was that, while the students obtained an excellent review of textbook diagnosis in Wartenberg's demonstrations, they also learned that the patient's problems in reality were usually much more complex. The use of laboratory diagnostic aids and therapy were stressed in addition to the supportive aspects of patient care and rehabilitation.

Going hand in hand with the tremendous political changes that have occurred in Germany as the result of two world wars and the Great Depression, plus the effects of biomedical scientific developments, German neurological teaching has changed considerably and can be illustrated in the career of Georges Schaltenbrand.

Georges Schaltenbrand (1897-1979)

The story of Schaltenbrand is an unusual one that well documents his courage and steadfastness under adversity. Following World War I, he emerged as the most outstanding of the young neurologists in Germany. When he finished his postgraduate studies abroad, he was considered for a major appointment at Johns Hopkins. With support from the Rockefeller Foundation, Johns Hopkins had planned a neurological institute, but the plan fell through with the onset of the Great Depression when the University could not fulfill its part of the plan. It was following this that Penfield, another Rockefeller Fellow, got his start at McGill University, Montreal.

After Nonne retired in 1934, Schaltenbrand was named as interim director of the Department of Neurology at the University of Hamburg. German universities, however, were dependent on government support, and with the rise of Hitler to the chancellorship in 1933, political considerations soon pervaded all appointments and, especially, prestigious ones, such as the Neurological Institute, Hamburg.

Schaltenbrand's early statements against the Nazis ruined his prospects at Hamburg, and he was fortunate to obtain a minor post in neurology at Würzburg. In spite of his setbacks, Schaltenbrand developed an excellent teaching and research unit in Würzburg. However, fate was soon to deal him still another blow.

The postwar period in Germany was not only chaotic but also saturated with the emotional issues inherited from the Nazi problem. Leading physicians were particularly suspect as possible collaborators in the deadly experiments of the German concentration camps. The Nürenberg trials, however, were conducted fairly, and Schaltenbrand was completely exonerated. Nevertheless, the disruption of this period and the suspicions it generated had a demoralizing effect on many careers. Again, Schaltenbrand's strength of character survived this ordeal.

The turning point came in 1952, when the State Department created traveling fellowships to compensate, in some measure, for the ordeal that had been inflicted on those exonerated. Schaltenbrand availed himself of this opportunity, and it was in this connection that I first met him. His old friend and co-worker, Percival Bailey, who was a fraternity brother of mine and whom I had known in Boston before he went to Chicago, wrote me about Schaltenbrand and requested that I welcome him. Some people were still antagonistic in a nondiscriminating fashion to all Germans, and Schaltenbrand's receptions varied. After receiving Bailey's letter, however, I had no hesitation in welcoming Schaltenbrand and showing him our research, clinical, and teaching facilities.* It was in this fashion that our friendship got off to a good start and grew through the years.

Schaltenbrand's reputation steadily grew following World War II. As a result of his dissertation on disturbances of motor function and his postgraduate work with Magnus, Schaltenbrand had a primary interest in this subject. With F. Hempl, he

---

*Those who know Percival Bailey will understand this. Bailey at times was blunt, but a more honest and forthright man would be hard to find. When he said that he had investigated Schaltenbrand's clinical setup and that clinical experiments were done with the full understanding and consent of the patients, I believed him.

developed an apparatus to measure the mechanical and electrical parameters of passive stretch and muscle extension (3). Another great interest was to establish an atlas for clinical and research stereotaxic studies of the human brain. This was started with Percival Bailey in the late 1950s and culminated in his publication with W. Wahren (4); he also published several texts of neurology, the last in 1969 (5). His neurology section at Würzburg was recognized as an independent university clinic in 1950. Several honors followed, including the highest German award, the Erb Medal, in 1952. A festschrift was published in his honor in 1977. His neurological institute at Würzburg, the Kopfklinikum, with his bust in the entrance, stands as a monument to his career and accomplishments.

Schaltenbrand's excellent English was unusual among the neurologists on the continent (other than Scandinavia) of that period, and this, plus his rich background of training and research, recommended him to me as a good prospect for our Visiting Professor of Neurology Program. I next saw Schaltenbrand at the International Congress of Neurology in Lisbon in early September 1953. Plans were initiated at that time, and he finally came with his wife, Lu, for 3.5 weeks in the spring of 1956. He proved to be an excellent neurologist and an effective teacher. Contrary to the ostentatious showmanship of some of the earlier German professors, Schaltenbrand's manner was simple and direct. One immediately sensed in Schaltenbrand that one was dealing with an exceptional person of great knowledge, wide experience, and critical insight. While with us as a UCSF visiting professor, he entered very fully into our teaching rounds, demonstrations, and bedside teaching. It was obvious that he agreed wholeheartedly with our system of student clinical assignments and follow through on student performance.

Over the years, we came to know Schaltenbrand, Lu, and their children quite well. We had dinner and luncheons with Schaltenbrand at medical meetings and visited the Schaltenbrands in Würzburg in both 1957 and 1968. On the latter occasion, his daughter, Elsi Li, and her husband, Oskar Boch, of Frankfurt am Main, flew to Würzburg to see us, and we all had a wonderful visit. We especially enjoyed the Schaltenbrands' new swimming pool with its amazing mechanical cover. Also, on this occasion, Schaltenbrand took great pleasure and some little pride in showing me the new Kopfklinikum, which he had so carefully planned and the development of which he had spearheaded.

My last contact with Schaltenbrand was in London in 1978. I had been invited to give a presentation at the Centennial Symposium for Gordon Holmes. Schaltenbrand was anxious that I complete an article on the electroencephalogram and its potential (written in collaboration with Bill Garoutte), and with his editorial help, I did this over a 2-day period (6). We had a fine visit on the side, and the article, published in his journal, *Neurologie*, proved to be a great hit—nearly 300 requests for reprints were received.

At heart, Schaltenbrand was a philosopher, and he delighted in "fathoming the depths of human thought," as H. C. Hopf has expressed it (7). At the same time, he possessed the objectivity of the true scientist, and his intense interests in research often assumed the proportions of his raison d'être. My contacts included more relaxed periods—our visits with his family in Würzburg, a motor trip to Yosemite National Park in California with both Schaltenbrand and his wife, a visit to his country home in Ronco, Switzerland, and our delightful visit in London. He had a good sense of humor, as may be illustrated by the following story (2).

Near the end of World War II, when the American army was sweeping across Germany, he realized that his home might be commandeered by officers because it was one of the few houses not demolished in the earlier bombing of Würzburg. They were helping as many of their neighbors as possible, and most were tense with fear. They were confused and depressed by the deceptions of Hitler and the terrible mess that he had contrived for them. As reports of the American advance were received, tensions grew, and to alleviate this critical situation, Schaltenbrand proposed a hoax that might save all from being ousted from the house. The men hauled large logs from a neighboring forest and propped them against the outside walls of the Schaltenbrand home. When the Americans arrived, the Schaltenbrand home was passed over because of its apparent unstable condition.

"Wasn't there some risk in doing that?" I asked him. "What if the Army inspected the house and found it sound?"

Schaltenbrand replied, "I believe the Americans would have seen it as a joke."

"Americans love jokes, all right," I said, "but an Army in wartime could be different."

"If they understood it as a measure to combat civilian fear and as a relief from a desperate situation, I believe they would have understood," he retorted.

"How a thing is presented is certainly important, and your excellent English might well have carried the day."

"The risk was well worth it," Schaltenbrand said. "It was a mild deception that was the source of great joy to our neighbors far and wide. It served as a release to their tension and fear and helped to normalize their subsequent contacts with the American occupation force."

This, of course, was not the usual American joke, but it did involve a sense of humor, as well as keen insight and understanding of a critical situation. I have always thought that Schaltenbrand's statement (referring to the advancing army), "I believe they would have understood," reflected, not only his understanding of America, but also his approval of it. This was evident in his reactions during many of our discussions. He had completely thrown off the old German approach to teaching and, as in America, combined teaching with basic research. As the leading neurologist of Germany, the editor of Neurologie, and founder of an important neurological institution, Schaltenbrand's impact was great, indeed.

THE BRITISH TRADITION

Bedside teaching was the hallmark of British neurological instruction and this reached a peak at the National Hospital, Queen Square, London, which was the center of neurological postgraduate teaching for the British Empire, before World War II. This has been highlighted in these essays by such outstanding examples as Sir Charles Symonds (as discussed in Chapter 16), Sir Gordon Holmes (Chapter 18),

Macdonald Critchley (Chapter 2), and several others. Another excellent example of this was Donald Macrae of our own staff, who had many years of training in British neurology, including 5 years at Queen Square. The British approach involved a critical analysis of the findings of each patient (both history and examination) with respect to the underlying pathology. This in addition to challenging student quizzing provided the essentials for understanding each condition as well as the variations and complications in individual patients.

Pride in their clinical analysis resulted in some deemphasis on laboratory findings in the early British period, when the scientific underpinnings of neurology were still in a developmental stage in the first half of the 20th century. This was exaggerated by the lack of neurological therapy, and the poor economic support of medical education in the United Kingdom over the same period did not help. Gordon Holmes has provided an excellent account of this early period at the National Hospital (8). He documented the slow progress of the physical plant and facilities of the National Hospital, always well behind in keeping pace with urgent clinical demands. The pathological laboratory and surgical and other facilities were limited and only belatedly added. The early archaic x-ray equipment was only finally updated by a gift from the Swedish Red Cross following World War II. The Medical Research Council aided with research facilities in 1922, but this was limited and interrupted by World War II. Even after this, the great majority of senior neurologists in Great Britain did not seem to be concerned about their belated "muddling through." It takes a generation to alter attitudes, and no doubt the interruptions of the two devastating world wars and the Great Depression played a major role in this. Certainly, the pride they took in their clinical diagnostic acumen, which often transcended laboratory aids, was a major factor. Nevertheless, several notable exceptions should be cited: Carmichael, Denny-Brown, and Dennis Williams at the National Hospital; Miller and Walton at Newcastle; Simpson in Glasgow; Harris in Edinburgh; and probably a number of others of whom I am not aware.

Perhaps an even more important factor was the lack of remuneration for the clinical staffs of the teaching hospitals in the United Kingdom (8). Before the National Health Service was started in 1948, the honorary medical staff at the National Hospital received no remuneration. Such appointments added great prestige, but the neurologists had to make their living on the side from private practice. Unless they had independent means, this was a heavy load. Furthermore, their reputations depended in large measure on the creative clinical work and writing that they did on the side. It was on this basis and their abilities as clinicians and teachers that they were selected for the hospital staffs, their appointments being made after years of training and service in the National Hospital itself. Understaffing was a chronic problem. Less than one appointment was made to the staff every 2 years on average, and only some 12 to 15 honorary physicians were on the active staff at any one time. Perhaps one half of these were outstanding as teachers and in their contributions. The result was that only the most persistent, dedicated, and brilliant neurologists achieved success in this strenuous and elite atmosphere.

Many fine qualities were involved in those who achieved success, but as consultants, their success in both teaching and practice depended almost entirely on their clinical abilities as diagnosticians. Until World War II, neurological therapy was very limited and depended largely on supportive and symptomatic measures. Research was almost entirely of a clinical nature and mainly involved clinicopathological correlations, or the descriptions of new clinical syndromes. In this climate, keen observation, memory, and deductive powers played major roles. Verbal abilities and showmanship were added requisites for successful teaching and demonstrating. That those who succeeded took pride in their clinical and teaching abilities was only natural, and their position in British medicine was accorded the highest recognition.

In this rigorous clinical climate, British neurology was not noted for its basic advances in the study of neurological disorders. In the earlier period, of course, and until the scientific techniques of study were developed, the basic approaches for investigation of disease processes could not be undertaken. In spite of much excellent, academic research in neurophysiology and other areas and with some exceptions, the factors discussed served to delay more basic approaches to the investigation of clinical disorders.

EDWARD ARNOLD CARMICHAEL (1896-1978)

Perhaps the most notable exception to the situation discussed was Dr. Carmichael, who was the pioneer in the development of the research arm of the National Hospital, Queen Square. His interests in neurological research showed up in his teaching, as I well remember in his discussion with Critchley of a lecture I gave on temporal lobe epilepsy at the National Hospital in 1957. His earlier background as a critical Scot may in part explain this. In his obituary on Carmichael, Critchley wrote "Queen Square held a strong contingent of residents and staff from remoter parts north of the Tweed, and Carmichael was closely associated with this clique— almost indeed to a chauvinistic degree" (9). If Carmichael's chauvinism included a stubborn Scottish will to have Queen Square keep pace with the great scientific advances of the past generation, Critchley certainly was correct.

As the son of a Scottish physician, Carmichael was educated in Edinburgh and graduated with honors in 1921 from the school of medicine at Edinburgh, having won the coveted Annandale Gold Medal. Because of his interests in neurology, after his service in World War I, he obtained the appointment of resident medical officer at the National Hospital, Queen Square, in 1923. Eventually, with staff appointments at both St. Bartholomew's Hospital and the National Hospital, Carmichael carried on in his clinical work but also became an exponent of basic research as an important aspect of neurology. His great opportunity came following World War II, when the Medical Research Council established a new research unit in the Rockefeller wing of the National Hospital, under his directorship. His analytical mind was well suited to this task, and he soon was surrounded by an able team of workers, many of whom later became outstanding in their own right. These included Professor George Dawson, Dennis Williams, Peter Nathan, J. A. V. Bates, Merion Smith, and others, as well as such foreign postgraduate clinical associates as Milton Shy of the New York Neurological Institute, Norman Geschwind of Harvard, and J. Doupe of Winnepeg. This constituted a major change of direction for the National Hospital and, secondarily, for British neurology in general.

Of Carmichael's 65 published articles that I have been able to find, clinical and clinico-pathological studies predominated. However, among these, were detailed observations of pain problems and vasomotor reactions under various conditions (10). They, also, included a number of articles on the effect of cerebral lesions on optokinetic and caloric nystagmus (11). Biochemical and experimental studies constituted about 20% of the total, and later, when he headed the Research Unit, the clinical effects of agents perfused into the cerebral ventricles predominated (12). These were pharmacological studies on cats, in which I was especially interested because of our own studies on the epileptogenic effect of intraventricular perfusions of hypertonic, isotonic, and hypotonic saline solutions (13). Previous findings had suggested that the hypothalamus (immediately adjacent in the walls of the lateral ventricles) was the most sensitive structure of the brain. The gentle perfusion studies done within millimeters of the hypothalamus (whose activity was simultaneously recorded) suggested that changes of cell membrane permeability were produced that altered the distribution of cellular-extracellular sodium and potassium ions. Our group had concluded that this probably explained the reactivity of the hypothalamus and its sensitivity in other experiments to low levels of x-rays (14).

It was in this later period that I came to know Carmichael more closely. He and Jeannette Carmichael came to visit one of their sons, who was a professor in the University of California, Berkeley. Two visits, however, were arranged under our Visiting Professor of Neurology Program to ensure that we might benefit from his lectures, demonstrations, and bedside teaching. He was particularly effective in the latter, and our residents insisted on a return visit in 1965, as I recall. This was in his early retirement period, not explained in his condensed curriculum vitae in Who's Who. It also was in this later period when Mrs. Aird and I visited the Carmichaels in Haywards Heath and that he advised us with respect to delightful spots in Scotland that we should visit.

Probably because of his critical stance, Carmichael did not receive as many honors as his clinically minded peers in Great Britain. However, this was compensated to some extent by the honors he received in America. He served as a visiting professor at the Montreal Neurological Institute, at the University of Pennsylvania School of Medicine, at Columbia, and twice at UCSF. He was an honorary member of several foreign neurological societies. He fulfilled several important named lectureships, was president of the Neurological Section of the Royal Society of Medicine, president of the British Electroencephalographic Society, and received an Honorary Doctor of Science degree from the University of Edinburgh.

Although the new National Health Service of 1948 constituted the greatest change in British medicine (as discussed under Brain in Chapter 16), there were additional factors that affected neurology in Great Britain, and Carmichael's push for basic research was one of them.

THE FRENCH TRADITION

In its heyday, French neurology boasted of such giants as Jean Martin Charcot, Armand Duchenne, Charles Laségue, Joseph Jules Dejerine, and Pierre Marie, as well as Claude Bernard and Louis Pasteur in allied fields. Charcot occupied the first chair of neurology ever established, and his dramatic lectures and demonstrations did much to center attention on the importance of the nervous system. He was an excellent neuropathologist as well as clinician and perhaps described more new neurological disorders than anyone else (15). It was a time when clinical "gold nuggets" were there to find, and the group mentioned were outstanding in their clinical discoveries. Their "gold mine" was the Hospice de la Salpétriere of Paris with its many thousands of welfare inmates. As the gold nuggets ran out, this remarkable period of neurology slowly subsided.

Large lectures and demonstrations were the rule in this older French school, but this has been superseded in more recent years as the scientific underpinnings of neurological research have transformed the field. Henri Gastaut (as discussed in Chapter 2), Jean Aicardi (Chapter 9), and Henri Laborit (Chapter 13) well typified the new order. The oratory of Gastaut harks back to the heyday of French neurology, but his real strength and position was rooted in his electroclinical research. Support for medical teaching and facilities had been vitiated by two world wars and the Great Depression. This was also true in Great Britain, but in France, it was exaggerated by the still earlier Franco-Prussian war and other circumstances. France is slowly improving its medical schools and teaching hospitals. In the case of Aix-Marseilles, this has developed since I was there as a Fulbright research scholar from 1957 to 1958. That France has done as well as it has speaks well for the abilities and promise of its human resources.

NEUROLOGICAL INSTRUCTION IN THE UNITED STATES

Starting with a British background, the United States has changed tremendously over the past 60 to 70 years as millions have migrated to America from all parts of the world. Graduate medical trainees turned to France and Germany in the 19th century and to Austria, Switzerland, and Scandinavia in the early 20th century, as well as to the United Kingdom. Many proprietary medical schools were established in the United States with limited libraries and basic science facilities. Large group lectures and demonstrations were the rule, and teaching hospitals were essentially unknown. The more thorough teaching experience provided by the German schools of medicine was introduced at Johns Hopkins in 1889, and this eventually was followed by Harvard and the other leading schools of medicine in the East and Midwest. However, it was not until after the Flexner Report of 1910 that more thorough, clinical instruction at the individual level became widespread. Much didactic instruction continued, of course, but the large and cheap clinical demonstrations of the past were slowly superseded by small group and individual instruction in the laboratory and at the bedside. I well recall this early transition period and can illustrate it by a few personal contacts.

As briefly mentioned in Chapter 7, my first brush with modern medical teaching occurred in my premedical courses at Cornell University. With adequate note taking, curricular subject material in the old days could be "regurgitated" with relative ease, and it was in this vein that I had enjoyed the course in psychology under the then-famous Edward B. Titchener. He was an English showman of the first order, who put on a most scintillating series of lectures and demonstrations. In the Old World style, he lectured in his full academic regalia and with his entire staff attending in the front row. His course was very popular, and the largest auditorium could scarcely hold his audience, which included many who audited his course as well as those who were formally registered. I have always had the impression that Hollywood and Madison Avenue learned a great deal from Titchener. Of course, there was much more to Professor Titchener than this, but I mention his teaching approach to contrast it with a second, which I also encountered at Cornell.

Comparative anatomy was one of the prerequisite courses for medical school, and I had greatly enjoyed it. On the side, I attended as many sessions as I could of another course in comparative neurologic anatomy. The course was given by James Papez, then an assistant professor. He did not object to my auditing his course, and it made a very stimulating supplement to my work in comparative anatomy. In retrospect, I believe this contact may have been what first stimulated my interest in the central nervous system. Certainly, it made me more fully aware of the central coordinating role of the central nervous system and its vital function in the brain-mind relationship.

Papez was a quiet and unassuming person but intense in his devotion to his work in neuroanatomy, and he worked closely with his students in the laboratory. The individual instruction and inspiration he gave, because of his great knowledge and correlation of function with anatomy, was a far cry from the flamboyant approach of Titchener. Both methods have their place, of course, but in my estimation, the more formal Old World method of instruction, at least in medicine, does not hold a candle to our individual "bedside" teaching or the quiet and in-depth type of instruction provided by Papez.

As described in Chapter 1, neurological instruction was impeded by still another factor—its ties to the old neuropsychiatry. However, as the new techniques of science were applied to neurology in the early decades of the present century and with the establishment of the National Institutes of Health (NIH) following World War II, the flowering of neurology really "took off." The great size and wealth of the United States inevitably made it the leader of post-World War II events. This involved the establishment of NIH and its neurological subdivisions with good support of both research and training grants. In addition, many migrant professionals from Great Britain, Germany, and other countries of Europe added to the enrichment and expansion of neurology in America. The result was a great upsurge of neurology, utilizing the best from the old world and the scientific advances of the first half of the 20th century. In our case, for example, we had Wartenberg, a great neurological scholar from Germany, and Macrae, a superb bedside teacher in the British tradition, in addition to our American staff. On top of this, I had initiated our visiting professor of neurology program, well before the NIH was established, which brought us more than 40 of the most outstanding English-speaking neurologists and neuroscientists of the world over a period of 17 years (1). Because their visits ranged from 2 to 6 weeks or more, they were effectively integrated into our teaching program, and we became well acquainted with them. For a period, we probably had the best teaching department of neurology in the country.

The striking changes in neurological instruction in the United States can best be illustrated by the first teaching service of neurology in America, the Harvard unit at the Boston City Hospital (as discussed in Chapter 2) and the career of Stanley Cobb, who organized and headed the unit.

STANLEY COBB (1887-1968)

Cobb and his development of the first neurological teaching unit in America had a great impact on American neurology, as recounted in Chapter 2. His inspiration and teaching was all the more remarkable in view of his severe stuttering defect. On first contact, this was the most obvious point about Cobb, other than his handsome and friendly mien. That he could overcome his impediment as a teacher at first brush seemed impossible, but he invariably succeeded. As I came to know him better at a later date, I concluded that he compensated for his stuttering defect by condensing his lectures. With fewer words, he made his subject both logical and lucid. His lectures went at a slower pace as compared with those of Zinsser, for example (as discussed in Chapter 11), and yet he seemed to cover as much ground. Furthermore, he sometimes acted out his lecture material. His dramatic portrayals of different seizure states, for example, were never to be forgotten. In addition, he skillfully simplified many points with blackboard sketches.

More background is essential if one is to grasp fully the impact of Cobb on both students and staff. His father was a well-known professor at Harvard College, and aside from some postgraduate work in physiology and psychiatry at Johns Hopkins University, Cobb was entirely a product of Harvard. He graduated from Harvard Medical School in 1914 and took a surgical internship under Harvey Cushing at the Peter Bent Brigham Hospital. After service in the Medical Corps in World War I, he became an instructor in physiology and neurology at Harvard Medical School and served as an assistant neurologist at the Massachusetts General Hospital. He was appointed Assistant Professor of Neuropathology in 1920 and was promoted to the associate professorship in 1923. As a Rockefeller fellow, he studied in Oxford, London, Paris, and Berlin. In 1925, he was awarded a substantial grant by the Rockefeller Foundation and became chief of service of a new neurology unit at the Boston City Hospital. In 1926, he was appointed Bullard Professor of Neuropathology at Harvard, and shortly, his unit became the focus of a notable neurological group. Studies on cerebral circulation were related to function and the cerebrovascular effect of drugs was studied. Continuing for a decade after 1928, he published some 50 articles on this subject. He was the editor of the volume *Circulation of Brain and Spinal Cord,* a publication of the Association for Research in Nervous and Mental Diseases (16). Other research projects included myasthenia gravis and the effect of neurological disorders on spinal reflexes and muscular tone. Also, he joined with Dr. William Lennox in a study of epilepsy, which initiated the remarkable advances achieved in this field in the 1930s (17), also discussed in Chapter 2.

Perhaps the most notable thing about Cobb was that, in spite of his academic appointment, he was not a neuropathologist in the traditional sense. Aside from his undergraduate course of neuropathology in the medical school, which used neuroanatomy and neuropathology to establish the scientific basis of neurology and neurosurgery, he was not interested in the neuropathological end point of disease processes. The formal aspects of traditional neuropathology were assigned to Charles Kubic. Instead, and this was the exciting thing about Cobb, his interests, teaching, and research were concerned with the pathophysiological processes that produced neuropathology. His enthusiasm and imagination with respect to neuropathophysiological processes had a great impact, attracted an amazing number of talented graduate students, and finally, produced one of the most outstanding neurological groups in history (as discussed in Chapter 2).

My reaction to Cobb's stance in neurological research, as well as my attraction to neurological subjects, led to spending my 4th-year elective period in Cobb's neurological unit at the Boston City Hospital. It was an excellent service, well supported by the Rockefeller Foundation. Here I came into contact with the cream of the neurological world of Harvard, and I found it most stimulating. In addition to Cobb, there was Tracy Putnam, Frank Freemont-Smith, William Lennox, Houston Merritt, and many others. Cobb's example and influence, no doubt, were determining factors in my own eventual choice of neurologic research.

Cobb's later clinical studies were almost entirely devoted to psychosomatic research; this was probably the main reason for his changing to the psychiatric service at the Massachusetts General Hospital. Although he accepted psychoanalysis[*] , he never shortchanged the possible role of organic factors in psychiatric conditions. As Nemiah has written, "First and foremost was his (Cobb's) pioneering investigations of psychosomatic phenomena. He was indefatigable in his attempts to understand how life stresses could lead to somatic dysfunction (18). *Borderlands of Psychiatry* (19) was one of his best books, and his earlier book *Foundations of Neuropsychiatry* went through six editions (20).

As a result of my research, I came to know Cobb quite well at a later date. He had found a protective effect with brilliant vital red in experimental epilepsy (21), which was explained by our studies, showing its effect on the blood-brain barrier (22,23). As I came to know Cobb more fully, it was obvious that psychosomatic research would be his approach. Psychosomatic research was one of the major preoccupations of neuropsychiatry before World War II. Because of Cobb's broad background in neurology and psychiatry, it was a subject that he was uniquely qualified to pursue.

Cobb continued as Bullard Professor of Neuropathology, holding this post as well as that of first chief of psychiatry at the Massachusetts General Hospital until his retirement in 1954. He received many awards and honorary degrees. I also remember him as president of the American Neurological Association. As Raymond Adams wrote in his obituary, "Stanley Cobb ranks as one of America's most distinguished men of medicine. He won renown as a naturalist, a scientist, a physician, a

---

*Cobb thought that psychoanalysis had helped his stuttering, but many of us debated this point, aside from its effect in affording understanding and support.

neurologist, and psychiatrist. Few men of this century have possessed such a wide breadth of knowledge of nature, medicine, and science" (24). He spent his final years of retirement in the study of avian neuroanatomy and paleontology.

Cobb's great impact on neurology resulted from his establishment of a neurological teaching unit that emphasized the importance of full-time teaching and research in an academic setting. The brilliant basic research accomplished on epilepsy constituted the first major surge in the flowering of neurology (as discussed in Chapter 2), and thanks to the generous NIH support of neurology following World War II, this ideal and trend came to its fruition over the next two decades. University appointments with adequate support of both teaching and research have been the rule, and this pattern has slowly spread to Great Britain, Europe, and elsewhere.

SUMMARY

Early neurological instruction followed the pattern in other medical fields—i.e., large group lectures and demonstrations. The British added small group and individual bedside teaching to this, but it remained for the United States to achieve widespread and adequately supported, full-time academic appointments for both neurological teaching and research. This was started by Stanley Cobb at Harvard and rapidly spread to other American medical schools following World War II, and more slowly, it is being adopted in other countries, as exemplified by the influence of Arnold Carmichael in Great Britain and Georges Schaltenbrand in Germany.

REFERENCES

1. Aird, R.B. *The History of Neurology*, San Francisco. History of Medicine Archives. San Francisco, University of California, San Francisco, 1979.
2. Aird, R.B. Some reminiscences. *Arch. Neurol.*, 45:1145-1155, 1988.
3. Schaltenbrand, G., and Hempl, F. Uber einer neuen myographen. *Dtsch. Z. Nervenheilkd.* 178:276-288, 1958
4. Schaltenbrand, G. *Atlas for Stereotaxis of Human Brain*. Stuttgart, Thieme, 1977.
5. Schaltenbrand, G. *Allgemeine Neurologie*. Stuttgart, Thieme, 1969.
6. Aird, R.B., and Garoutte, B. Some recent advances in electroencephalography. *J. Neurol.*, 212:185-204, 1976.
7. Hopf, H.C. Georges Schaltenbrand (1897-1978). *J. Neurol.*, 223:153-158, 1980.
8. Holmes, G. *The National Hospital, Queen Square*. London, E. & S. Livingston, 1954.
9. Crichley, M. Edward Arnold Carmichael. *Lancet*, 1:398-399, 1978.
10. Uprus, V., Gaylor, J.B., Williams, D.J., and Carmichael, A.E. Vasodilatation and vasoconstriction in response to warming and cooling the body: study in patients with hemiplegia. *Brain*, 55:448-455, 1935.
11. Carmichael, E.A., Dix, M.R., and Hallpike, C.S. Lesions of cerebral hemispheres and their effects upon optokinetic and caloric nystagmus. *Brain*, 77:345-372, 1954.
12. Carmichael, E.A., Feldberg, W., and Fleischauer, K. Methods for perfusing different parts of the cat's cerebral ventricles with drugs. *J. Physiol.* (Lond.), 173:354-367, 1964.
13. Sams, C.F., Aird, R.B., Adams, G. Ellman, G., and Endo, S. Central Nervous System Response to Low-Level X-Irradiation. Final Report to Public Health Service. Washington, D.C., Department of Health, Education, and Welfare, 1965, pp. 47-56, 57-73.
14. Sams, C.F., Aird, R.B., Adams, G.D., Ellman, G.L., and Endo, S. A functional response of the central nervous system to low-level radiation. *Trans. Am. Neurol. Soc.*, 89:129-132.
15. Wechsler, I.S. *Jean Martin Charcot* (1825-1893). In: Haymaker, W., and Schiller, F. (eds.). Founders of Neurology. Springfield, IL, Charles C. Thomas. 1970.

16. Cobb, S. Circulation of Brain and Spinal Cord. New York, *Association for Research in Nervous and Mental Disease*, 1937.
17. Lennox, W.G., and Cobb, S. Epilepsy from the standpoint of physiology and treatment. *Medicine,* 7:105-290, 1928.
18. Nemiah, J. An appreciation of Stanley Cobb. *Harvard Med.*, 59:45-48, 1985.
19. Cobb, S. *Borderlands of Psychiatry*. Cambridge, MA, Harvard University Press, 1943.
20. Cobb, S. *Foundations of Neuropsychiatry*. Baltimore, Williams & Wilkins, 1941.
21. Cobb, S., Cohen, M.E., and Net, J. Brilliant vital red as an anticonvulsant. *J. Nerv. Ment. Dis.*, 85:438-441, 1937.
22. Aird, R.B. Mode of action of brilliant vital red in epilepsy. *Arch. Neurol. Psychiatry*, 42:700-723, 1939.
23. Aird, R.B., and Strait, L. Protective barriers of the central nervous system: an experimental study with trypan red. Arch. Neurol., Psychiatry, 51:54-66, 1944.
24. Adams, R. Stanley Cobb, In: Denny-Brown, D. (ed). American Neurological Association (1875-1975). New York, Springer, pp. 253-258, 1975.

A Few Outstanding Teachers
of Neurology

As documented in the previous chapters, the true flowering of neurology was based on the scientific advances made in the first several decades of the 20th century. The application and teaching of the new techniques to the next generation mainly depended on the organically minded instructors of the old neuropsychiatry, before and during World War II. In many instances, as might be expected, there was a considerable overlap of teachers and research workers. However, it was the teachers who led in the actual flowering of neurology. As a rule, they also constituted the role models for the younger generation and combined their backgrounds of science with the art of bedside medical instruction and patient care. For this reason, these essays have been dedicated to the teachers as well as to the research workers who made the flowering of neurology possible.

The careers of Stanley Cobb, Arnold Carmichael, and Georges Schaltenbrand were presented in the previous chapter to illustrate some of the essential features involved in medical teaching and the different approaches that historically have been tried in neurological instruction. In addition, the teaching abilities of many others included in these essays have been mentioned. The purpose of the present chapter is to emphasize the qualities that are vital to successful teaching. Again, this can be done by considering a few outstanding neurologists who were superb teachers and who should be included because of their great contributions to the flowering of neurology.

RAYMOND ADAMS (1911-   )

Superior teachers, as a rule, have a broad basis of knowledge, in addition to an in-depth experience and understanding of their particular areas of interest and expertise. The evolution of a superb teacher is well illustrated in the case of Adams. Starting with an interest in psychology at the University of Oregon, Adams gravitated to the medical school of Duke University to obtain background training on the central nervous system. Initially drawn to psychiatry, he was disappointed in the lack of a scientific approach to psychiatric disorders. After 2 years of graduate training in general medicine at Duke, he obtained a Rockefeller Fellowship for 3 additional years of graduate training. He spent the 1st year with Dr. James Ayer in neurology at the Massachusetts General Hospital. The 2nd year was devoted to psychiatry and neuropathology with Stanley Cobb and Charles Kubic at the Massachusetts General Hospital. His 3rd year was in psychiatry with Eugene Kahn at Yale.

In 1941, Adams joined Houston Merritt and Dr. Denny-Brown at the neurological unit at the Boston City Hospital. His association with the latter continued for 10 years. He was put in charge of the neuropathological laboratory and, with Denny-Brown, undertook a series of studies on alcoholic, cerebrovascular, and muscle disorders. With Denny-Brown and Carl Pearson, a classic book, *Diseases of Muscle*, was completed (1). His continuing correlative studies of neuropathology and neurology produced a broad series of reports and established the basis for his later teaching.

In 1951, Adams succeeded Kubic at the Massachusetts General Hospital as chief of the neurological service and neuropathology. He quickly expanded the service in several directions, but with neuropathology as a unifying basis for the clinical disciplines of neuromedicine and child neurology, he established the laboratories of neuropathology, neurochemistry, immunology, and behavior. Electron microscopy was added to neuropathology. The neuropathology course of Stanley Cobb was continued as a medical undergraduate course in the neurological sciences.

Dr. Wilder Penfield recognized Adams as a potential successor to himself as director of the Montreal Neurological Institute and bidding for Adams developed between McGill and Harvard. When appointed the Bullard Professor of Neuropathology at Harvard and offered excellent support for his services at the Massachusetts General Hospital, Adams stayed on in Boston. He was made director of the Joseph P. Kennedy, Jr., Memorial Laboratories for the study of Mental Retardation at the hospital; this later became a major independent research unit. He also was made director of the Shriver Research Laboratories at the Fernald State School, which concentrated on metabolic and developmental disorders of childhood. Also, through his initiatives, departments of neurology were started at the University of Lausanne and the American University of Beirut.

As might be expected, a host of research studies followed, such as those on chronic idiopathic polymyositis (with Walton) (2), central pontine myelinolysis, Korsakoff's syndrome, cerebellar degeneration in alcoholism (with Victor and Mancall) (3), experimental allergic polyneuritis (with Waksman) (4), chronic hepatic encephalopathy (with Victor and Cole) (5), and normal pressure hydrocephalus (with Fisher and others) (6).

As a teacher, Ray Adams stood apart. His vast knowledge and in-depth discussions often bordered on the incredible. His impact was overwhelming to many. I well recall on one occasion, when we happened to be in Stockholm at the same time, we joined forces to visit the neurological service at the huge City Hospital, which was under the direction of the superintendent of the hospital. Without intent to embarrass, Adams dumbfounded the director and his staff by raising questions concerning the neurological diagnosis of some of their patients. I later wondered if this sort of reaction in foreign clinics may have been a factor in Adams not being elected president of the World Federation of Neurology in 1982. I believe he did not always realize his impact on others. His well-meant and brilliant discussions were not done in a vain or hypercritical fashion. It all seemed very obvious and natural to him.

Another facet of Adams was his great hospitality to foreign guests, and this extended to foreign visitors at meetings. On one memorable occasion he almost did me in with his "gentle kindness," as his colleague, C. Miller Fisher, has termed it. For a number of years following World War II, Russian neuroscientists would schedule articles on the program of the American Neurological Association. Almost invariably these were canceled for reasons that were never explained. However, on one occasion, the Russian speaker did show up. His subject concerned the central nervous system effects of changes in the permeability of the blood–brain barrier. I could not understand a word he said, and I am fairly sure that others also did not understand. At the end, a long pause followed, as the Chair asked if there were comments or questions. Finally, Ray arose and, in a most diplomatic fashion, regretted that I was not present to discuss the article. At this point, three acquaintances made an energetic show of pointing me out. I was trapped! I made a few general comments, such as that cerebrovascular permeability changes in the regions of central nervous system lesions constitute a common basis for neuropathological staining and concerning cerebral localization by means of radioactive isotopes and focal neurophysiological changes as shown by electroencephalography, which latter in susceptible patients might produce epileptogenic seizures. I finally asked the author about the blood–brain barrier conditions that were involved in obtaining the slide he had shown on the brainstem. The Russian appeared delighted with my comments and spoke again in his incomprehensible fashion. Whether Adams was satisfied with this odd exchange I never found out, but I believe that he was, inasmuch as it at least satisfied the immediate needs of medical diplomatic protocol.

The career of Adams especially well illustrates the combination of a superb clinical teacher with neurological research that goes beyond the clinical descriptive level.

CHARLES PUTNAM SYMONDS (1890-1977)

Symonds was often rated as the shining light of that great center of neurological training for the British Empire, the National Hospital, Queen Square, London. He had a keen appreciation of the changes that were under way in neurology during and following the 1930s and kept up with them in his practice. Nevertheless, he was a transitional figure, having been trained in the proud traditions of British neurology. He well exemplified the hardships, limitations, and glories of neurology in Great Britain, as noted in Chapter 15.

Steeped in the old traditions, Symonds was certainly one of the most outstanding neurologists of the mid-20th century. He added considerable works to the neurological literature and was a superb teacher. His keenness of mind, however, was well aware of the changes going on in neurology, and he joined in these to the extent that he could. As Air Marshall of Great Britain, with the neurosurgeon, Hugh Cairns, he headed a study of head injury at Oxford during World War II. Following the war, he organized a comprehensive research team, working mainly on temporal lobe epilepsy in the Guy's Hospital Epilepsy Unit at the Maudsley Hospital, London. It was to this center that Murrary Falconer was drawn in 1950 and which proved so productive (as discussed in Chapter 8). Symonds's story is an interesting one.

He was the son of Sir Chartres Symonds, a London surgeon. Following graduate training at the National Hospital, Queen Square, London, in 1920, he obtained a staff appointment at Guy's Hospital and Medical School, London. His service was the first complete neurological unit in a general hospital in Great Britain. A traveling fellowship permitted him further postgraduate study with Adolf Meyer at Johns Hopkins and with Cushing at Harvard.

According to Denny-Brown, who worked with him, Symonds "inherited the mantle of Gowers and Gordon Holmes in the great tradition of bedside teaching" and was considered by many to be the foremost neurologist of his time (7). His meticulous studies, keen analysis of clinical problems, and remarkable memory made him outstanding. His articles covered the whole field of neurology and a selection of his most important contributions was published in book form under the title *Studies in Neurology* (8). He included in this ten articles on head injury, the last being in 1945 (9). The last of his seven articles on epilepsy in 1955 suggested several approaches to classification (10). It was his studies on head injury, however, and his heading the Oxford research project on head injury that led to his being knighted in 1946.

I have always thought of Symonds as a neurological Sherlock Holmes. This line of thought, no doubt, was the result of my meeting Arthur Conan Doyle in Paris in 1925, as discussed in Chapter 2. I had become fascinated by Doyle's use of the methods of detection and deductive reasoning, as exploited in the Sherlock Holmes stories, inasmuch as they were based on his own medical training and are basic to medical diagnosis. Then, too, Symonds in appearance could pass as a Sherlock Holmes of sorts. It was always a pleasure to observe his meticulous examinations. Better still was his deductive reasoning, which was buttressed by his "computerized" recall that lent the support of long experience to his current findings. The end result was an outstanding diagnostic acumen. These qualities, plus his clarity of thought and analysis, made him a superb teacher.

My acquaintance with him extended over a period of 25 years. He was most helpful as a visiting professor, and I greatly enjoyed his accounts of neurology in England and his experiences in both world wars. In turn, Symonds seemed interested in my experimental research and clinical studies on epilepsy, which involved prolonged follow-up and a comprehensive therapeutic approach (drugs plus regulation of demonstrated seizure-inducing factors) (11). However, these seemed to be aspects of neurology that were foreign to his English background.

We hit the ornithological jackpot on one of his visits. Like Sir Russell Brain (later Lord), Symonds was a devoted bird watcher. As luck would have it, he spotted several Allen's hummingbirds in our garden. These were new to him because hummingbirds are not found in Great Britain. When we drove him to the top of Mount Tamalpais for a view of the Bay Area, there was another flock of hummingbirds. A few days later in the garden of the Carmel Mission, we encountered even more. He and my wife exchanged ornithological observations for many years.

Another episode will illustrate his remarkable memory for clinical detail. While Mrs. Aird and I were motoring in southwestern England in 1969, our rented small automobile developed a knock that ominously increased from day to day. When we reached Porlock on the Bristol Channel, we stopped at a garage to have the car checked before venturing onto Exmoor Downs. The mechanic advised that we not proceed "a foot further." The owner of the garage heard me call the nearest office of the car rental agency in Bristol and, realizing that I was a doctor, told me of his wife's illness. She had developed a pituitary tumor, was referred to a neurologist in London, and had made a good recovery from her neurosurgery, which followed. By way of showing interest, I asked him who the neurological consultant was.

"A remarkable chap, sir. He had been knighted, and his name was Sir John Symonds."

"Oh! You must mean Sir Charles Symonds."

"Why yes. You are quite right, and do you know him?"

"We are now on our way to visit him at his home in Ham."

"What a coincidence!"

"And who was your surgeon?"

"Mr. Murrary Falconer."

"He, also, is an old friend and we will be seeing him shortly at a meeting in New York City."

This exchange and my further explanation of his wife's condition led the garage owner to insist on entertaining us, inasmuch as the new automobile would not arrive from Bristol for some 3 hours. He drove us to the nearby village of Selworthy that has been preserved by the National Trust. It is a most quaint, old English village, one that we thoroughly enjoyed visiting.

When we later recounted this story to Symonds, who was then retired, he immediately rose to the occasion and, after asking a few questions, recalled the lady and her condition. He provided a much better history than the husband and then managed to correct certain details of my own hasty second-hand diagnosis.

Symonds's memory for old details was also shown in his article on the birthplace of Sir Thomas Willis. It was in Great Bedwyn, a neighboring town to Ham. Symonds took much pleasure in driving us over to Great Bedwyn and pointing out the chimney and other features of the ancient house that matched the old illustration of Willis's home. Because of the great interest that Professor Erik Ask-Upmark of Uppsala, Sweden, had in Willis, which he conveyed to us on a trip to Gotland, Sweden, 4 years earlier, I was well aware of much of the background of Willis, and this helped to save the day for us with Symonds.

When Dr. Gooddy of the National Hospital, London, informed me of Symonds's last days, I felt somewhat guilty in not alerting some of my English friends, who might have kept an eye on him. I had visited him only months before and wondered about his condition and situation. When Sir Charles and Lady Symonds gave up their home in Ham, he had wanted to go to Oxford but, finally, acceded to her wish to return to London. An apartment on Baker Street, however, was a far cry from a cottage in Oxford, where he had old associations from the World War II period.

Luckily, Gooddy recognized Symonds on the wards of one of the London hospitals, and his transfer to the National Hospital ameliorated to some extent, his sad end.

HENRY MILLER (1913-1976)

The English have a penchant, if not a strong flair, for public speaking. This was especially well exemplified in the case of Miller. Not only was he a fine neurologist in the British tradition, but also, he was a great orator of the University of Newcastle-upon-Tyne, as well as its Vice Chancellor. He brought still other aspects to neurological teaching—humaneness, joy, and understanding. His unusual personality was coupled with diplomacy, sound judgment, and considerable organizational ability. Fully aware of the importance of basic research in neurology, he developed two research and clinical units at Newcastle. Because of his wit, humor, and remarkable showmanship, an account of neurological teaching would not be complete without his inclusion.

Born and raised in Chesterfield, Derbyshire, he studied medicine at the Newcastle College of Medicine, which at that time, was part of the University of Durham. Over the next 2.5 years, he received graduate training in the Royal Victoria Infirmary, Newcastle, in the Johns Hopkins Department of Pathology, Baltimore, and then in the Hospital for Sick Children, Great Ormand Street, London. Working under Professor Nattrass at Newcastle, he developed an interest in neurology and qualified for the M.D. and membership in the Royal College of Physicians. He married Eileen C. Baird, a member of the Royal College of Obstetrics and Gynecology, in 1942, and then was caught up in World War II, serving in the Royal Air Force. It is especially interesting to note that, in this early period, Miller came under the influence of Sir Charles Symonds in the Royal Air Force, when Symonds was Vice Air Marshal. This proved to be a lifelong influence, which he fully acknowledged (Miller, H., personal communication, 1964). Directly after World War II, he did further graduate training in neurology at the National Hospital, Queen Square, and the Hammersmith Hospital, London.

By 1947, he was back at the Royal Infirmary with Professor Nattrass. In 1953, he was elected to fellowship in the Royal College of Physicians, and in 1961, he was appointed a reader in neurology at Newcastle. The next year, he was instrumental in establishing a new medical curriculum at Newcastle, and in 1961, he served as a Visiting Professor of Medicine at the University of Queensland, British Australia.

When the University of Newcastle-upon-Tyne was established, Miller was made its public orator. In March 1964, he came to us as a visiting professor of neurology, and in that same year, he advanced to a professorship of neurology at Newcastle. In the following years, he served as secretary-general of the World Federation of Neurology, dean of medicine at Newcastle, director chair of the Planning Unit of the British Medical Association, and chair of the Medical Panel of the Multiple Sclerosis Society of Great Britain and North Ireland.

In 1968, he was made vice chancellor of Newcastle and, over the next 6 years, fulfilled numerous appointments in Great Britain, served as a visiting professor in

Canada, and received various honors and awards. Except for his untimely death in 1976, he would have gone on to still higher honors, lectureships, and appointments.

Miller was author of some 155 medical articles. They involved a wide variety of subjects, but from 1944 on, essentially all of his articles related to neurology. His first one on multiple sclerosis appeared in 1953, and over the next 22 years, he was author or co-author of over 30 articles on this subject, which had become a central research theme for him by 1960 (12). Nevertheless, for years, he and R. Daley published summary reviews of Progress in Clinical Medicine, as well as many articles on the economic and political aspects of medicine. His other main interests were on pain problems, head injury, and accident and compensation neurosis. In addition, he wrote regularly for the journals Listener and Encounter on medical subjects of interest to the lay public.

Although I knew Miller for a scant 12 years, they were the peak years of his career. Two or three episodes will convey some understanding of his brilliance and spirit.

We had invited the Millers in March 1964 to come to San Francisco. Two main objectives for him involved his participation in an extension division course in neurology for graduates and a lecture before the San Francisco Neurological Society at Carmel, California. It so happened that Dr. Macdonald Critchley was on a medical trip to Vancouver and could be with us over the period of the extension division course. I proceeded to develop honoraria for both and drove with Professor Sigvald Refsum to Vancouver and back to fetch Critchley. Miller was spending 2 weeks with us and was scheduled for many more lectures, conferences, and rounds in the UCSF Department of Neurology.

On the morning of the extension division course in our largest auditorium, UCSF, Critchley held forth in his usual stellar fashion, demonstrating, diagnosing, and discussing patients with aphasia, parietal lobe syndromes, and dyslexia. In the afternoon session, Critchley sat next to me in the front row as Miller was examining and discussing a patient with multiple sclerosis. Perhaps, due to the circumstances, Miller outdid himself. As Andrew Smith, an old friend and lecturer in family medicine at the University of Newcastle-upon-Tyne, has described Miller, "He spoke quickly but distinctly, carrying one along by the sheer pace with which he developed his theme. His fluency, wit, and verbal extravagance left one informed, astonished and roaring with laughter by turn" (13). So it was on this occasion—his wit and stories had the large audience in excellent humor and keen attention. As Miller made some telling point with great showmanship, Critchley leaned over and whispered, "Why this chap is good!" In amazement, I whispered back, "Well, you must have known that through your meetings in England." "I have never seen him perform," replied Critchley. Here were two of the best showmen of Great Britain together on our program, and the older one could not recall seeing the younger. It was hard to believe, but Miller in discussing it later, may have had it right when he said, "My time at Queen Square was before Critchley returned from his naval service in the Second World War and he is so busy with his practice and own lectures, I doubt if he hears anyone else, except those right in London." Mrs. Aird helped me repay Miller and Critchley for their outstanding extension division performances by putting on a lovely reception with Chancellor Saunders and many other local dignitaries and neurologists in attendance.

We had taken the Millers to Carmel on the previous weekend. Our arrival at the Pine Inn was somewhat late but in time for a late dinner. Following this, I discovered the reservation desk had given our reserved rooms to others, the excuse being that we had arrived late. Mrs. Aird and I did not mind our substitute rooms, and at first, I thought they had done the Millers a favor. They were given what appeared to be a lovely suite in a penthouse. However, to get to, it was a climb of two floors—there was no elevator! Ellinor and I had preceded to inspect it, and it did not occur to me that portly Miller might find this a difficult climb. He made it all right but with much puffing. In spite of two or three rests, his face had a distinctive reddish glow, and he was perspiring. I was alarmed, and the next morning saw to it that we were given more acceptable accommodations.

On the weekend, we drove the Millers to Point Lobos and the Big Sur coast. I stopped to show them the house of Henry Miller, the writer. The house was in a dramatic location on a rocky ridge, extending above a cove from the Pacific Ocean. At first, Miller thought I was joking, but when finally convinced, said "This is pretty high class—a writer living like a king in this beautiful spot! We Henry Millers in England are a rummy lot in comparison—mere peons, flotsam on the tides of time." His talk at the meeting was very well received. By the time the Millers left, his rounds and conferences swelled in the numbers attending, and I received favorable comments from attending physicians for weeks afterward.

Miller had several jaundiced opinions on subjects that he did not always suppress in the presence of those sensitive to them. The specialty teaching hospitals of Great Britain and, in particular, the National Hospital, Queen Square, came in for critical appraisal and with much more emphasis than in my discussion in Chapter 15. Certain aspects of psychiatry and academic neurophysiological studies were other subjects. He must have known of my research interests, but like Sir Francis Walshe, he seemed to accept them when they came up in our discussions. Our discussions were free and far ranging, and the warmth of our reception in Newcastle makes me believe that his reported blasts must have been reserved for special studies, which perhaps did involve dubious features. Of course, Miller was an orator, and perhaps like Walshe when holding forth in fervent declamation, spirited verbiage may have prevailed at moments to make a point. However, I never detected this trait in him, as I had in Walshe. On the other hand, Miller, unlike Walshe, was not a profound critic. Some, who knew him better than I, like Jack Foster, have written that he could be indiscretely critical and that this blunted the enthusiasm of his many admirers (14). On checking with another associate about this, he admitted the charge but added that it only occurred on very lively exchanges and after considerable tippling. Another possibility is that these incidents may have been done in the spirit of his address to the World Psychiatric Association in 1969 (15). His title was "Psychiatry—Medicine or Magic," in which he announced his founding of the Society for the Abolition of Psychiatrists. Only Miller could get away with such extravagances, a point I am convinced he well understood and, on occasion, used to great advantage. How much was jest and good fun, carried off in his inimitable fashion (sometimes with an underlying purpose), must remain one of the imponderables. Certainly, he succeeded in keeping everyone "on their toes."

In spite of his reported aversion to academic neurophysiological work, Miller had a real interest in research that went well beyond the usual clinical research. He went to great lengths with the university and research council to obtain space and funding for research and developed the support of paramedical societies to this end. Between himself and Walton, two outstanding research teams were established with excellent equipment and facilities. Both Miller and Walton took great pride in showing me this aspect of their setup. However, the multiple sclerosis laboratory was headed by E. J. Field, Miller's contributions being in clinical research.

Miller's interest in research was shown, again, in the serious inquiry he made on one of my projects. Because of the "sink" effect of cerebrospinal fluid absorption from the subarachnoid spaces, I had always questioned the central effect of agents injected by lumbar or cisternal puncture. Library investigation, however, showed that there were about 100 articles of such trials per year involving innumerable agents, and this had not diminished over many years—in fact, since salvarsan was thus used in 1913. In the late 1960s, one of my research projects evaluated the early claims that seemed to justify this approach, e.g., to bypass the blood–brain barrier in obtaining effects aimed at the central nervous system. Anesthetic levels could be well regulated by the rates of infusion of selected barbiturates. Miller was particularly interested in the cisternal perfusion studies that produced identifiable, steady-state central nervous system effects. These effects could be reproduced by sustained, slow intravenous injections at dose rates that were identical to the cisternal perfusion dose rates. The cisternal perfusion effects, however, were delayed and could only be explained in terms of a vascular effect following venous reabsorption from the cerebrospinal fluid (16). This explained the poor results obtained in the many reports in the literature and suggested that the intrathecal route is not an effective one for injections aimed at producing central effects. Incidentally, the matching of venous and cisternal perfusion dose rates for steady-state central nervous system effects proved to be a better control than blood levels, although this might not be true for substances that readily pass through the blood–brain barrier.

Miller was especially interested in these results because of his own therapeutic studies in multiple sclerosis, which had shortly antedated this discussion.* He had published eight articles on the experimental therapy of multiple sclerosis between 1961 and 1965 and touched on the subject again in an article on intrathecal steroid therapy at the annual meeting of the American Neurological Association in 1969. My discussions with him on this were at the 1969 occasion and, again, when I visited him in Newcastle in 1976.

The story of Miller's turbulent career would not be complete without mention of Eileen, his wife. Less verbal than her husband, she more than made up for this by

---

*Although the studies were done in the late 1960s, the analysis of results and final report were interrupted by other activities.

her great charm, understanding, and practical efficiency. As A. G. Ogilvie, an Honorary Consulting Physician to the Royal Victory Infirmary, has said, "things always ran smoothly, when Eileen was in charge" (17).

One cannot gather the many fascinating facets of this extraordinary man from the few comments recorded here. I would strongly recommend readers to delve into that delightful compendium *Remembering Henry*, edited by Stephen Lock and Heather Windle and published by the British Medical Association, 1977 (quoted in references 13, 14, and 17).

DEREK DENNY-BROWN (1901-1981)

Another great teacher, trained in the Queen Square tradition, but devoting most of his career to teaching and research in the Harvard Medical School, was Denny-Brown. As a colonial, he was not tied to Mother England and, in this respect, was like Foster Kennedy, whose origin was in Ireland. Furthermore, Denny-Brown was steeped in neurophysiology, realized that the great challenge of neurology was research, perceived the limitations of the National Hospital in this respect (as discussed under The British Tradition in Chapter 15), and fully grasped the opportunity afforded by Harvard.

Dr. Macdonald Critchley has described Denny-Brown's training as "completely self-sufficient" (18). Using the laboratory facilities of Dr. Greenfield at the National Hospital, he personally handled all stages of the staining and pathological study of his patients, including the slide preparation and microphotography. Other postgraduate students might learn the techniques but usually turned the procedures over to Greenfield and the laboratory staff as quickly as possible. Denny-Brown had been equally meticulous in his neurophysiological studies and was the one, along with Lidell, who introduced John Eccles, a later Nobel prize winner, into research on the cerebellum. This was in the Oxford laboratories of Sir Charles Sherrington. When Sherrington organized his book on the researches of the Oxford school of neurophysiology, he chose Denny-Brown, along with Lidell, Eccles, and Creed as collaborators in this effort (19). Later, Denny-Brown published the *Selected Writings of Sir Charles Sherrington* (20).

In 1935, Denny-Brown obtained appointments at the National Hospital and St. Bartholomew's Hospital, London. One year later, apparently stymied in carrying on with his interests in basic research in the clinical world of neurology in London, he obtained a Rockefeller Fellowship with John Fulton at Yale from 1936 to 1937. This led to many contacts with American neurologists and neuroscientists. In 1939, he was appointed a professor of neurology at Harvard and director of the neurological unit at the Boston City Hospital when Putnam went to New York City (as discussed in Chapter 2). This appointment, however, was delayed because, as a British citizen, he was inducted into the Royal Army when World War II started that same year. He was released 4 years later but again was reactivated in the final war effort. In May 1946, he finally resumed his appointment at Harvard.

Over the next 21 years, his postgraduate training program produced an outstanding group of neurologists. His research involved almost all phases of neurology but with an emphasis in basic studies on the basal ganglia, related to tremors, posture, and movements (21,22). With Adams and Pearson, he published *Diseases of Muscle* (1).

Denny-Brown won many honors, including several honorary degrees. He was an officer of the Order of the British Empire, president of the American Neurological Association, and president of the Association of Neuropathologists. In 1969, his students and colleagues published a festschrift in his honor (23).

I have always categorized Denny-Brown as an American neurologist, inasmuch as it was in this guise that I knew him. My first impression of Denny-Brown was not too favorable because of his apparent decimation of the previous professional staff at Cobb's neurological unit at Boston City Hospital, many of whom were old friends of mine. Also, I wondered about his development of a one-man clinical and research unit. His staccato speech and New Zealand accent were added hazards to my Western ear. However, as I came to know him better, I found a highly critical mind tempered with a breadth of understanding, a kindly disposition, and a sense of humor that was quite fascinating to me. One could not but admire his extensive background in neurophysiology, neuropathology, research, and neurology and the depth of his discussions in these fields. Visits to his unit at Boston City Hospital lent further perspective with respect to the administrative vicissitudes of a highly disciplined man in a large, chaotic city hospital with its political problems and frustrations. We became good friends and, over a period of years, regularly had luncheons or dinners together at the meetings of the American Neurological Association and on other occasions.

Critchley has described him as "not a great communicator on paper" and added "... once (Denny-Brown) had a postcard from FMR Walshe which read 'Dear Denny, I see you have a paper in *Brain*. When is the English version coming out?'" (18). He was at his best and definitely an excellent communicator in his teaching of postgraduate students. He gave much time and effort at this level in his unit at the Boston City Hospital, and this showed up in those trained. It was in this unit that Ray Adams, taking full advantage of its neuropathological and clinical resources, developed his outstanding qualities as a teacher. Denny-Brown also attracted many British postgraduate students, in preference to their going to France or Germany.

When Denny-Brown was with us as a visiting professor in 1963, he put on stellar performances in both his patient rounds and more formal presentations. He drew a considerable number of neurologists from the outside, as well as from within the medical school. This was at a period when the University of California at San Francisco was having growing pains and its own political problems that struck me as childish and most distasteful. Denny-Brown's reaction was identical with my own, and his advice was most helpful. At a later date, I recommended him for consideration to the Nobel prize committee for his pioneer work on the dyskinesias when my advice was sought on this matter, but nothing came of it.

KARL GUNNAR WOHLFART (1910-1961)

As a representative of Scandinavian neurologists, Professor Wohlfart illustrates still other aspects of teaching. With his youthful vigor, enthusiasm, and brilliance, he was an inspiration, and at the same time, he possessed unusual administrative abilities. As the first professor of neurology at Lund, Sweden, when still only 40 years of age, he established excellent graduate and research programs and strongly emphasized the neurological aspects of rehabilitation and occupational medicine.

The son of a professor of music at the University of Stockholm, Wohlfart was an accomplished musician and a man of unusual cultural background. His medical training was in the Karolinska Institute, Stockholm, where he earned doctorates of medicine and philosophy. He achieved early recognition by his clinical studies on carbon monoxide poisoning, a complication of the substitute fuels used in automobiles in Sweden during World War II. He was an outstanding histopathologist and became well known for his studies on neuromuscular disorders (24,25). His contributions in this developing field were most promising but, unfortunately, were interrupted by his early death.

As a visiting professor in our program, Wohlfart was very effective, both at the graduate and undergraduate levels of teaching. He enlivened his lectures with stories that the students would never forget. For example, to illustrate the cardinal symptom of myasthenia gravis, its abnormal fatiguability of muscles, he told about one of his patients, who was a hunting-lodge keeper for the King of Sweden. When the king arrived, all attendants stood in line to welcome him. Invariably, the head of Wohlfart's patient drooped very low. The king interpreted this as a sign of respect and loyalty and duly remunerated him with extra awards. This perhaps is the only instance in which myasthenia gravis served to help one of its victims!

When I was invited by the Swedish Medical Council, Stockholm, as a visiting professor of neurology in 1953, Mrs. Aird and I were astounded by the warmth of Swedish hospitality and have always wondered if our good Swedish friends, such as Wohlfart and Ask-Upmark, were responsible for this behind the scenes. My problem was how to join in their festive dinners and yet minimize the effects of their amazing number of drinks so that I could function effectively day after day. I did not have the excuse of being a driver, so I quickly had to learn to skoal with reasonable aplomb but with minimal imbibing. I had been prepared for their formalities by my good friend, Sigvald Refsum (as discussed in Chapter 12), and once over these hurdles, I managed fairly well, even to performing our six thank-yous after each gala event. On a later trip to Monterey, California, I asked Wohlfart if he thought that the explanation for Swedish social formality might lie in its protective effect against people getting on each other's nerves during the long and dark Swedish winters. He had never thought of this but finally agreed that it was a reasonable possibility (1).

I was always careful to have our piano tuned before Wohlfart came on his visits, and it did not take too much prodding to involve him in delightful concerts. I have copies of his father's compositions, and he helped me with some of the technical aspects of my own amateurish efforts at composition.

An insight into Swedish social life and justice was gained on one occasion when we were invited to a luncheon held by one of Wohlfart's residents, whose wife was of the nobility and who owned a castle not far from Lund. The conversation had turned to skiing, and I asked the resident where they would be going over the

Christmas holidays. His astonishing answer, "I will be going to prison," was explained by his arrest on driving after a dinner. Someone had observed him take a drink and reported him. Incriminating blood levels of alcohol were far more strict in Sweden than in the United States, and he would have been declared sober in the United States. Because the resident was an essential person, he was allowed to serve his sentence on weekends and during the Christmas holidays, still 2.5 months away! Both Wohlfart and the resident seemed to accept this, and no effort had been made to alleviate or avoid Swedish justice. I could not help but contrast this situation with our own at that time—who would have reported a person for taking one drink in America? Would the verdict have been accepted so meekly?

I obtained a grant from the former Poliomyelitis Foundation (now the National Foundation for Infantile Paralysis) for a fellowship for one of our staff, Bertram Feinstein, to spend 1 year with Wohlfart. Dr. Feinstein was the husband of Dianne Feinstein, who later became mayor of San Francisco and, still later, a California senator. He, unfortunately, died a few years after his fellowship. Feinstein had a good background in electromyography with Alexander G. Weddell at Oxford, in addition to training in neurology and some neurosurgery. The plan was to combine this background with Wohlfart's background in muscle pathology and then to undertake basic studies of neuromuscular disorders. This was in 1951, when such studies were still in an embryonic stage. Three articles resulted from their studies, the one with D. Fex perhaps best illustrating the purpose of the project (26).

Wohlfart's untimely death in 1961 was a great tragedy to neurology in Sweden. His organization at Lund was outstanding, and his connections with physiology, pathology, and rehabilitation medicine were close. His comprehensive teaching in neurology touched on all these fields and was outstanding. He was an early pioneer in neuromuscular disorders and did much to establish neurology on a firm footing in Scandinavia.

SUMMARY

A review of the characteristics of the neurologists used to illustrate teaching in this section permits the following summary of the attributes of gifted teachers. Above all, they were a verbal group, whose wit and humor commanded the interest and cooperation of their students and colleagues. This was vital in both clinical demonstrations and beside teaching. Second, they had developed a background that historically, scientifically, and neurologically added perspective and depth to their teaching. Third, they were good role models for their students. Their ability at history taking, examination, and summarizing the pertinent facts in arriving at a logical diagnosis was outstanding. Perhaps even more important in this category was their considerate handling of patients and follow through to ensure further studies as necessary, developing a proper therapeutic regimen, and preparing a full report to the referring physician. In addition, when necessary, they advised as to the mobilization of the resources of the patient's local community to ensure a comprehensive plan of care and follow-up. Fourth, they were good organizers and developed strong teaching setups. Judgment as to the selection of associates and service and research facilities were involved in this category.

Beyond all these basic qualities, a fifth category can be added. In one way or another, they were able to take advantage of the developing phase of the flowering period of neurology and by utilizing the new scientific techniques of study, contributed to the advancement of their field.

Small wonder that this notable group constituted a great impetus to the flowering of neurology, They were gifted persons of vision, who gave direction to the great changes that developed in the period of their active careers. They were role models for the next generation that put neurology on a firm basis as an independent, clinical discipline.

REFERENCES

1. Adams, R., Denny-Brown, D., and Pearson, C. *Diseases of Muscle*. New York, Paul Hoeber, 1953.
2. Walton, J.N., and Adams, R. *Poliomyelitis*. Edinburgh, Livingston, 1938.
3. Adams, R., Victor, M., and Mancall, E. A restricted form of cerebellar cortical degeneration occurring in alcoholic patients. *Arch. Neurol.*, 1:579-688, 1959.
4. Adams, R., and Waksman, B.H. Experimental allergic neuritis produced in rabbits with nerve and adjuvants. *Fed. Proc.*, 13:516, 1954.
5. Adams, R., Victor, M., and Cole, M. The acquired (non-Wilsonian.) type of chronic hepatocerebral degeneration. *Medicine*, 44:345-396, 1965.
6. Adams, R., Fisher, C.M., Hakim, S., Ojemann, R,G., and Sweet, W.H. Symptomatic occult hydrocephalus with "normal" cerebrospinal fluid pressure. *N. Engl. J. Med.*, 273:117-126, 1965.
7. Denny-Brown, D. Sir Charles Symonds. *Ann. Neurol.*, 6:137, 1979.
8. Symonds, C.P. *Studies in Neurology*. London, Oxford University Press, 1970.
9. Symonds, C.P. Prognosis in closed head injuries. *Br. Med. Bull.*, 3:14, 1945.
10. Symonds, C.P. Classification of the epilepsies. B.M.J., 1:1235, 1955.
11. Aird, R.B. The importance of seizure-inducing factors in the control of refractory forms of epilepsy. *Epilepsia*, 24:567-583, 1983.
12. Schapira, K., Poskanzer, D.C., Newell, D.J., and Miller, H. Marriage, pregnancy and multiple sclerosis. *Brain*, 89:418-428, 1966.
13. Smith, A. *Comments*. In: Lock, S., and Windle, H. (eds.). Remembering Henry. London, British Medical Association, 1977, p. 80.
14. Foster, J. *Comments*. In: Lock, S., and Windle, H. (eds.). Remembering Henry. London, British Medical Association, 1977, p. 26.
15. Miller, H. Psychiatry—medicine or magic. Br. J. Hosp. Med., 3:122-126, 1970.
16. Aird, R.B. A study of intrathecal-to-brain exchange. *Exp. Neurol.*, 86:342-358, 1984.
17. Ogilvie, A.G. *Comments*. In: Lock, S., and Windle, H. (eds.). Remembering Henry. London, British Medical Association, 1977, p. 48.
18. Critchley, M. The Ventricle of Memory. New York, Raven Press, 1990.
19. Sherrington, C.S. *The Integrative Action of the Nervous System*. revised edition and final bibliography. New Haven, Yale University Press, 1947.
20. Denny-Brown, D. *Selected Writings of Sir Charles Sherrington*. London, Oxford University Press, 1939.
21. Denny-Brown, D. *The Basal Ganglia and Their Relation to Disorders of Movement*. Liverpool, Liverpool University Press, 1966.
22. Denny-Brown, D. *The Cerebral Control of Movement*. Liverpool, Liverpool University Press, 1966.
23. Locke, S. (ed). *Modern Neurology Papers in Tribute to Derek Denny-Brown*. Boston, Little Brown, 1969.
24. Wohlfart, K.G. Dystrophia myotonica and myotonia congenita: histopathologic studies with special reference to changes in the muscles. *J. Neuropathol.* Exp. Neurol., 2:109-124, 1951.
25. Wohlfart, K.G. Collateral regeneration from residual motor nerve fibers in amyotrophic lateral sclerosis. *Neurologie*, 7 1:124-134, 1957.
26. Wohlfart, K.G., Feinstein, B., and Fex, D. The relation of electromyographic to anatomical findings in healthy muscles and neuromuscular diseases. *Arch. Psychiatry Berl.*, 191:478-482, 1954.

CHAPTER

17

Statesmen of Neuroscience

Another theme, not addressed in the previous sections, concerns the contributions of a small but distinguished group whose impact on the teaching, training, and research potential of neurology was great. Working in either academic or other institutional settings, they significantly influenced the advances that have been made in neurology and aided its establishment as an independent discipline. Several leaders previously considered, such as Penfield and Percival Bailey, might well have qualified as statesmen of neuroscience, but because of their outstanding accomplishments in the categories already considered, they have not been included here.

Inasmuch as the leadership influence of this select group depended on their insight with respect to the importance of research in advancing our knowledge of the nervous system and in postgraduate training of neurologists to deal better with its disorders, a review of a few of the outstanding members of this group deserves consideration.

HERBERT McLEAN EVANS (1882-1971)

In some respects, Dr. Evans is the most controversial individual that I have included in these essays. His great accomplishments, however, cannot be denied. As the instigator and director of the first large-scale research institute in the United States that contributed to the flowering of neurology, he merits inclusion in this special category.

Dr. Evans was one of the first biomedical scientists to establish comprehensive research projects involving large numbers of workers, necessary to obtain the interdisciplinary collaboration of several specialties. This involved biochemists to extract and purify the various hormones and vitamins and to test their physico-chemical properties and experimental biologists to test the effects of the purified extracts in animal experiments and to determine their physiological effects. In addition, pathological control studies were necessary, and finally, in some instances, their application to human disorders followed. All this involved a large setup and considerable administrative detail. Earlier, American scientists had worked either alone or in small groups in a particular field. Evans did not invent "big science," but he was among the first to develop it in America. For some 25 years, his Institute of Experimental Biology was the largest and best organized endocrinological laboratory in the United States. Evans received many honors but fewer than might have been expected, considering his major contributions. As in the case of Walter Cannon (as discussed in Chapter 5), but for entirely different reasons, Nobel prizes have been awarded for lesser achievements than were made by these two.*

Born in Modesto, California, Dr. Evans graduated from the University of California, Berkeley, in 1904 and from Johns Hopkins School of Medicine in 1908 (1). His early studies on the development of the vascular system from capillaries were published in 1909. He continued on at Hopkins until 1915 and advanced to the level of associate professor of anatomy. For a number of years, he also was a research associate at the Carnegie Institute in Washington, D.C.

The main accomplishments of Evans may be listed as follows:

1. As a student, Evans studied the blood supply of the parathyroid glands and, with Halsted, emphasized how these glands, vital to the metabolism of calcium and phosphorus, could be preserved in operations on the neighboring thyroid (2).
2. He developed Evans blue, widely used for estimating blood volume. This was later used by T. Broman and others for studies on the blood-brain barrier. Evans used other analine dyes in his studies of the vascular system, and he has been credited for the first systematic investigation of this system (3).
3. His studies on the estrous cycle of the rat and the role of the pituitary gonadotropins in reproduction were basic and have stood the test of time (4). These were done in a long series of studies with J. A. Long and were summarized in a monograph published by the University of California, Berkeley, in 1922.
4. With collaborators, including Miriam Simpson and Choh Hao Li, he discovered and purified growth hormone, another basic contribution, which only recently is attaining its full clinical significance (5) (as discussed under Li in Chapter 10).
5. With G. O. Burr, he discovered vitamin E and described its initial characteristics (6). Although an earlier study by Evans and K. S. Bishop had recognized a dietary factor that was essential for reproduction, the credit for the discovery of vitamin E is attributed to Evans and Burr. G. A. Emerson and Evans later obtained a purified extract from wheat germ oil, which was recognized as alpha tocopherol (7).
6. His elucidation on the number of human chromosomes aided early genetic studies.

---

* Chauncey Leake, a former UCSF Professor of Pharmacology and past president of the American Association for the Advancement of Science, strongly felt that Evans should have been awarded the Nobel prize and following Evans' death wrote , "The recent death of fourfold Nobel-latent Herbert M. Evans." (1)

7. With many collaborators, he initiated studies to identify the various hormones of the anterior pituitary body. These studies were summarized in his Harvey Society lectures in 1924. My use of their thyrotropic and other extracts used as controls are mentioned in Chapter 2. By the time of his retirement, all had been identified and purified and their properties studied.

8. Early studies were made on adrenocorticotropin with Choh Hao Li and M. Simpson (8). Similar investigations were being made in a number of laboratories more or less simultaneously. Later, Li showed that the responsible steroid was due to a polypeptide, and the amino acid sequence was determined (also see studies on endorphins under Li in Chapter 6).

It so happened, as the result of several circumstances, that I came to know this unusual person in ways that were different from those of his colleagues and students in Berkeley. Friends have suggested that my judgment of Dr. Evans may have been biased by the fact that my original introduction to him came by way of Dr. Naffziger, an influential person in the medical school and community, whom Evans respected. There also was the point that, later on, my wife and Evans discovered that they were second cousins. However, I am sure there was much more to it than these aspects. More pertinent were the background factors of two of my research projects. The first concerned my use of the pituitary extracts of Dr. Evans' group in a study to determine the cause of malignant exophthalmos. Dr. Naffziger had developed an operation for the relief of this condition and, in order to determine its cause, had obtained the promise of extracts from Dr. Evans for experimental use. Using small animals (guinea pigs), because of the expense and difficulty of obtaining the extracts, I developed a camera lucida technique for measuring eye protrusion levels and proceeded to undertake the long-term treatments that were necessary. Control studies were made, using different pituitary extracts. It was the thyrotropic hormone that produced exophthalmos, and the malignant form appeared in the myxedematous period following prolonged hyperthyroidism (9). It was this study that won the confidence of Dr. Naffziger in my ability and led to my being put on the staff as an instructor in the middle of the Great Depression. Evans, too, was pleased with the result.

It was a second study, however, that won the respect and greater approbation of Dr. Evans. This involved my use of the supravital dyes, brilliant vital red and trypan red, to modify the permeability of the blood-brain barrier in an explanation of the protective effect that brilliant vital red had in the experimental epilepsy studies of my former professor, Stanley Cobb of Harvard (10). Needless to say, both Cobb and Evans were delighted with my results, following which I became more fully acquainted with these outstanding men. It was on subsequent visits to Evans's home that the relationship between Dr. Evans and my wife was discovered. However, a second cousin relationship did not greatly impress either Herbert or Ellinor.

This contact did have one other beneficial effect. I discovered that Dr. Evans was a bibliophile and had a wonderful collection of Western Americana. This included an early report of the Lewis and Clark expedition from the Midwest to the Pacific

Ocean and their return in 1804 to 1806. I was interested in this because they described a thriving Indian village on an island in the Columbia River, which is now known as Miller Island, but which has had no inhabitants in more recent history. Funds had been given to the Anthropological Department of the University of California, Berkeley (UCB), to find this old village and study its artifacts. It so happened that a former roommate at Cornell University, Julian Steward, who was doing postgraduate work in anthropology at UCB at that point, was put in charge of the project. He asked me to join him as an assistant in the summer of 1926, just before I started at the Harvard Medical School.

The study had been successful. We found the village, and many artifacts of this study are now in the anthropological collection at UCB. I had always wanted to check the report of Lewis and Clark on this and to study the Indian background more carefully but had never had the time to do so. Thus, the unexpected discovery of the Lewis and Clark report in Dr. Evans's library was a most pleasant surprise.

All this was equally intriguing to Dr. Evans. It turned out that he had been on a somewhat similar expedition in his student days at UCB—a paleontological trip to Idaho, which resulted in his first publication and added to the collection of the Department of Geology (11). These old recollections aroused a responsive chord in him, perhaps overtones to a more harmonious youth. In any case, it was through these connections that I came to know him more fully. Once his protective front was pierced, he was a delightful person, whom both Ellinor and I grew to like and highly respect.

In addition to the great impact that Evans had on American research, as well as through his neuroendocrine, nutritional, and other contributions, he also was innovative in other respects. His instigation of research projects for 1st-year medical students had a stimulating effect, which has been continued ever since and specifically emphasized by my associate Dr. Bill Garoutte in neuroanatomy. Evans also started the History of Science Club at UCB, a society that later was named in his honor and that has continued. Dr. Evans's dedication to teaching was demonstrated in his faithful organization of postgraduate seminars three times per week. These seminars, which involved his commuting from Berkeley to San Francisco, were conducted for years, and I was happy to participate in them.

The controversial aspects of Evans have mainly centered on his entrepreneurial style and his "ruthless competitiveness" and failure to designate research credit properly in some instances. There is no denying his entrepreneurial style, as judged by those in the early decades of the present century. Having lived through both periods and known Evans for 33 years, it is my belief that his conduct as the first "tycoon of science" would now be considered well within the limits of normal activity for directors of large institutions. However, the competition now has added side effects, which Evans would never have tolerated. In a sense, he was ahead of his time and he jarred on the nerves of some of the scientists of the older generation.

It is true that the pace of science considerably accelerated with the large coordinated approach of Evans's institute, but in retrospect, this charge also can be seen to be the result of the transitional period in which he worked. No charge of ruthless competitiveness has stood up, and the Rockefeller Foundation continued to support his institution loyally for years. Instead, his comprehensive approach greatly added to the depth and productive yield of biomedical research.

Charges of failing to give proper research credit are common in large coordinated projects in which many research workers are engaged. Someone has to make decisions. In short, the charges against Dr. Evans have not stood up, and this has been corroborated in a careful report of one of Evans's associates, Dr. Leslie Bennett (11). The account of E. C. Amorosa and G. W. Corner in Evans's biographical memorial of the Royal Society also deals with this problem and should be consulted by those interested (12).

At least one other factor was involved in Dr. Evans's predicament. He was a highly cultured person, and his encyclopedic knowledge at times was daunting. This highly intellectual stance, combined with his great polish and impeccable politeness, was commonly interpreted as a "false front" by many of his more unsophisticated Western contacts.* False charges gained credence in this dubious atmosphere.

Although Dr. Evans was always a challenge, in my many dealings with him over many years, I never thought that he was untrustworthy or deceitful. On the contrary, he was always forthright, supportive, and most generous. This opinion fits in with the known reactions of his staff and collaborators, many of whom worked with him for years.

Evans was a transitional figure who was a leader in comprehensive large-scale neurobiological research. He was ahead of his time in one sense and was criticized by some competitors of an earlier and more simple era and, also to some extent, for his "high falutin" manners. In retrospect, however, one can only agree with the detailed and fair analysis provided by his Royal Society biographers, Amorosa and Corner (12). Chauncey Leake was correct; Evans's contributions were outstanding.

DETLOV WULF BRONK (1897-1975)

Bronk played a leading policy-making role in both private and governmental institutions involved in the medical sciences. This came at a crucial time, when the stage was set for the scientific advances in the biomedical sciences but still needed the strong germinating support of government and foundation agencies, as well as the policy-making decisions to achieve this safely.

There are occasional individuals, who by dint of their intellect and clarity of thought and expression, dominate any group with which they become associated. I have always thought of Paul Bucy and Bronk as good examples of this. Both were men of short stature, commanding miens, and deep sonorous voices who spoke with eloquence and great conviction. One of the old definitions of oratory was that it is the ability to make deep sounds from the chest sound like inspired messages from heaven. Williams Jennings Bryan, in the early part of the century, was the first in this category that I heard. Bronk, I believe, would be a close second. He may have inherited this from his father, who was a Baptist minister, or again from his Pilgrim

---

*As one nonmedical acquaintance put it, after meeting Evans, "His high falutin' ways are greater than real."

ancestor, William Brewster, of Mayflower fame and Governor of New Plymouth, of whom he was proud. In any case, I well recall that I always dreaded following him on scientific programs. His was a hard act to follow.

On one occasion, while working in the Johnson Foundation of Medical Physics at the University of Pennsylvania in late 1939, I recall that Bronk was scheduled to give a talk at some scientific meeting in New Orleans. For some reason, he and his co-author, Martin Larrabee, had not completed the necessary studies for their article. Nevertheless, Bronk took off ahead because of some other appointment, leaving poor Larrabee working day and night to complete the research. Much to the amazement of everyone in the laboratory, this continued until the very morning of the presentation. With minutes to spare before the scheduled presentation, Larrabee telegraphed the final results. I asked Larrabee if he thought Bronk could assemble the data into a final presentation so quickly. Thoroughly exhausted, Larrabee managed a smile and replied, "You don't know Det; of course he can." I later heard that he had given a masterful and smooth presentation. Of course, he knew his subject, the background, and methods used in the study. He probably even knew the approximate answers and only had to plug in the specific data. Nevertheless, it seemed like a most extraordinary performance to my young mind.

Following Swarthmore College, Bronk obtained M.S. and Ph.D. degrees in physics and physiology at the University of Michigan. From 1928 to 1929, he was a National Research Council Fellow and studied with Adrian at Cambridge, England, and with A. V. Hill in London. In 1930, he was offered the post as director of the Johnson Foundation for Medical Physics at the University of Pennsylvania. He also was the Director of the Institute of Neurology and professor of Biophysics. As Adrian has written, it was here that Bronk "gained his spurs as a scientist." It was during this period, when I worked in the Johnson Foundation, that I came to knew him. The Johnson Foundation had been established shortly before the Institute of Experimental Biology of Herbert Evans, but the two laboratories were entirely different. Bronk's laboratory was a neurophysiological setup, and he operated it in a benign fashion, which encouraged cooperative projects, but primarily involved independent research. When I was there, in late 1939, some 30 M.D.s and Ph.D.s were working in the laboratory, including such later distinguished scientists as H. K. Hartline, M. G. Larrabee, R. F. Pitts, J. C. Lilly, F. Brink, and Carl Pfaffmann. It was with the last named that I did my study on pressure stimulation of peripheral nerves (as discussed in Chapter 3). An electronic laboratory in the foundation maintained the cathode ray oscilloscopes and amplifiers. Bronk's setup was the neurophysiological paradise of which I had dreamed in connection with my plan to study vagus and other nerve fiber conduction in the disorders of organ and other body structures (as discussed in Chapter 5). Unfortunately, my time was limited on a sabbatical leave from the University of California, San Francisco (UCSF). This was shortly before World War II, when Bronk broke the "sound barrier" in his aviation studies and went "jetting" off into the peak of his extraordinary career. From 1940 to 1942, he was a professor of physiology at Cornell Medical College in New York City. During World War II, he served in various advisory capacities in federal offices, which included scientific advisor to the President. He was chairman of the National Research Council (1946 to 1950) and president of Johns Hopkins University (1949 to 1953). From 1950 to 1962, he was president of the National Academy of Science. In addition to several other positions, he reorganized the Rockefeller Institution for Medical Research into Rockefeller University, a graduate school of medicine and research, of which he was president from 1953 to 1958.

Aside from his many publications as an administrator and "statesman of science," there were some 54 scientific publications in Bronk's bibliography. One of his main concerns was the autonomic nervous system. His initial five studies, mainly on respiration, were with Gassell (13). His collaboration with Martin Larrabee started in 1936, and over the next 12 years, they produced 13 articles, one of the most important being on the synaptic excitation of sympathetic ganglia (14). Other important articles were published with Pitts and Brink (15,16). At an earlier period, he published four neurophysiological articles with E. D. Adrian (17). One of his innovations was the shielded electrode, which permitted nerve recording without room shielding.* During World War II, in his capacity as advisor to the Air Force, Bronk also produced several publications (18).

In his research, Bronk is usually credited with establishing the science of biophysics (19). He was an early molecular biologist, and as indicated in the sample references cited, he studied nerve cell structure and the changes in cells that occurred with nerve stimulation and nerve activity (20). He measured the oxygen concentration of nerves and investigated their chemical excitation (21).

As would be expected, Bronk received many honors and awards and fulfilled a number of prestigious lectureships. The National Medal of Science and the Presidential Medal of Freedom were awarded to him for his development of science as a major concern of the government. In 1963, a mountain in Antarctica was named in his honor. His creative genius was reflected in the new buildings and establishments that housed his expansions wherever he went—Philadelphia, Baltimore, New York, and Washington, D.C. He was particularly proud of the new Rockefeller University, New York, and the National Academy of Science in Washington.

During and after World War II, Bronk was the guiding light of science in its contacts with government and obtaining financial support (22). He became recognized as an outstanding university administrator and eventually was referred to as the "Statesman of Science." I have listed only the main features of his career. Needless to say, he was the recipient of endless honors and awards. He received at least 55 honorary degrees and was elected to the Royal Society in 1948. Lord Adrian, who wrote his memoirs for the Royal Society, summarized Bronk's career as follows, "In fact for the eighteen years, from 1950, when he became President of the National Academy of Science, until 1968, when he retired from his official position at the Rockefeller University, Detlev Bronk played a leading role in the organiza-

---

* In my special project (see under Erlenger, Chapter 5), I had developed a shielded needle for nerve recording, but never reported it.

tion of scientific research in the United States. By his work as Chairman of the National Research Council and of the National Science Board from 1956-1964, he had become the accepted leader in the campaign for expanding the influence of scientists in the federal policy of the government"(23).

LORD RUSSELL BRAIN (1895-1966)

One of the great neurologists of the past generation was Lord Russell Brain, the unquestioned leader of British neurology during the middle decades of the 20th century. He was not the superb neurologist that Sir Charles Symonds was, nor was he the inimitable teacher that his British colleagues Macdonald Critchley or Henry Miller were. He was not an experimental neurologist who broadened the field of neurology, as in the case of Evans, Bronk, Wilder Penfield, Percival Bailey, or many others included in these essays. He also lacked the kindly touch that marked the doctor–patient relationship of Swithin Meadows, Dalsgaard-Nielsen, and others, which in America we call the art of medicine.

Brain's leadership, like that of Bronk and the other distinguished men of this authoritative group, was one of sheer intellectual power, encyclopedic knowledge, and ability in medical organizational work, which went well beyond his field of neurology. He invariably ended up the head of all commissions or groups in which he took an interest and in whose affairs he participated. He was president of the Royal College of Physicians from 1950 to 1957. He was president of the Association of Physicians, the Association of British Neurologists, the Standing Committee on Drug Addiction, the Family Planning Association, and many other governmental commissions. As a member of the House of Lords, he had great influence in high places and used this to excellent advantage in many sociomedical causes, such as improving the facilities for care and treatment of epileptic patients.

He was an imposing man, courteous, impeccable, and never ruffled. I never knew him well because his diffidence made him hard to know. However, I have gained some insight through my friend, Dr. Ronald Henson, who was his close associate and successor at the London Hospital. According to Henson, behind this imposing facade and his "famous" and "formidable" silences was an amiable man with a broad range of interests and hobbies. I knew of his bird-watching interest, inasmuch as his terms for coming as a visiting professor to UCSF involved time for birding. Except for our wonderful birds that were new to him, I wondered if we could have attracted him at all! Although my wife was a good amateur ornithologist, I never dreamed of putting him in her charge, or inevitably, as it would be, in the reverse order! I wheedled the aid of one of our prominent ornithological staff at UCB. Whether this turned the trick or not, or just his interest in birds did it, I do not know, but on our expeditions, he seemed to be a different person, who more closely fit the description of Dr. Henson. He kept a life list and between the land birds and, later, the sea birds at Point Reyes, he added 80 new birds to his list while he was with us.

The background of this inscrutable man was that he was the son of a Reading solicitor, who read history at New College, Oxford. In World War I, he served with the

Friends Ambulance Unit, and following the war, he entered Oxford to study medicine. He won prizes in physiology and, later, the Price Entrance Scholarship to the London Hospital Medical College. Following various junior appointments at the London Hospital and Maida Vale Hospital for Nervous Diseases, he was elevated to the staff of Maida Vale in 1925. In 1927, he was elected to the staff of the London Hospital, where he worked with Hugh Cairns, George Riddoch, Dorothy Russell, and others.

Brain was a steady worker from 1926 to 1927 on. His popular book with E. B. Straus, *Recent Advances in Neurology*, was first published in 1929 and went through six editions, as well as Italian and Spanish translations (24). Perhaps the best known text of neurology for years was his *Diseases of the Nervous System* (25). This was first published in 1933 and, by 1962, had gone through six editions and, again, Italian and Spanish translations.

Of his 141 medical publications, those on epilepsy, cervical spondylosis, exophthalmos, various aspects of aphasia, and the mind-brain theme were the most common, each subject being dealt with 8 to 12 times. Otherwise, he wrote widely in the field of neurology, and his productiveness was maintained at 28 to 29 articles per decade from the 1930s through the 1960s, except for 37 publications in the 1930s. However, in the 1950s, he also published four books.

Brain was a philosopher. In addition to some 11 articles on the mind-brain problem, he wrote several others, such as "The Need for a Philosophy of Medicine"and "Neurology, Past, Present and Future" On top of all this, he was a historical critic and a poet.

According to G. W. Pickering, who wrote Russell Brain's biographical memoirs for the Royal Society, his neurological contributions to clinical neurology can be attributed to his keen "power to observe, his urge to collect, ability to discern logical relationships, and his capacity for scholarship and lucid writing." Beyond this, however, in "his interpersonal contacts were his impressive mien and reserve, his excellence in public speaking, and his ability as an organizational person to accomplish cherished objectives in committees, on commissions and in the House of Lords" (26).

His clinical observations on the carpal tunnel syndromes, exophthalmos, and even the neurological effects of cancer, were not original (27-29). What he and his collaborators added was the collection of cases, clear delineation of all their clinical aspects, and repeated publicity, which eventually assured them broad recognition and confirmation.

Perhaps his greatest accomplishment was in his work with organizations to guide the Royal College of Physicians and other councils and committees to pursue a critically constructive role with respect to the development of Great Britain's National Health Service, instead of blindly opposing it (26). The post-World War II era was a crucial period for medicine in Great Britain when the National Health Service was vehemently opposed by the British Medical Association. However, conditions in Britain had reached intolerable proportions, including the lack of adequate medical care for the poor. Socialistic thinking had gained ascendancy, the Labor Party was in control, and the other two parties were committed to a national health program.

Under these conditions, Brain's policy made sense, and this was slowly recognized by the medical profession. The real question was to keep a medical delivery system that was as efficient as possible for the public and that at the same time properly utilized and rewarded the services of the medical profession, both the specialist consultants and the general practitioners. As usual with the social and economic problems of Great Britain, its health system has muddled through since 1948 and still is slowly adjusting. People like Sir Francis Walshe refused to join the system and were sharply critical of it (as discussed in Chapter 18).

As with the other members of this distinguished group, Brain received many honors, lectureships, and degrees. The honor that Brain probably prized the most was his election to the presidency of the British Association for the Advancement of Science (1963 to 1964). This honor was last conferred on a British physician or surgeon, Lord Lister, around the turn of the century. Brain was knighted in 1952, made a Baronet in 1954, and a Baron in 1962.

ABRAHAM BERT BAKER (1909-1988)

Baker was born in Minneapolis and spent his entire career there. He was an intense and dynamic person, whose keen vision and tenacity added much to the flowering of neurology. He obtained his undergraduate education at the University of Minnesota and, by the age of 23, had received four degrees. On completion of his training in neuropsychiatry, he acquired a fifth degree, a Ph.D. in neuropathology.

By 1946, he was made head of a new and independent department of neurology at the University of Minnesota and, in the next 31 years, built this into one of the leading departments of the country. His teaching was said to be of a "dogmatic," forceful style, but it was carefully prepared and highly successful. I can well believe this on the basis of one of my encounters with him. He had invited me as a visiting professor in 1951 to present some cerebrovascular material in a postgraduate course. My main recollection of this concerned the "ice-age" conditions of Minnesota in January. My California clothing was entirely inadequate, and I almost froze in one sortie from the postgraduate center. Another distinct recollection was Baker's being upset when I countermanded one of his teachings. This was not done intentionally, nor directly, of course, but was contrived by one of his own residents. The resident thought that Baker was wrong in not permitting arteriograms on patients with mild hypertension. At the end of one of my sessions, the resident asked if I considered mild hypertension on patients otherwise in good condition to be a contraindication for arteriography. I emphasized that it depended on the patient's condition and the urgency for obtaining arteriographic studies in the particular case, but that mild hypertension in many patients would not be considered a contraindication. The resident joyfully informed Baker of my "heretical" stance. Much to my astonishment, Baker accosted me on this point, and I believe it took him another 2 or 3 years to alter his position. Baker's "dogmatism," however, was not of a venomous type. It was on this trip that he asked me to sign the Founding Charter of the American Academy of Neurology and also requested that I write a chapter for his proposed text of neurology (30).

Baker's principal studies were on the neuropathology of patients with bulbar polio and cerebrovascular atherosclerosis (31,32). Baker's great contribution to neurology was lobbying the politicians in Washington, D.C., to establish training and research grants in neurology. When this was extended to other fields and supported by the medical profession and universities, the National Institutes of Health (NIH) was finally established. The National Institute of Neurological Diseases and Blindness (NIND&B) was the neurological portion of this, and again, Baker fought to have the NIND&B properly represented and budgeted. An important preliminary aspect of this involved the neurological training program of the Veterans Administration. Pearce Bailey was the chief neurologist in the Veterans Administration, and he was able to demonstrate the need for neurological training more broadly, taking advantage of the generous funding of this administration in the immediate post-World War II period.

Between the training grants, the research funds, the development of many new departments of neurology, and the expansion of the preexisting departments, the development of neurology was tremendously expanded (as discussed in Chapter 1). This came at a propitious time, inasmuch as the scientific basis of neurology was well established by the late 1940s. This constituted the background on which the organically minded members of the old neuropsychiatry were able to capitalize. Although involving many facets, there is no question but that Baker played an important role in this—and so, he repeatedly proclaimed. On one occasion, Houston Merritt downplayed Baker's part in the NIH development to me. However, having served on five committees of the NIH, starting before the NIND&B was established, I saw enough to make me believe Baker's role was significant. Much of his work was lobbying on the side with Congressmen, of which Merritt may not have been aware or discredited the effect. Certainly, Baker had the vision, and it was my impression that his forceful persistence made him a powerful catalyst in the development of the NIND&B. Furthermore, it was a role that few of us in neurology had the taste, gumption, and time to play. Baker was a unique individual, and one had to know him and to see him in action to understand the impact he had. His aggressive approach to attain an expanded neurology and to gain governmental support has been emulated by the American Academy of Neurology, and I believe this still carries on.

RICHARD L. MASLAND (1910-   )

A very different type of career from Baker's is exemplified by that of Dr. Masland. His quiet efficiency and persistent emphasis on achieving desired, long-range goals won out in a hectic political and bureaucratic milieu, which quickly made mincemeat of bombastic advocates displaying prejudiced or self-serving schemes. It was this stance that Merritt feared in Baker, but in the political arena in which Baker operated, I believe he managed to escape it. In the case of Masland, for 10 years, he worked in an environment of shifting pressures—neuromedical, neuroscientific, political, administrative, and bureaucratic, which required the ultimate degree of patience and diplomacy, as well as knowledge and ability. In this environment, the brilliance of a Bronk or Brain might well have won a few or many "battles" and yet, in the long run, have lost the "war." No one person could manage the complex situation single-handedly, but he who could win and maintain strong allies in Congress and in the other factions that were involved in the program of the NIH and his own NIND&B was the one who finally prevailed. Because Dr. Masland possessed the unique qualities necessary for this complex type of operation and because the program was so vital to the flowering period of neurology, he well deserves a place in this category of leaders.

Masland was a product of Haverford College (1931) and the University of Pennsylvania School of Medicine (1935). Postgraduate training in neurology and psychiatry followed, and he was certified in both subjects by the American Board of Neurology and Psychiatry. From 1939 to 1946, he advanced from assistant neurologist to associate in neurology at the University of Pennsylvania. During World War II, Masland made five reports on altitude chamber flights and the neurological sequelae of decompression anoxia. These studies were done on various projects in the School of Aviation Medicine (33). In the next 10 years, he advanced from assistant professor to the full professorship of neurology in the Bowman-Gray School of Medicine, Wake Forest College, at Winston-Salem, North Carolina.

From 1955 to 1957, he took a leave of absence from Bowman-Gray to conduct a survey on research related to mental retardation for the National Association for Retarded Children. The results were summarized in a book entitled *Mental Subnormality: Biological, Psychological, and Cultural Factors* (34). This same movement led to a vast collaborative project in the NIND&B, entitled "Collaborative Project for the Study of Cerebral Palsy and Related Disabilities." Pearce Bailey, the first director of the NIND&B, had done some initial programming of this project with the assistance of Henry Imus, but Masland was brought in to develop the study design with the help of Jacob Yerushalmy, an epidemiologist who previously had experience with clinical investigations, The project involved 13 institutions and studies on over 40,000 subjects. Dr. Masland's role in this, in addition to planning the program, involved endless time and effort defending the program against critics. To handle this great and prolonged effort, which extended beyond his leave of absence from Bowman-Gray, Masland was made assistant director of the NIND&B under Bailey. In 1959, when Bailey retired as chair and director, Masland was made director of the NIND&B and ran it for the next 9 years.

Masland has always given great credit to Pearce Bailey for his earlier efforts of developing training centers in neurology in the Veterans Administration and for his initial work in the NIH. The research training programs were started under Bailey and aided by a committee of the American Neurological Association and the efforts of Mary Lasker. Neurology study sections were developed separately from the initial mental health study section. I was well aware of this change inasmuch as I served on the study sections both before and after this administrative reorganization. The actual work of selecting and promoting the neurological study sections was done by Gordon Seger.

The principal achievements of Dr. Masland's directorship of the NIND&B can be summarized as follows:

1. Many new training centers were established in the 1950s and 1960s, which involved a tremendous increase in the NIH budgets. This was the peak period for both the neurological research grants and training programs (35).

2. Because of Masland's interest in and acquaintance with the main pediatric neurology centers of the country, training centers in pediatric neurology were established, a move that definitely put this neglected field on the map. There had been great resistance to this as mentioned in the section on pediatric neurology (as discussed in Chapter 9). This move, finally recognized by the American Boards, gave a great impetus to this important field.

3. Improvements in the quality of drug evaluation were affected, especially with respect to the design of projects involving drug trials. Another problem concerned the pharmaceutical companies' neglect of the so-called orphan drugs, which affected several important areas of neurological therapy. The problem involved ways and means whereby this difficulty might be corrected. As chair of one of the committees that made recommendations on this, I was aware of Masland's continuing support, which eventually helped with this problem.

4. Because of the importance of epilepsy and the great advances that were made in this field, an epilepsy branch of the NIND&B was established. Drs. William Caveness and Kiffin Penry were appointed to head this branch, and they effectively handled its program.

5. The program on kuru was established. This had been initiated by Dr. Joseph Smadel, but he had been strongly criticized by those who opposed Gajdusek's brain culture approach. This included the Fish and Wildlife Service and some groups in Australia. Masland protected Gajdusek, and this brilliant project finally led to a Nobel prize for Gajdusek (as discussed in Chapter 11).

6. Great efforts were made to improve the quality of both the intramural and extramural research programs. This was brilliantly achieved with the result that the period between 1956 and 1960 were the "golden years" of the NIND&B (35,36).

This sustained period of growth and improvement in quality could not have developed without the strong financial support of Congress, and in this, Masland closely worked with Congressman Fogerty and the NIND&B lobbyist, Luke Quin, to present the needs and opportunities of the institute before Congress. This was especially important inasmuch as the budgets of the institute were initiated in the House of Representatives. Masland served the same role with Lister Hill in the Senate, which body finally passed on the funding bills.

In 1968, Dr. Masland was offered the chairmanship of the Department of Neurology, College of Physicians and Surgeons, Columbia University, as well as the directorship of the neurological service of the Presbyterian Hospital, New York. He served in these capacities until 1974 when he retired because of his age, but he retained the title of the Houston Merritt Professor of Neurology, Emeritus.

From 1976 to 1977, Masland was the executive director of a special commission of the Department of Health Education and Welfare concerning the control of epilepsy and its consequences. Much of the findings of this commission were incorporated into the text on epilepsy that we wrote with Dr. Dixon Woodbury (37).

From 1982 to 1989, Masland served as clinical professor of neurology at the University of Medicine and Dentistry of New Jersey, Rutgers Medical School. In 1988, he was elected president of the World Federation of Neurology and served an international role in neurology for the next eight years.

His bibliography contains 80 publications. These include 3 books, 25 chapters of books, and over 50 articles. Twenty-nine of his scientific publications were on epilepsy, and 20 dealt with disorders of language, reading problems, and dyslexia. Twenty-two were related to pediatric neurology.

The honors that came his way are too numerous to list. Eight awards were related to the problems of childhood and 5 to epilepsy, in addition to 13 other awards. The most notable were an honorary degree from Haverford College, the William Lennox award (American Epilepsy Society), and the Samuel T. Orton Award (dyslexia).

In spite of his great attainments, Masland has remained his quiet and unpretentious self. In particular, he could well qualify as an outstanding example of the art of medicine in neurology. Because of my long friendship with him, extending back to 1939, when he was an assistant neurologist in the University of Pennsylvania School of Medicine, innumerable anecdotes come to mind, but I will limit my comments to one.

Directly after Masland was inducted as President of the World Federation of Neurology in Kyoto, Japan, in 1981, he and Mrs. Masland (Molly) joined our group in an exchange program and neurological study tour of China. I had organized this trip over the previous year, and it involved meeting the top medical officials of China, as well as China's leading neurologists and neuroscientists. This gave Masland, as the new President of the World Federation of Neurology, a chance to work diplomatically on their top people to induce China to become a member of the World Federation of Neurology. This he adroitly did, but to no avail. Communist China was dominated by overriding political considerations. They had sent a delegation to the World Federation meetings in Japan, but it had been called back when they discovered that a delegation from Taiwan was attending. This event, of course, had nothing to do with our neurological study tour, but it did thwart Masland's diplomatic efforts.

In addition to his diplomatic efforts, Masland was kept very busy with our heavy tour schedule. He had agreed to give one of the talks in our exchange program and also prepared some of the reports of our tour study. His main report was on the talk of Professor Huang Chia-Ssu, President of the Chinese Academy of Medical Science, which involved a thorough analysis of China's two systems of medical education and medical practice.

From these exalted heights, the Maslands plummeted to a low and ignominious level as we departed from Guangzhau to Hong Kong. It was a train trip, for which the visitor forms for departure from China were required. The Maslands had packed these important documents, and the baggage had been checked through! We almost lost them at this point, but at the last moment "the officials were persuaded to recognize the dilemma and allowed them on the train" (J. Kofman, excerpt from the Neurological Study Tour of the People's Republic of China).

Masland could hardly be expected to oversee such mundane details while operating at lofty levels. I had him writing a report on the Chinese Academy of Medical Science at this point, as I recall. His report, along with others, went into the final summary account of the *Neurological Study Tour of the People's Republic of China*. He was a thoughtful man of great composure, but the shock of this incident briefly had an effect that I had never seen in him before. The possibility of their being detained in communist China was too much! Perhaps, Masland envisioned headlines, such as "President of World Federation of Neurology Detained by Communist China." In any case, I suspect that this episode was more traumatic than his earlier bouts with the politicians and bureaucracy of Washington.

SUMMARY

It will be apparent that the men that I have included under the designation "Statesmen of Neurology" were a widely varied group. Aside from their being men of great vision and abilities, they do not neatly fit into characterizations as suggested in some previous chapters. Their times and opportunities were important factors, and yet perhaps, their most important aspect concerned their qualities of leadership. They had the ability to grasp the opportunities of their times and to mold events along constructive lines. This was personified most strongly in Bronk and Brain. Evans's comprehensive approach to biomedical science and his remarkable accomplishments place him high in this group. The widely different approaches of Baker and Masland illustrate in still other ways how success could be achieved. The aggressiveness of Baker was resented by many, and yet his vision, drive, and tenacity were sufficient to mold significantly the events of his time. Masland accomplished the same thing from the inside through quiet diplomacy in establishing goals and winning the cooperation of key people in Congress, who determined policy and support.

REFERENCES

1. Leake, C.D. Herbert M. Evans. *Science*, 172:1084-1085, 1971.
2. Halsted, W.S., and Evans, H.M. The parathyroid glandules. Their blood supply and their preservation in operation upon he thyroid gland. *Ann. Surg.*, 46:489-506, 1907.
3. Dawson, A.B., Evans, H.M., and Whipple, G.H. Blood volume studies: III. Behavior of large series of dyes introduced into the circulating blood. *Am. J. Physiol.*, 51:232-256, 1920.
4. Evans, H.M. The oestrous cycle in the rat. *Anat. Rec.*, 18:241-245, 1920.
5. Li, C.H., Simpson, M.E., and Evans, H.M. Isolation and properties of the anterior hypophysis growth hormone. J. Biol. *Chem.*, 159:353-366, 1945.
6. Evans, H.M., and Burr, G.O. The anti-sterility vitamin fat soluble E. *Proc. Natl. Acad. Sci.* U.S.A., 11:334-341, 1925.

7. Emerson, G.A., and Evans, H.M. The effect of vitamin E deficiency upon growth. *J. Nutr.*, 14:169-178, 1937.
8. Li, C.H., Simpson, M.E., and Evans, H.M. Isolation of adrenocorticotropic hormone from sheep pituitaries. *Science*, 96:450, 1942.
9. Aird, R.B. Experimental exophthalmos and associated myopathy induced by thyrotropic extract. *Arch. Ophthalmol.*, 24:1167-1174, 1940.
10. Aird, R.B. Mode of action of brilliant vital red in epilepsy. *Arch. Neurol. Psychiatry*, 42:700-723, 1939.
11. Bennett, L.L. Herbert McLean Evans. *Bull. Alumni Assoc.* School of Med. U.C.S.F., 27:3(special issue),1-17, 1983.
12. Amorosa, E.C., and Corner, G.W. *Herbert McLean Evans.* vol. 18. In: Biographical Memoirs of Fellows of Royal Society. London, Royal Society, 1976, pp.83-186.
13. Bronk, D.W., and Gassell, R. The regulation of respiration: X. Effects of carbon dioxide, sodium bicarbonate and sodium carbonate on the carotid and femoral flow of blood. *Am. J. Physiol.*, 82:170-180, 1927.
14. Larrabee, M.G., and Bronk, D.W. Prolonged facilitation of synaptic excitation in sympathetic ganglia. *J. Neurophysiol.*, 10:139-154, 1947.
15. Bronk, D.W., Larrabee, M.G., and Brink, F. The effect of chemical agents on the excitability of ganglion cells. *Am. J. Physiol.*, 126:361, 1939.
16. Bronk, D.W., and Pitts, R.F. Excitability cycle of the hypothalamus-sympathetic neuron system. *Am. J. Physiol.*, 135:504-522, 1941-1942.
17. Adrian E.D., and Bronk, D.W. The frequency of discharge in reflex and voluntary contractions. *J.Physiol.*, 67:119-151, 1929.
18. Bronk, D.W. *Human Problems in Military Aviation.* Washington, D.C., Smithsonian Institution, 1946, pp. 401-411.
19. Bronk, D.W. The relation of physics to the biological sciences. *J. Appl. Physics*, 9:139-142, 1938.
20. Bronk, D.W. Cellular organization of nervous function. *Trans. Stud. Coll. Physicians*, 6:102-117, 1938.
21. Bronk, D.W., Davies, P.W., Brink, F., Jr., and Larrabee, M.G. Oxygen supply and oxygen consumption in nervous system. *Trans. Am. Neurol. Assoc.*, 70:141-144, 1944.
22. Bronk, D.W. The genesis of the President's science advisers and the National Science Foundation, science advice in the White House. *Science*, 186:116-121, 1974.
23. Lord Adrian. Detlev Wulf Bronk. vol. 22. In: Biographical Memoirs of the Fellows of the Royal Society. 1976, pp. 1-9.
24. Brain, R., and Strauss, E.B. *Recent Advances in Neurology.* London, J. & A. Churchill, 1933.
25. Brain, R. *Diseases of the Nervous System.* Oxford, Oxford University Press, 1933.
26. Pickering, G.W. *Walter Russll Brain.* vol. 14. In: Biographical Memoirs of the Fellows of the Royal Society. 1968, pp. 61-82.
27. Brain, R., Wright, A.D., and Wilkinson, M. Spontaneous compression of both median nerves in the carpal tunnel. *Lancet* 1:277-282, 1947.
28. Brain, R., and Turnbull, H.M. Exophthalmic ophthalmoplegia. *Q. J. Med.*, 7:293-323, 1938.
29. Brain, R., and Henson, R.A. Neurological syndromes associated with carcinoma. The carcinomatous neuropathies. *Lancet*, 2:971-974, 1958.
30. Baker, A.B. (ed). *Clinical Neurology.* 2nd ed. New York, Harper & Brothers, 1962.
31. Baker, A.B., Matzke, H.A., and Brown, J.R. Poliomyelitis II. Bulbar poliomyelitis: a study of medullary function. *Arch. Neurol. Psychiatry*, 63:257-281, 1950.
32. Baker, A.B. An Outline of Neuropathology. Dubuque, IA, Brown, 1949.
33. Masland, R.L. Injury of the central nervous system resulting from decompression to simulated high altitudes. *Arch. Neurol. Psychiatry,* 59:445-456, 1948.
34. Masland, R.L, Sarason, S.B., and Gladwin, T. Mental Subnormality: *Biological, Psychological, and Cultural Factors.* New York, Basic Books, 1958.
35. Masland, R.L. The impact of the training program of the National Institute of Neurological Diseases and Blindness on the specialty of neurology. *Neurology*, 13:315-320, 1963.
36. Masland, R.L. *National Institute of Neurological Diseases and Blindness: development and growth* (1960-1968). In: Tower, D.B. (ed.). The Nervous System. New York, Raven Press, 1975, pp. xxxii-xivi.
37. Aird, R.B., Masland, R.L., and Woodbury, D.M. *The Epilepsies: A Critical Review.* New York, Raven Press, 1984.

Legendary Neurologists

If one accepts the dictionary definition of legendary as "a romanticized or popular myth of modern times," there would be few legendary figures in science and, more specifically, in neurology (1). Nevertheless, neurology has had its Merrill Moore, the inimitable specialist on limericks at Harvard, its absent-minded Graeme Robertson of Australia (as discussed in Chapter 14), and its James Risien Russell of lightning diagnostic fame, not to mention its Jean Charcot, Weir Mitchell, and Hughlings Jackson of the past. Neurosurgery has had its Geoffrey Jefferson, who had little or no sense of time, and its Temple Fay, who ranged far afield in his enthusiasms—his ideas on the origin of epilepsy and his cryogenic treatment of cancer. Pediatric neurology has had its eccentric Frank Ford (as discussed in Chapter 9), and the list could be extended in several other directions. They were all outstanding men in their respective fields, and yet, they were men who possessed an added luster, which set them apart. The six examples I have selected were not bizarre in any way but were men of unusual talent and sparkle or men who responded heroically to difficult circumstances. My use of the term "legendary," therefore, is based on the simpler definition of a person of very unusual characteristics or one who struggled so successfully against great odds that stories were evoked, which eventually gave the individual legendary status. Neither romantic nor mythical factors need be invoked in this.

Legendary is a category, as in the preceding four chapters, which gives scope to factors beyond the usual clinical or scientific skills and, yet, because of its unique and lustrous aspects, makes a fitting close to this series of essays. I will start off with Bernard Sachs, an extraordinary figure by any method of evaluation.

BERNARD SACHS (1858-1944)

Sachs was one of the best educated American neurologists of his time. After graduation from the medical school of the University of Strasbourg (when the city was part of Germany), he did postgraduate work for 2 years with the most outstanding neurologists of Europe—Jean Charcot, Hughlings Jackson, Theodor H. Meynert, and C. F. O. Westphal. His early recognition of Tay-Sachs disease and his interest in child neurology led to his being made the director of the Child Neurology Research Fund in New York. Although primarily a clinician, he also was active in research and teaching, and he played an influential role in the early 20th century. He was twice elected president of the American Neurological Association (1894 and 1937), was president of the First International Congress of Neurology, Bern, Switzerland, in 1931, and was president of the New York Academy of Medicine in 1933.

The background of Sachs should be mentioned. His parents migrated from Germany in 1847. Three of his brothers became famous—Sam and Harry in banking and Julius in education. The latter had a great influence on Dr. Sachs, which led to his going to Harvard, where he studied under William James and read for him when James's vision was failing. The bankers loyally supported him in obtaining his education and later projects.

Two aspects of Sachs's extraordinary career are not well known. Because it was with these aspects that I had contact, both contributing greatly to his legendary fame, they may be worth recording.

In the period from 1938 through 1940, I was concentrating on the effect of changes in the permeability of the endothelium of the cerebrovascular system (blood–brain barrier) as produced by cerebral pathology (2). This involved observations on alterations of convulsive susceptibility and the electroencephalographic changes associated with such changes. However, it was a very bleak period from the standpoint of research support. This period predated the National Institutes of Health by a dozen years, and the Great Depression had dried up what meager funds were available. It was at this point that I heard that Sachs controlled funds, which he could award for studies he deemed to be of promise. Application involved personal contact, and it was in this way that I came to know him. Three of my projects were completed with the support of the Child Neurology Research Fund that he administered. His mind was still keen and his questions, penetrating. It also became obvious that he highly prized his contacts with younger, research-inclined neurologists.

For several years in the 1930s, Sachs was at the center of the placement activities for refugees from Hitler's Germany, and this was the second aspect with which I had contact. Through his banking brothers and other wealthy connections, he controlled considerable money, which aided the refugees until they could be placed. In the case of the University of California School of Medicine at San Francisco, an opening for a neuropathologist was decided on in 1935. In some mysterious way, Dr. Robert Wartenberg, who was under Sachs's tutelage at that point, was dispatched to San Francisco. This seemed like a major mistake to the involved departments because, as a neurologist, Wartenberg was thrust onto the neuropsychiatric division of the Department of Medicine, while the Department of Pathology still lacked a neuropathologist. The situation deteriorated even further when Wartenberg found the neuropsychiatrists quite inadequate, and he was shortly at swords' points with the chairman of the Department of Medicine and, still later, with the dean of the medical school. Except for the generous and continuing local support of refugee funds, plus the intervention of a number of us, Wartenberg could not have survived for long in this precarious situation. To top it off, Wartenberg undertook detailed criticisms of neurological articles and books on an international scale, and his critiques were published under the guise of raising the standards of neurology. Needless to say, this caused widespread resentment among the recipients of his devastating critical reviews (3).

At a later date, I was able to wean Wartenberg away from this behavior. I realized that he was intensely unhappy and thrashing out at the world for being displaced in midlife for no other reason than that a small portion of his blood was Jewish (an eighth was enough for Hitler). Eventually, as chair of the Department of Neurology, I was able to strike a bargain with him and get him to undertake creative work of his own. With encouragement and support, his last years were very happy ones, and we became close friends. It was in an earlier period, however, while these developments were still in an embryonic stage, that through Wartenberg and his charming wife, Isabella, I learned more about Sachs. My admiration for Sachs blossomed considerably as I came to understand his work more fully among the refugees. Again, it was not Sachs as a neurologist (although this also was legendary), but his broader vision and impact that made him outstanding. Inevitably, as the stories of his activities circulated, his legendary status grew.

GORDON HOLMES (1876-1965)

It is easy to understand the legendary aspect of Mogens Fog, who was the head of the underground resistance movement of Denmark during the German occupation of World War II (see later section), but how can this be explained in the case of such a man as Gordon Holmes? It seems unlikely that it could be based on his tall, commanding presence, his brusqueness, his formidable austerity, his demanding discipline of his clinical clerks, or even his personal modesty and reticence. Possibly, it was a mixture of these characteristics combined with his remarkable bedside teaching ability. Certainly, the latter was legendary. Postgraduate students flocked to his service from all quarters, not deterred by his martinet qualities. Instead, they were attracted by his no-nonsense, high-quality service and, especially, by the lucidity of his clinical teaching.

I had planned to go as a postgraduate student to his service in 1932 or 1933, as explained elsewhere in these essays, but the Great Depression and an offer in the West changed these plans. I still harbored such hopes as late as 1939, the first opportunity I had to leave my new post, but World War II and Holmes's departure unfortunately intervened. Because of this old background, I was overjoyed when I was asked to give one of the articles at the centenary celebration of Holmes's birth in 1976 (4). This was held at the Charing Cross Hospital, London, where he had served for many years. It afforded me the opportunity to learn more about him from his colleagues and students.

Of Irish-English stock, he was born in Castlebellingham on the eastern sea coast of Ireland, some 15 miles south of Northern Ireland. His mother died when he was still very young, but his abilities were recognized by the village schoolmaster. With his aid, Gordon obtained a sound primary and secondary education. At Trinity College, Dublin, he developed an interest in botany and biology as a result of his hikes in the Wicklow Hills just south of Dublin. On various scholarships, he continued at Trinity in medicine and graduated in 1897. Following his service as a resident medical officer in the Richmond Asylum (now St. Brenan's Hospital), he studied briefly in Berlin on prize funds. Two years of postgraduate study in neuroanatomy followed with Carl Weigert and Ludwig Edinger at Frankfurt-am-Main. He then took a house physicianship at the National Hospital, Queen Square, London, in 1902 and qualified for the M.D. degree in 1903. At the National Hospital, he progressed through the stages of resident medical officer, pathologist, director of research, and in 1909, he was made an honorary member of the staff. He qualified for the M.R.C.P. in 1908. His consulting posts were at the Charing Cross Hospital, Seaman's Hospital, and Royal London Ophthalmic Hospital (Moorfields Eye Hospital and, now, the Institute of Ophthalmology).

It should be noted that his service at these institutions was on a voluntary basis, inasmuch as none of the hospitals had stipends for their consulting staffs. He, like the other physicians of his day, had to depend on private practice for a living. Under these circumstances (private practice and three consulting and teaching posts), his opportunity for research was limited. This, of course, explains the primary, clinical nature of Queen Square and its late adoption of laboratory and research facilities (as discussed in Chapter 15). That Holmes and his colleagues managed to do considerable clinical research and publish outstanding articles on the side says a great deal for their superior quality, fortitude, and stamina. During his early period before World War I, Holmes and Henry Head published their classic article, "Sensory Disturbances from Cerebral Lesions," in Brain in 1911 (5). This required much refinement of the sensory examination and marked the introduction of precise methods of mapping skin sensations. It also was the first significant account of thalamic functions and the relation of the thalamus to the cortex.

Holmes volunteered for the Royal Army Medical Corps in World War I but was rejected on the basis of his myopia. His outstanding service in a Red Cross Hospital in France was finally recognized by the medical authorities, and he was commissioned in the medical corps in spite of his myopia. His study of the neurological effects of brain and spinal cord wounds resulted in several reports. His studies on spinal cord injuries were summarized in the Goulstonian lecture in 1915 (6), on vision in the Montgomery lectures in 1919 (7,7a), and on the cerebellum in the Croonian lecture in 1923 (8,8a). In all of these, there was great emphasis on the underlying physiology to explain clinical symptomatology, and it was this background that made him an outstanding neurologist. This, combined with his analytical aptitude, resulted in his superb ability as a teacher.

From 1920 to 1939 (when Holmes' career was again interrupted, this time by World War II), his reputation as a teacher and consultant steadily grew, and by the late 1920s, his international fame was well established. In spite of his age, when World War II began, he served as a consultant to the Emergency Medical Service and, in this, did much to establish an adequate neurological service.

Holmes was elected to the Royal Society in 1933 and was knighted in 1951. He received honorary degrees from four universities in Great Britain and Ireland, was an honorary member of many foreign neurological societies, was an honorary fellow of the Royal Society of Medicine, and was its Gold Medalist. He was selected for the most prestigious of the medical lectures of Great Britain, including the Ferrier Lecture of the Royal Society (1944) and the Hughlings Jackson Lecture of the Royal Society of Medicine (1951).

An important ingredient of the legendary aspect of Holmes derived from the hardiness and toughness of fiber that he developed as a result of his early privations and his continued struggles throughout his career. Great achievement in the face of a heavy schedule of teaching and service without remuneration, and above and beyond making a living in private practice, constituted a killing agenda that only a dedicated person of unusual ability and stamina could accomplish. The secondary molding of his character against this background undoubtedly explained his expectation of diligence and superior effort from his postgraduate students. He was one of the last of that old, dedicated group, almost all of whom were outstanding men. His long life, however, carried him through the early flowering period of neurology, and in my presentation at his centenary celebration, I referred to his keen observations on electroencephalography and epilepsy (4). Except for his legendary status, he might well have been included in the chapter on teachers (Chapter 15).

FRANCIS MARTIN ROUSE WALSHE (1886-1973)

Another towering figure of neurology in Great Britain was Sir Francis Walshe. Although trained in neurophysiology, as well as in clinical neurology, he was not an outstanding leader in either field. However, as a critic, whose logic was usually impeccable and whose sharp tongue could be devastating, he had no peer and did much to establish British neurology on the high plane it enjoyed throughout the flowering period of neurology.

Of mixed parentage, like Holmes, his father was Irish from County Mayo and his mother was English from Devon. Born and raised in London, his higher education was at University College and University Hospital and Medical School, London. He served as a Resident Medical Officer of the National Hospital, Queen Square, from 1912 until the start of World War I. During the war, he served as a neurologist to the British Army in Egypt and gained considerable experience with polyneuritis and beriberi, which stood him in good stead in his later controversy with Gowland Hopkins. Hopkins held that peripheral neuritis was a vitamin deficiency disorder, while Walshe stressed an added toxic factor.

Walshe was appointed to the consulting staff of the National Hospital in 1921 and also was a member of the medical unit at University College Hospital. When he left the Medical Unit in 1924 to become a consultant to the University College Hospital, he started a private consulting practice and made his living in this fashion until he retired. He had been a sharp critic of the National Health Service, and from its inception in 1948 on, he refused its remuneration. With the aid of Dr. Critchley and a few others, Sir Francis carried on in his consulting work long after retirement because of his age, which had been extended to 70 at the National Hospital.

Walshe won the highest awards and positions in British medicine. He was president of the Association of British Neurologists, president of the Royal Society of Medicine, editor of Brain, and a Fellow of the Royal Society. He was knighted in 1953. Few figures in neurology have had a more striking career.

Walshe was entirely different from his contemporary neurological colleagues, such as Sir Charles Symonds. Fundamentally, he seemed to me to be a philosopher, and this may be the reason that he tolerated me so well. Over a period of years, I accumulated a small library of his reprints and other historical articles that he was kind enough to send me. I always wondered about this because, after all, I was one of those meddling people who did experimental research, which he felt too often missed the mark in human neurology.

Although very good in his demonstrations and lectures while with us as a visiting professor of neurology in 1959, he lacked the diagnostic acumen of Sir Charles Symonds and the showmanship of Critchley and Henry Miller (as discussed in Chapters 2 and 15).

Because of his training in physiology, Walshe was interested in showing that tonic neck reflexes, as experimentally demonstrated by Magnus and De Kleijn in animals, also existed in humans and were exaggerated by the spasticity of hemiplegia and quadriplegia. He also took delight in showing that the Babinski response could be modified by head turning and shifts of posture in the legs and trunk.

His principal role was that of a logician, critic, and philosopher. It was his abilities in these respects, buttressed by his masterful English and adroit witticisms, that raised him to the highest echelons of British neurology and finally made him a legendary figure.

As a critic, he attacked the theory of Henry Head that protopathic-epicritic sensation had developed in two stages, the older being relatively crude in comparison with the younger and more discriminating form. Another controversial issue concerned poliomyelitis during its earlier, devastating epidemic period. In this, he tilted with his esteemed colleague, James Collier of the National Hospital and with Sister Kennedy of Australia. Walshe also had running battles with those who found spirochetes in the cerebrospinal fluid of patients with poliomyelitis, including Purves Stewart of London. With John Fulton, he argued about the precise definition of the prefrontal cortex. Still other debates involved psychogenic headache, the miraculous cures of Lourdes, and so forth. However, it was his bouts with Wartenberg and Penfield that I observed first hand, and these may be worth recording because both illustrated different aspects of Walshe.

The bout with Wartenberg was an emotional tilt over Walshe's textbook, *Diseases of the Nervous System* (9). In spite of the fact that he had chided authors of student textbooks for years, in 1940, he came out with his own. Wartenberg, while a member of our staff, published one of his criticisms of this text, the sixth edition in 1949, as I recall. As mentioned in my comments on Sachs in an earlier section,

Wartenberg did this with the best intent "to raise the standards of neurology." However, his detailed criticisms, which often included punctuation and grammar, were not always well received, and so it was with Walshe, who prided himself on his use of the English language. Criticisms from a German refugee in far away San Francisco may have been too much. Wartenberg was trembling when he brought me Walshe's unprintable letter of protest and could not understand why Walshe had taken his "constructive" criticism so poorly. Having been accosted by many other neurologists, who were upset by "that demon out there," I was not surprised. Wartenberg did not know what to do. I told him to frame the letter and hang it on his office wall if he thought that this would help, but under no circumstances was he to reply to it.

A few years later, when I invited Walshe to come to San Francisco as a visiting professor, I promised him that we would "banish" Wartenberg at the time of his visit. Walshe agreed to come but, unfortunately, was not able to make it. When he finally did come in 1959, Wartenberg was dead. This experience has always made me wonder if Walshe dished it out better than he received it. Both men had assumed the role of critic, but this floundered on an emotional level, when they clashed, rather than on the high intellectual level where they usually operated.

A much greater engagement was Walshe's attack on Penfield's concept of his "centrencephalic system." When Sir Francis came to San Francisco in 1959, he had just completed a critique of this, and we received the full blast of his critical ideas of Penfield's theory of the "highest cerebral center." Two of Penfield's students made feeble attempts to defend him, but they were brushed aside by the forceful rhetoric of Walshe. I discounted much of this, because I had already formed the opinion that, when Walshe got to his feet, he became somewhat hypnotized by his own oratory and valiantly charged ahead with his criticisms, which on occasion could be devastating. Twice, following such outbursts, I recall that he pursued a more moderate tone, and I suspected that he sometimes regretted the ardor of his public statements. There can be no question, however, as to his honesty, the depth of his analytical powers, and the rigor of his logic.

Following this episode, I went out of my way in 1960 to invite Penfield, to be a visiting professor of neurology, which indeed he was. Although I had my own reservations about his centrencephalic system, it seemed important to hear his side of the argument (10). When Penfield came in 1960, he put on a good show, was entirely open about his theoretical postulations, and was quite ready to admit their error when so proved. It is true that several of Penfield's theories have not panned out, but there is no question that these, along with his meticulous neurosurgical observations on humans, have played a major role in stimulating a tremendous amount of good research. Being right in some instances can be less important than stimulating research that demonstrates what is right.

Our group, undoubtedly, saw Walshe well after his prime in 1959, but he still had much spark and put on a good show for us. He later retired to the village of Huntingdonshire, near Cambridge. According to his son, John, of Cambridge, who visited me several years later, Walshe still had considerable "spunk and fire."

As Dr. Critchley has written, "Every neurologist of that era had his own 'Walshisms' to narrate and to chuckle over, or sometimes to deprecate" (11). This is the sure path to legendary fame.

For those interested in further reading about this legendary character, the biographical memoirs of Professor C. G. Phillips is a must (12). Walshe's striking career is covered in detail and with much astute discernment.

GEORGE H. MONRAD-KROHN (1884-1966)

It was through my acquaintance with Professor Sigvald Refsum that I came to know Monrad-Krohn. Monrad-Krohn was his mentor and, in an earlier period, had raised neurology in Norway from its fledgling, provincial status in the 1920s to a high level, comparable with neurology in England by the end of World War II. This was a great accomplishment, considering that he had to contend with the unfavorable conditions of the Great Depression, World War II, the German occupation of Norway, and their aftermaths, an essentially continuous period extending from 1930 to almost 1950. It was this and his early textbook of neurology that made him a legendary figure to a previous generation.

Monrad-Krohn's early life was spent in Bergen and his medical training, in Oslo. At the age of 28, he took graduate training at the National Hospital, Queen Square, London, where he worked with Victor Horsley, E. F. Buzzard, F. Batten, J. S. Collier, Purves Stewart, and S. A. Kinier Wilson. He also studied in Paris with J. J. Dejerine, Pierre Marie, J. F. F. Babinski, and A. A. Souques. He returned to Oslo in 1917 and was appointed professor of neurology in 1922.

His main interests were in reflexes, facial innervation, aphasia, prosody, and leprosy; altogether, he published some 200 articles. His text, *Clinical Examination of the Nervous System* became internationally famous (13). First published in 1917 in Norwegian, it was soon translated into English (12 editions), French, Spanish, and German.

He was one of the founders of the Norwegian Neurological Association (1920) and the Scandinavian Neurological Association (1922). He received many honors, including Doctor Honoris Causa of the University of Göteborg, Fellow of the Royal College of Physicians, London, Chevalier de la Légion of Honneur, and the highest awards of the Scandinavian countries. He was elected honorary president of several international and Scandinavian societies and fulfilled innumerable posts in public health, mental hygiene, multiple sclerosis, and others.

Refsum had come to the United States shortly after World War II and spent a year with us (November 1951 to November 1952) while waiting for a department to be built for him at the University of Bergen (Norway). He has visited us several times since, and I have lectured in Norway on several occasions. The cordial bonds established in this fashion gave me an excellent introduction to Monrad-Krohn. Even so, my impressions are based on glimpses obtained in his later years and may not do full justice to a remarkable man.

Norwegian budgets were frugal in the period before the discovery of oil in the North Sea, and honoraria for visiting lecturers were limited. Like my own efforts before the Jet Age, when I had to improvise to obtain the funds necessary to support our visiting professor of neurology program, Monrad-Krohn had developed potent techniques to encourage such exchanges. He had persuaded the board of directors of the Norwegian American Steamship Line to extend first-class passage between Oslo and New York for invited guests of the University of Oslo during the off-tourist season. His second device involved consultations with his Norwegian patients. I was the recipient of both strategies but will confine my comments to the second.

In January 1958, Monrad-Krohn asked me to see one of his patients, the head of a large steamship line, who lived on an estate several kilometers out of Oslo. A recent snowstorm in early January had blocked the roads, so I was surprised when Monrad-Krohn proposed going the following day. We were picked up by a car with very large snow tires and successfully made the trip through beautiful snow-covered hills and valleys. The patient's problem was one of supportive measures for a degenerative disease complicated by spasticity.

Monrad-Krohn's earlier training had made him a top-notch diagnostician but helped little with the therapeutic and supportive follow-up aspects of neurologic disorders. It was this phase of neurology in the early days that held back its development as an independent specialty. The history of medical disciplines clearly indicates that they evolved into well-developed and independent specialties only when they could offer therapeutic as well as diagnostic services. The simple symptomatic and supportive measures that were available in earlier periods for incurable conditions could be applied by local referring physicians as well or better than the diagnosticians in distant centers.

Although Monrad-Krohn had learned a great deal since his days in England and France, he was still not aware of the latest neuropharmacologic developments, and it was this aspect that may have helped his patient. In any case, it was this phase of neurology that we discussed on our return trip. Monrad-Krohn fully agreed with the limitations of neurology, as formulated, and I gathered that it was for this reason that he had favored Refsum's trip to America—to learn to use the electroencephalogram, the new antiepileptic drugs, and other neuropharmacologic forms of therapy, which were then being developed.

Monrad-Krohn was unable to attend my lecture that evening. His angina pectoris had flared up, and I suspect that our consultation trip under difficult circumstances was the cause. It was probably one of the last of such consultations that he arranged. He was 74 years old at the time and died a few years later. He was Refsum's mentor, and his obituary is well worth reading (14).

During the German occupation of Norway in World War II, Monrad-Krohn served in a sensitive position as dean of the medical faculty in Oslo. It was this, plus his many connections and honors, that made him a legendary figure. His "struggle for neurology" extended for over four decades and did much in the critical pre- and post-World War II period to establish neurology as a separate discipline. As with the other men that I have included in this category, Monrad-Krohn was more than just a neurologist. He was a well-organized individual of superior intelligence who could hold his own in any group. His leadership role in Norway went well beyond neurology and the University of Oslo. It was inevitable that he would become a legendary figure in Scandinavia and that his reputation would spread worldwide because of his textbook.

WARREN S. McCULLOCH (1898-1968)

To emphasize the point that all legendary figures were not neurologists, I have included McCulloch in these essays. He was one of the most notable neurophysiologists of the past generation, who led the modern conceptual changes of how the neuronal networks of the brain function, and whose career centered in the flowering period of neurology.

McCulloch's career can be divided into two distinct phases, or perhaps three, if his early, more floundering background is separated out. Born in Orange, New Jersey, his early years were not unusual for a bright youth raised in one of the better suburbs of New York City. His education followed the usual pattern, B.A. from Yale in 1921, M.A. in 1923, and M.D. in 1927 from Columbia. Internship followed at the Bellevue Hospital in New York, and still further training was obtained in physiology, psychology, and psychiatry between 1928 and 1934 in various institutions in the New York City area.

Perhaps the change into the second phase of McCulloch's career started at Yale, where he worked with Dusser de Berenne. He learned a great deal about neurophysiology from de Berenne, and he always prized him as his teacher. He had become a research fellow in the Physiological Institute of Yale in 1934 and was a Sterling Fellow from 1935 to 1936. Academic appointments followed at Yale, and he was an assistant professor by academic year 1940 to 1941.

In 1941, he accepted an associate professorship of psychiatry at the University of Illinois in Chicago, and in 1945, he was promoted to the full professorship. When the Illinois State Psychiatric Institute was started in 1951 under the direction of Percival Bailey, Warren obtained better space and facilities for his neurophysiological research and was made head of research. His earlier studies involved the usual anatomical and physiological investigations of primate cortex, as had been initiated with Dusser de Berenne in the 1930s (15,16). This earlier work was summarized in 1944 (17). However, his thinking changed in the 1940s and 1950s to a more integrated and functional approach to the study of cortical neuronal systems. This developed in association with a number of leading neurophysiologists in a series of conferences supported by the Macy Foundation. Bob Pitts, whom I had known in Bronk's laboratory at the University of Pennsylvania in 1939, was prominent in this, as was John Neumann (18).

The role of Norbert Wiener should be mentioned in this same connection, inasmuch as he was also one of the leaders in the Macy Foundation conferences. It has been said that his concept of cybernetics grew out of these conferences. This concerned control mechanisms and the transmission of information (feedback) and was central to the new functional approach of the cerebral neuronal network (19). Wiener's background in the development of high-speed electronic computers was important to this new neurophysiological approach. Wiener was a child prodigy who became a mathematician and expert on the Fournier analysis of wave form, by the time I met him at an electroencephalographic congress in 1953. He had obtained his Ph.D. degree from Harvard at the age of 18 and was a professor at the Massachusetts Institute of Technology by the age of 25.

McCulloch's role, as chair of the Macy conferences, was to coordinate these various inputs into an integrated whole, and this he did very well (18). He summarized much of his theories and work in *Embodiments of the Mind* (20). He also was very pleased with his application of these new concepts in his studies on the vision of the frog (21).

A notable aspect of McCulloch was his bearded countenance and informal dress. Ralph Gerard has described him as a socially rebellious person, who started the hippie movement (22). However, I have always doubted this. When I went on an ethnological expedition to the Columbia River in 1926, the Berkeley graduate students in anthropology were well advanced in these outer manifestations of "hippiness," and many of them outdid Warren. I attributed their worn Levi Straus apparel and informal manners to their field work. In both cases, however, it is difficult for me to bridge the gap between brilliant and hard-working graduate students or teaching staff and the inchoate and incoherent, drifting hippie movement of the 1960s.

That Warren delighted in soaring from the known factual basis to ethereal heights of fancy there is no doubt. He was a superb raconteur and invariably dominated the "bull sessions," in which he held his students and colleagues in an hypnotized state of wonderment. It was hard enough to follow him in his scientific work, but to discern where facts fell off and soaring imagination took off could often be a fascinating, but insoluble puzzle. In short, Warren was a brilliant character, striking in his cultivated informality of dress and manner, but extraordinary in his abilities as a raconteur and dazzling neurophysiological speculations. His colorful speech is what made Gerard term him "an off-beat philosopher" (22). This even showed up in his titles to articles and books (only the more regular have been included in the references). In spite of these latter, legendary aspects, Warren was a superb neurophysiologist, whose visionary ruminations never tripped him up in the laboratory. I may be wrong, but it was my impression that Warren enjoyed his hippie and raconteur roles, which expressed his disdain for the rigid thinking of the past and his efforts to explore the complex physiology of the cerebral networks of the brain–mind complex. It required no great perception to predict the legendary mantle that soon enveloped Warren.

MOGENS FOG (1904-1990)

Professor Fog is the youngest and yet the most legendary neurologist that I have included in this section. He was an extraordinary man, who did unusual things and whose entire career touched on the dramatic.

Born in Fredriksberg, Denmark, his father was a Ph.D. in library work. His mother was born in Greenland, the daughter of an engineer. He had a quick mind and driving personality. His early education was excellent, and he started medical studies at the age of 18. His interests, however, seemed innumerable, and he became involved in many activities, which included political reform, better conditions for young physicians, and improved public hygienic conditions. He became noted for his fantastic work capacity and his ability to analyze complicated situations. His strong will, brilliance, and good humor were other attributes. These personal characteristics were highlighted by his informality of dress and manner in an age when this was unusual and, especially so, in academic and intellectual circles in Denmark. In short, Fog was a firebrand, and except for the fact that he excelled in everything he undertook, he would not have been tolerated. He was a member of the executive committee of the Association of Young Physicians from 1930 to 1934 and, later (1939 to 1969), was editor of the Danish Weekly Journal for Physicians. As editor of the Science and Practice Column from 1939 to 1967, he maintained a high scientific standard for the journal.

Through his many interests, he developed far-ranging contacts, often well beyond his own background of experience. Politically, he was a "pink" but never a member of the Danish Communist Party. Nevertheless, his social and political views were on the radical side. Although I lectured and visited Copenhagen on several occasions, my friends "protected" me from more than casual contacts with Fog, fearing that, if I communed with such a radical, it might become known in America and, in the McCarthy period, might have deleterious effects. This, of course, was nonsense but developed as the result of our sensational press, which greatly magnified the influence and power of McCarthy. I learned of this later, after Russia invaded Hungary in 1956, and Fog had reacted strongly against this. His neurological colleagues now thought that he had "seen the light," and because he was no longer a communist-leaning threat, Fog was invited to receptions and meetings, which allowed us to become better acquainted.

Aside from his work in the Danish underground movement during the German occupation, other details of Fog's background can be summarized as follows:

1. He completed his M.D. thesis in 1934.
2. He had residency training in neurology at the University Hospital starting in 1935 and was a member of the Executive Committee of the Danish Association of Physicians from 1935 to 1938.
3. In 1938, he was made professor of neurology in the University of Copenhagen and head physician of the Neurological Department of the University Hospital, positions he retained until retirement.
4. He was a member of the Danish Society of Medicine from 1939 to 1942 and a member of the Council for Medical Specialists in the National Board of Health and Welfare from 1941 to 1966.

Fog's reaction to the German occupation, starting in 1940, was immediate and intense (23). He was one of the founders of the illegal newspaper Frit Danmark (Freedom for Denmark) and was searched for illegal activities in December 1942. He wrote many letters to his friends, students, colleagues, and associates in his many causes, arguing against any cooperation with the Germans and explaining the necessity of underground resistance activities, which the Nazi considered illegal. Fog became the center of formulating a line of social and political resistance that historically was very effective in disrupting German shipping and communication. In 1943, he was one of the founders of the Council for Denmark's Liberation and, finally, was arrested by the Gestapo in October 1944. In the hope of avoiding the bombing of the Gestapo headquarters in the Shell building of Copenhagen, the Nazis confined Fog and other prisoners in its upper floors and notified the British of their action. The British bombed anyway. The first bomb was an indirect hit. Another prisoner, a former policeman in Copenhagen, managed to convince the German jailer to give him the keys. Quickly, the prison doors were unlocked, and the prisoners escaped. Fog went to a barber shop across the street, got them to call his underground allies, and then, went incognito by having a shave. This worked well, and he was soon spirited off to Sweden and safety. He indeed was lucky; a second bomb hit a nearby school and killed 270 children. A third bomb struck the Shell building directly and demolished it. I vaguely recall an account of this in the *Reader's Digest* some 30 to 40 years ago. The preceding account was given to me by Rosa Muller, who worked with Dalsgaard-Nielsen, when he, also, was a member of the Danish underground (as discussed in Chapter 14).

Later in 1945, after Denmark was liberated by allied troops, Fog served for 5 to 6 months as State Secretary of Special Offices in the Government for the Freedom of Denmark. It was following this that he became a member of the Folkefinget, i.e., a governing body of a movement associated with Denmark's Communist Party. It was this connection that led his colleagues to believe that he was a communist and to protect me from him over the next several years. It was at a dinner given by Margaret Lennox and Friz Buchthal in 1965 that I really became better acquainted with Professor Fog and his wife, Dr. Elin Edwards Fog. It was a jolly party with the Dalsgaard-Nielsens, the Professor of Psychiatry at Copenhagen, and Dr. E. M. Trolle, who had spent several months with me in San Francisco in 1954. Professor Fog was most charming and invited us to visit them at his home (an "old ruin") near Antibes on the French Riviera, a delightful area that we knew fairly well. Obviously, Fog had mellowed from his younger days, and Elin Fog seemed to be at her peak, as well. It would have been a wonderful experience, but it was not to be. I had started my campaign to get out of administrative detail and was fed up with the political aspects of the University of California, San Francisco, at that juncture. The basic pattern of the department was well established. After 19 years to protect the interests of neurology (the so-called struggle for neurology, as expressed by Monrad-Krohn), I was anxious to get back to my research. Fog seemed to understand this, and we departed, realizing that we probably would never see each other again.

Professor Fog served in several capacities in later life, including the Presidency of the University of Copenhagen from 1966 till 1972. He received several prizes, including the 500-year Jubilee Medal of the University of Copenhagen in 1979. He was an honorary member of several neurological societies and was given the Doctorate Honoris Causa by both the Universities of Oslo and Aarhus.

The legendary aspect of Mogens Fog perhaps developed mainly from his role in the Danish underground resistance movement during World War II. His brilliance, drive, radicalism in shaking up old traditions, in addition to his substantial work as professor and chief of neurology, well merited the title of a book about him, The *Charismatic Working Man* (23). Perhaps, the personal description of Fog by my friend Professor Olle Höök (discussed in Chapter 19), who knew Fog while secretary and later president of the Swedish Neurological Association, is as good as any of this complex and remarkable man. "He was far from being a teetotaler...but even here he had an extremely good capacity! He was a fascinating and intense living person. I will never forget the sparkling fire in his eyes under dark heavy eyelashes" (personal communication, 1992). However, Fog was far more than this. Basically, I have always considered him to be a man of unyielding moral fiber. He saw through the shams and pretenses of his society, and his earlier flirtation with radicalism was toned down as he came to grips in furthering his many causes. The end result was a series of reforms: social, political, and academic. He was an intense, positive force, who impressed his more sedate countrymen as a " whirlwind," but one who also won their respect and who often was successful in inspiring them to achieve important goals.

In his obituary, Povl Riis has stated in summary that, " the key-words to Mogens Fog's personality were talent, courage and humor, but also charisma and warmth" (24).

SUMMARY

Holmes, Walshe, and Monrad-Krohn differed in their characteristics, abilities, and interests but shared in their determination to advance neurology and possessed the capabilities that enabled them to do so. They were extraordinary men, who actually were more than neurologists and were leaders in other respects. Their unusual genius and success in handling difficult situations created the luster of supermen, which led to stories and their legendary status. They all overlapped into the flowering period of neurology.

Two younger men, McCulloch and Fog, were at their peaks in the flowering period of neurology. Both were informal in dress and manners and did their best to transcend the cut-and-dried conceptual patterns of their times. In this respect, they were more unusual than the three preceding characters but shared with them a legendary status. All were vital men of genius, whose lives excelled in sparkling accomplishment.

REFERENCES

1. Morris, W. (ed.). *The American Heritage Dictionary of the English Language.* Boston, Houghton Mifflin,1970.
2. Aird, R.B. Mode of action of brilliant vital red in epilepsy. *Arch. Neurol. Psychiatry.*, 42:700-723, 1939.
3. Aird, R.B. Some reminiscences. *Arch. Neurol.*, 45:1145-1155, 1988.
4. Aird, R.B. *Some observations of clinical interest on the pathophysiology of epilepsy.* In: Rose, F.C. (ed.). Physiological Aspects of Clinical Neurology. London, Blackwell Scientific Publications, 1977.
5. Head, H., and Holmes, G. Sensory disturbances from cerebral lesions. *Brain* 34:102-254, 1911.

6. Holmes, G. On the spinal injuries of warfare. *B.M.J.*, 11:769-774; 815-821; 855-861, 1914.
7. Holmes, G. The Montgomery Lecture in Ophthalmology, 1919: I. The cortical localization of vision. *B.M.J.*, vol. II:193–199, 1919.
7a. Holmes, G. The Montgomery Lecture in Ophthalmology, 1919: II. Disturbances of visual space perception. *B.M.J.*, :230-233. Vol. II:230–133, 1919
8. Holmes, G. Clinical symptoms of cerebellar disease and their interpretation: Croonian Lecture, Royal College of Physicians. Part I. *Lancet*, 1:1177-1182, 1231-1237, 1922.
8a. Holmes, G. Clinical symptoms of cerebellar disease and their interpretation: Croonian Lecture, Royal College of Physicians: Part II. *Lancet*, 1:59-65, 111-115, 1922.
9. Walshe, F. *Diseases of the Nervous System*. Baltimore, Williams and Wilkins, 1949.
10. Aird, R.B., and Woodbury, D.M. *The Management of Epilepsy*. Springfield, IL, Charles C. Thomas, 1974, pp. 26-28.
11. Critchley, M. *Sir Francis Martin Walshe* The Ventricle of Memory. New York, Raven Press, 1990, pp. 195-206.
12. Phillips, C.G. *Francis Martin Walshe* (1886-1973). In: Biographical Memoirs of the Fellows of the Royal Society. vol. 20. London, the Royal Society, 1974, pp. 457-481.
13. Monrad-Krohn, G. *Clinical Examination of the Nervous System*. New York, Paul B. Hoeber, Inc., 1921.
14. Refsum, S. G. H. Monrad-Krohn (1884-1966). *Arch. Neurol.*, 13:104-105, 1965.
15. Ward, A.A., Jr., and McCulloch, W.S. Projection of frontal lobe on hypothalamus. *J. Neurophysiol.*, 10:309-314, 1847.
16. Bailey, P., von Bonin, G., Garol, H.W., and McCulloch, W.S. Functional organization of temporal lobe of monkey (Macaca mulatta) and chimpanzee (Pansatyras). *J. Neurophysiol.*, 6:121-128, 1943.
17. McCulloch, W.S. The functional organization of the cerebral cortex. *Physiol. Rev.*, 24:390-407, 1944.
18. McCulloch, W.S., and Pitts, W.H. *A Logical Calculus of the Ideas Imminent in Nervous Activity*. vol. 5. Chicago, University of Chicago Press, 1943, pp. 115-133.
19. Wiener, N. *Cybernetics, or Control and Communication in the Animal and the Machine*. New York, J. Wiley & Sons, 1948.
20. McCulloch, W.S. *Embodiments of the Mind*. Cambridge, MA, The M.I.T. Press, 1963.
21. Maturano, M.R., Lettvin, J.Y., McCulloch, W.S., and Pitts, W. Anatomy and physiology of vision in the frog (Rana pipiens), *J. Gen. Physiol.*, 43(suppl):129-175, 1960.
22. Gerrard, R.W. Warren Sturgis McCulloch: rebel genius. Trans. Am. Neurol. Assoc., 94:344-345, 1970.
23. Bredsdorff, E. (ed.). Det Karismatiske Arbejdsmenneske. Vennernes bog om Mogens Fog griber ikke dybt, men den er sober (The Charismatic Working Man). Copenhagen, Forlaget Speiktrum, 1991.
24. Reis, P. Mogens Fog. Ugeskr. Laeger, 152:2692-2694, 1990.

Epilogue

The flowering period of neurology was a very exciting era in which the traditional neurological fields were cross-fertilized by many new scientific advances. Its illustration by means of biographical sketches seemed to me to have advantages over the usual scholarly methods of history. After all, this revolution was accomplished by people who were very extraordinary and intensely interesting as individuals. My objective, therefore, has been to portray my *personae dramatiques* as vividly as possible—their personalities, traits of character, interests, and goals. At the same time, a primary objective has been to emphasize the unifying theme of these essays, which concerns the great progress achieved in the neurological fields as a result of the scientific advances in the early decades of the 20th century.

My biographical approach, however, has its pitfalls, one of which concerns the variable and diversionary approach to its desired primary objective. It is for this reason that I have added summaries to each chapter, and to this same end, it now seems appropriate to attempt a summary of the summaries.

Not only did the progress of neurology and the neurosciences have to await the advances of science before and during World War II, but also the support of society in the form of National Institutes of Health research and training programs following World War II. It is this sequence of determining events that explains the flowering of neurology in the mid-decades of the 20th century (about 1935 to 1965).

The initial scientific advances primarily involved neurophysiology and neurochemistry, as attention became focused on the processes that transformed normal anatomy and function to pathophysiology and pathology. Although Stanley Cobb was by no means alone in promoting this vision of biomedical investigation, he was one of the pioneers, and because of his setting and support, he had a great impact in shifting American medical research in that direction. It was the gains in our understanding, diagnosis, and control of epilepsy that gave the initial and crucial impetus to modern neurology. Although this was accomplished by Lennox, Putnam, Penfield, and their many colleagues, the scientific underpinnings were established by such neuroscientists as Erlanger, Berger, and Adrian. Corresponding gains were achieved by Quastel, Daley, and others (aided by the isotopes of Lawrence) in neurochemistry and neuropharmacology.

Advances in related fields quickly followed, such as by Evans and Li in neuroendocrinology, Zinsser and Meyer in neuroinfectious disorders, Lysholm and many others in neuroimaging, and Cushing and the other pioneers of neurosurgery. It was an electrifying era that witnessed the "explosive" transformation of the neurological fields into their modern forms.

Neurological advances continue, of course, as exemplified by the research of Gajdusek and Prusiner in the delayed infectious processes and some genetic degenerative disorders. The great advances now occurring in neurogenetics and the progress made in behavioral neurology are other examples of the continuing research advances in neurology.

A final section was added to emphasize the basic importance of teaching and the art of medicine in neurology, as well as the neurological statesmen who have guided the advances of neurology and its allied fields at the social and political levels. Finally, for the fun of it, I have added a few extraordinary neurologists and neuroscientists who achieved legendary status.

Because of my age, with contacts extending back nearly 70 years, I have enjoyed this undertaking, in spite of the laborious library research and effort it has involved. No doubt some readers will want to add other worthies to illustrate the aspects covered and perhaps other aspects not covered; some may want to shift the emphasis here and there. Providing constructive criticisms and suggestions develop, and my memory and health hold out, perhaps an improved second edition might be attempted in the future.

Person Index

Subject Index